The Sublime Object
of Psychiatry

International Perspectives in Philosophy and Psychiatry

Series editors: Bill (K.W.M.) Fulford, Katherine Morris, John Z. Sadler, and Giovanni Stanghellini

Volumes in the series:

Portrait of the Psychiatrist as a Young Man: The Early Writing and Work of R.D. Laing, 1927–1960
Beveridge

Mind, Meaning, and Mental Disorder 2e
Bolton and Hill

What is Mental Disorder?
Bolton

Delusions and Other Irrational Beliefs
Bortolotti

Postpsychiatry
Bracken and Thomas

Philosophy, Psychoanalysis, and the A-Rational Mind
Brakel

Unconscious Knowing and Other Essays in Psycho-Philosophical Analysis
Brakel

Psychiatry as Cognitive Neuroscience
Broome and Bortolotti (eds.)

Free Will and Responsibility: A Guide for Practitioners
Callender

Reconceiving Schizophrenia
Chung, Fulford, and Graham (eds.)

Darwin and Psychiatry
De Block and Adriaens (eds.)

Nature and Narrative: An Introduction to the New Philosophy of Psychiatry
Fulford, Morris, Sadler, and Stanghellini (eds.)

Oxford Textbook of Philosophy and Psychiatry
Fulford, Thornton, and Graham

The Mind and its Discontents
Gillett

Thinking Through Dementia
Hughes

Dementia: Mind, Meaning, and the Person
Hughes, Louw, and Sabat (eds.)

Talking Cures and Placebo Effects
Jopling

Schizophrenia and the Fate of the Self
Lysaker and Lysaker

Responsibility and Psychopathy
Malatesti and McMillan

Body-Subjects and Disordered Minds
Matthews

Rationality and Compulsion: Applying action theory to psychiatry
Nordenfelt

Philosophical Perspectives on Technology and Psychiatry
Phillips (ed.)

The Metaphor of Mental Illness
Pickering

Mapping the Edges and the In-between
Potter

Trauma, Truth, and Reconciliation: Healing Damaged Relationships
Potter (ed.)

The Philosophy of Psychiatry: A Companion
Radden

The Virtuous Psychiatrist
Radden and Sadler

Feelings of Being
Ratcliffe

Values and Psychiatric Diagnosis
Sadler

Disembodied Spirits and Deanimated Bodies: The Psychopathology of Common Sense
Stanghellini

Essential Philosophy of Psychiatry
Thornton

Empirical Ethics in Psychiatry
Widdershoven, McMillan, Hope and Van der Scheer (eds.)

The Sublime Object of Psychiatry: Schizophrenia in Clinical and Cultural Theory
Woods

The Sublime Object of Psychiatry
Schizophrenia in Clinical and Cultural Theory

Angela Woods
Lecturer in Medical Humanities,
Durham University, UK

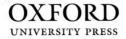

OXFORD
UNIVERSITY PRESS

OXFORD
UNIVERSITY PRESS

Great Clarendon Street, Oxford ox2 6DP

Oxford University Press is a department of the University of Oxford.
It furthers the University's objective of excellence in research, scholarship,
and education by publishing worldwide in

Oxford New York

Auckland Cape Town Dar es Salaam Hong Kong Karachi
Kuala Lumpur Madrid Melbourne Mexico City Nairobi
New Delhi Shanghai Taipei Toronto

With offices in

Argentina Austria Brazil Chile Czech Republic France Greece
Guatemala Hungary Italy Japan Poland Portugal Singapore
South Korea Switzerland Thailand Turkey Ukraine Vietnam

Oxford is a registered trade mark of Oxford University Press
in the UK and in certain other countries

Published in the United States
by Oxford University Press Inc., New York

British Library Cataloguing in Publication Data
Data available

Library of Congress Cataloging in Publication Data
Data available

Typeset in Minion by Cenveo, Bangalore, India
Printed in Great Britain
on acid-free paper by
CPI Antony Rowe, Chippenham, Wiltshire

ISBN 978–0–19–958395–9

10 9 8 7 6 5 4 3 2 1

Whilst every effort has been made to ensure that the contents of this book are as complete,
accurate and up-to-date as possible at the date of writing, Oxford University Press is not
able to give any guarantee or assurance that such is the case. Readers are urged to take
appropriately qualified medical advice in all cases. The information in this book
is intended to be useful to the general reader, but should not be used as a means of
self-diagnosis or for the prescription of medication.

Acknowledgements

The ideas in this book have been inspired, developed, tested, and extended through extensive dialogue, and I count myself lucky to have been in conversation with so many sparkling minds. It is a privilege to be published in the Intellectual Perspectives in Philosophy and Psychiatry series, and I thank K. W. M. Fulford and the editorial board, and the editorial team at Oxford University Press, for giving me the opportunity to reach such a distinguished readership.

From the University of Melbourne, where this project began in 2002, I would like to thank David Bennett, Marion Campbell, Bret Farmer, and Stephanie Trigg. Alex Murray at the University of Exeter and Robert Eaglestone from Royal Holloway were instrumental in helping this project find a home, and I thank them heartily for their encouragement. To my wonderful colleagues at the Centre for Medical Humanities at Durham—Martyn Evans, Jane Macnaughton, and Bethan Evans—special thanks for giving me the support to see this book to completion.

Claire Colebrook, now at Penn State, I thank for her exceptional feedback on an earlier version of *The Sublime Object of Psychiatry*. Amelia Douglas and Matt Pritchard are cherished friends and astute critics, and I thank them for their incisive feedback, emotional intelligence, and intellectual flair. Matthew Ratcliffe I thank for his generosity, originality, and invaluable advice throughout the later stages of this project; Pat Waugh likewise has been a beacon of wisdom. To Louis A. Sass, at Rutgers University, I owe a tremendous debt of gratitude. Not only has his work been an inspiration to me for many years, his engagement with and advocacy for *The Sublime Object of Psychiatry* has been decisive in helping realize its final form.

Writers do not emerge from or exist in a vacuum. Throughout the lifetime of this book, my family, Gay, John, and James Woods, and Rebecca Jenkin, an honorary family member for the duration, have been incredible sources of strength, support, and humour. Finally, to my partner David L. Martin—reader, lover, fiery interlocutor, and intellectual inspiration—a thank you that I hope will resonate for years to come.

Contents

Introduction *1*

Part 1 **Clinical theory**

1 Psychiatry on schizophrenia: clinical pictures of
a sublime object *13*
Cats, mice, and modern psychiatry *13*
Madness and Civilization: insanity and scientificity *16*
Approaching a disciplinary sublime *25*
Schizophrenia and sublimity *29*
Clinical psychiatry and dementia praecox *34*
From dementia praecox to schizophrenia *46*
Schizophrenia today *54*

2 Schizophrenia: the sublime text of psychoanalysis *63*
The schizophrenic symptom and its secret *63*
Tackling dementia praecox: Jung and Abraham *67*
Freud on Schreber *76*
Reading Schreber *85*
A sublime Schreber *100*
Lacan: the sublime structure of psychosis *107*
Schizophrenia and the problem of the father *118*

Part 2 **Cultural theory**

3 Antipsychiatry: schizophrenic experience and the sublime *125*
A brief overview of antipsychiatry *127*
Thomas Szasz and anti-sublime schizophrenia *132*
Between two sublimes: schizophrenia and *The Divided Self* *136*
Schizophrenia as sublime experience *139*

4 *Anti-Oedipus* and the politics of the schizophrenic sublime *145*
Introducing schizophrenia and capitalism *148*
Sidelining and sanitizing schizophrenia *150*
Deleuze, Guattari, Schreber *153*
A politics of the sublime *157*

5 Schizophrenia, modernity, postmodernity *162*
Dementia, regression, Dionysus: three tropes of madness *163*
Schizophrenia and hyperreflexivity *168*
Schizophrenia, modernism, and modernity *171*
The question of postmodernity *175*

6 Postmodern schizophrenia *183*
Introducing the figure of 'the postmodern schizophrenic' *186*
Schizophrenia and 'The Cultural Logic of Late Capitalism' *189*
Beyond Jameson *195*
The postmodern *stimmung* *199*

7 *Glamorama*, postmodernity, and the schizophrenic sublime *203*
The town crier of postmodern consciousness *205*
A postmodern Schreber? *212*
Glamorama and the schizophrenic sublime *215*

Conclusion *220*
References *225*
Author Index *249*
Subject Index *255*

Introduction

The word 'schizophrenia' first appeared in print 100 years ago, in Swiss psychiatrist Eugen Bleuler's *Dementia Praecox* or *The Group of Schizophrenias* (1950). Throughout the last century, it has been used to describe some of the most severe forms of human suffering and some of the most extraordinary thoughts, sensations, and feelings the human subject can experience. 'Schizophrenia' describes states in which thoughts are broadcast, families re-peopled by imposters, bodies emptied of organs and operated mechanically; states in which divine persecution and messianic duty commingle, feelings are flattened, and speech is inaccessible; states in which the world, engulfed in an indescribable brightness, smashes the syntax of the sentence. The word 'schizophrenia' is used, too, in the less remarkable realms of the everyday, in struggles prosaic, painful, and purposeful, in the relationships that sustain us in the search for health and happiness. We encounter the word 'schizophrenia' in clinical settings—early intervention psychosis units and outpatient facilities, doctors' surgeries and psychiatric hospitals—and in clinical research contexts, genetics and pharmaceutical laboratories, randomized control trials, and academic conferences. We read it, or its abbreviation SZ, in the hundreds of thousands of peer-reviewed journal articles reporting and debating developments across this ever-widening field of research. The term 'schizophrenia' is defined in diagnostic manuals, legal statutes and guidelines, in mental health policies, and in the work of advocates seeking an end to stigma and discrimination. But the word 'schizophrenia' is also routinely opened up—used and abused in the mass media, re-imagined, for better or for worse, in cinema and literature, music and art. In contexts intimate and individual, the word 'schizophrenia' circulates in memoirs and testimonies, in survivor and patient meetings and publications, in virtual worlds, embodied protests, and proliferating networks of support. By international agreement the term is held to describe people in every country and in every culture, yet around the world there are those who declare it stigmatizing, culturally insensitive, and scientifically illegitimate; a relic to be rejected and from which we must move on.

Convention dictates that one should begin a book by defining its object of inquiry. I have chosen instead to emphasize the complexity of my key term.

If we acknowledge that the word 'schizophrenia' is meaningful in each of the very different contexts mentioned above, then we can also acknowledge the relevance of a variety of approaches, methodologies, and interpretive frameworks in analysing what 'schizophrenia' means in and across these spheres. This observation, which applies to all diagnostic categories, serves to underline the importance of interdisciplinary inquiry.[1] But 'schizophrenia' is, as I will go on to argue, a special case, in part because its complexity bears the unmistakable stamp of conflict. One of the reasons this book begins by treating 'schizophrenia' as a word and foregrounding the complexity of its semantic contexts is that there is no consensus regarding how it might further be defined. To write and speak about 'schizophrenia' is to enter a highly contested discourse. Does the word 'schizophrenia' refer to a 'disabling and baffling brain disease' (Meyer-Lindenberg, 2010, p. 194), a 'multidimensional psychotic syndrome' (van Os et al., 2010, p. 203), or a scientific fiction and a stigmatizing label (Bentall, 2004, 2009)? No one disputes that some people experience anomalous and often distressing changes in their sense of self and world, in their thoughts and feelings, bodies, and behaviour. But a growing number of people argue that to continue to refer to these changes as 'schizophrenia' 'is extremely damaging to those to whom it is applied' and serves 'to perpetuate the myth that when talking about "schizophrenia" we are discussing something that actually exists' (Hammersley and McLaughlin, 2010).[2] This conflict is not about how best to understand, treat, research, or cope with the clinical reality of a condition designated 'schizophrenia' (although all of these things are strenuously debated); it is, at a deeper level, a conflict about whether it is legitimate to use the term at all.

My aim is neither to inflame nor to resolve these conflicts, but to shed some light on how and why they developed. *The Sublime Object of Psychiatry: Schizophrenia in Clinical and Cultural Theory* is a study of schizophrenia in theoretical texts: a study of how the concept of 'schizophrenia' is represented in specific disciplines, and of how, at the meta-discursive level, these representations reveal some of the complex relations between disciplines. As its title suggests, one of my key arguments will be that psychiatry frames schizophrenia as its sublime object or disciplinary limit point. And as my subtitle makes clear, this book's two major areas of focus will be texts in clinical and cultural theory.

* * *

---

[1] And in particular, work in the medical humanities—an emerging interdisciplinary research field that seeks to demonstrate the value of the arts, humanities, and social sciences in improving and interrogating 'medical' practice and understanding.

[2] This is discussed in more detail on pp. 42–5.

In 1984, American Marxist literary critic Fredric Jameson published his most famous essay 'Postmodernism, or the Cultural Logic of Late Capitalism'. In this essay, Jameson argued that postmodern culture has fundamentally altered our experience of ourselves. He suggested that transformations in our experience of time, language, agency, and identity could be understood through the French psychoanalyst Jacques Lacan's theory of schizophrenia. 'Postmodernism, or the Cultural Logic of Late Capitalism', confirmed the figure of the 'schizophrenic', to use Jameson's term, as the representative postmodern subject.[3] The article, re-published in a 1991 book of the same name, has since been cited in peer-reviewed publications over 7650 times.[4]

I began writing this book because the central question raised for me by Jameson's analysis could not be easily answered. Why did schizophrenia—or notions thereof—come to be seen as holding the key to understanding the everyday experience of postmodern life? My research led quickly to a series of discoveries: that schizophrenia has long been one of psychiatry's most contested clinical categories; that the schizophrenic patient was mobilized as a central symbolic figure in the political opposition to psychiatry and psychiatric practices; and that the phenomenology of schizophrenia has been understood to illuminate (and to be illuminated by) the structures of modern art and thought. 'Schizophrenia', I realized, had become one of the most potent and politicized topoi, or themes, in the cultural theory of the late twentieth century. But so far no attempt has been made to analyse how this theoretical topos had developed, or to explore its relationship to clinical accounts of schizophrenia.

This book is a study of representations of schizophrenia in the texts of a wide range of disciplines and discourses: biological and phenomenological psychiatry, psychoanalysis, critical psychology, antipsychiatry, and postmodern philosophy.[5] The terms 'clinical' and 'cultural' theories are descriptive rather than technical, and should not be interpreted as referring to narrow or internally

---

[3] See Chapter 7 for a more detailed account of Jameson's claims, his intellectual and political debts, and his influence on postmodern cultural theory.

[4] Citation search conducted using Google Scholar, 17 November 2010.

[5] Almost all of the texts I examine in detail were written by an elite class of European and American white men, many of whom sought to grasp the essence of a universal form of human experience. Questions of gender, race, and sexuality are seldom if ever foregrounded in their accounts of schizophrenia. Jonathan Metzl's powerful study of the way schizophrenia was transformed during the American civil rights era into a disorder of black, male hostility, has brought renewed urgency to the task of analysing the way 'anxieties about racial difference shape diagnostic criteria', as well as to understanding schizophrenia's 'ongoing clinical–cultural dialectic' (Metzl, 2009, p. xi, 197). I hope that the analysis offered here can contribute to future feminist and postcolonial scholarship on the category of 'schizophrenia' in clinical as well as cultural theory.

consistent bodies of work. I use 'clinical theory' to refer to work that aims to achieve a clinically meaningful outcome, whether by increasing our scientific understanding of schizophrenia or seeking more directly to alleviate the suffering of people who receive the diagnosis. This kind of theory is developed largely through the analysis of the patient, whether that patient is viewed primarily in terms of their psychology, neurochemistry, genetic profile, physiology, behaviour, or, in the case of epidemiological studies, as a statistically meaningful part of a population. By contrast, cultural theory, as I use the term, refers to works in which theorists have drawn on conceptions of schizophrenia to interpret aspects of (mostly twentieth-century Western) culture. The apparently unlikely assortment of philosophers, literary critics, Marxists and post-Marxists, psychologists, futurists, sociologists, and social historians who make up the field of cultural theory vary considerably in their approaches to schizophrenia (or to what they call 'schizophrenia'). Some have very little declared interest in the clinical realities of schizophrenia; others have extensive clinical training and experience. What unites them is their conviction that the phenomenon of schizophrenia—as they understand it—gives us insight into *something more than* conventional clinical theory would allow.

The dialogue between clinical and cultural theories has so far been fairly one way. Cultural theorists, most famously those associated with the antipsychiatry movements of the 1960s and 1970s, have mounted passionate and powerful critiques of mainstream psychiatry, showing, among other things, how scientific descriptions of mental disorders reflect the cultural values and assumptions of the day. Clinical theorists have, for the most part, preferred to attend to the arguably more pressing tasks of caring for those they consider to be mentally ill. My hope is that this book will help facilitate a greater exchange between thinkers in these theoretical fields, and with it the realization that cultural theory, although not always digestible or even palatable, deserves recognition for the quality of its critique of clinical theory and its analysis of the cultural meanings of schizophrenia.

* * *

Among many other things, the International Perspectives in Philosophy and Psychiatry series has shown that classical psychiatry is not the only discipline interested in and indeed capable of defining and interpreting the mind and its disorders. Recent studies in the philosophy of psychiatry and the phenomenology of psychopathology have explored crucial questions about the nature and definition of mental disorder, the conceptual underpinnings of mental health care, and the subtle changes to bodily feelings and perception that characterize certain experiences as exceptional (Bolton, 2008; Ratcliffe, 2008; Stanghellini, 2004; Thornton, 2007). In her famous book *Illness as Metaphor*, cultural critic Susan Sontag observed that 'Any important disease whose causality is murky, and for which treatment is ineffectual, tends to be awash in significance' (Sontag, 1991, pp. 59–60).[6] If psychiatry is dedicated to making causality less murky and treatments more effective, philosophers of psychiatry focus more often on interrogating the key concepts that intersect with our accounts of normal and pathological (concepts such as rationality, personhood, beliefs, emotions, and values), addressing the ethics of the psychiatric encounter, and deepening our understanding of the phenomenology of health and illness. Being neither a psychiatrist nor a philosopher of psychiatry, but coming from the perspective of literary and cultural studies, my interest, like Sontag's, is in understanding how schizophrenia came to be 'awash in significance'.[7]

This book is an analysis of theoretical texts—textbooks, diagnostic manuals, philosophical treatises, monographs and journal articles, books written for specialists, and books written to appeal to a broader public. I also look in detail at one autobiographical work, Daniel Paul Schreber's *Memoirs of My Nervous Illness* (1955), and, in the final chapter of the book, one novel. As evidenced by the number and treatment of direct quotations in what follows, my reading of clinical as well as cultural theories proceeds from an attentiveness to language, to the gaps and fissures, the passions and politics that find their way into even the most technical of texts. My interest is not in essences, but effects: I do not seek an answer to the question 'what is schizophrenia?', rather, my work seeks to understand how schizophrenia is described and conceptualized, how it is represented in specific clinical and cultural contexts, but perhaps more importantly, how it *functions* across these discourses. In this it contributes to larger medical–humanities inquiries into how culture structures knowledge production in medicine, and how medical, in this case psychiatric, terms are in turn used to interpret cultural phenomena.

In *The Psychiatric Team and the Social Definition of Schizophrenia*, psychiatrist and anthropologist Rob Barrett states unequivocally that in his book 'no one view of schizophrenia is accorded priority. In particular, it is neither an apology for nor an attack on psychiatric definitions of schizophrenia' (Barrett, 1996, p. 4).

---

[6] Gillian Beer makes a similar point with respect to science in general in her essay 'Forging the Missing Link: Interdisciplinary Stories' (1996). Beer argues that 'placeholder terms' for concepts and conditions for which there is little satisfactory causal explanation tend to accrue highly charged and conflicted cultural meanings. My thanks to Pat Waugh for introducing me to Beer's work.

[7] As is well known, the focus of Sontag's work is tuberculosis, cancer, and then HIV/AIDS. These diseases of the flesh, however, derive their power as metaphors from difference and differentiation, from a capacity to demarcate the Other from the self. What is so striking about the representation of schizophrenia in cultural theory, by contrast, is that it is used to speak to and of the structures of contemporary experience *for us all*.

Albeit from a very different disciplinary perspective, these statements capture sentiments I share. It is not my intention to attack or to valorize any aspect of psychiatric practice or cultural theory, nor to posit or defend a single account of schizophrenia, and I am careful throughout this book to use language that highlights my critical distance from the works being discussed. My commitment to ambivalence—an openness to multiple ways of understanding schizophrenia— necessitates the suspension of a common assumption, namely, that the terminology of today is inherently more accurate, value-free or uncontested than the terminology it has displaced. There is a wide and distinguished body of work documenting shifts in the vocabularies of madness, mental health, and mental illness, and examining the values and politics, intended and otherwise, of terms such as 'lunatic', 'mad person', 'schizophrenic', 'person with schizophrenia', 'person having schizophrenia', 'schizophrenia-sufferer', 'mental health service user', 'consumer', 'client', 'patient', 'survivor', and the compound 'consumer/ survivor/ex-patient' (Crossley, 2002; 2004; Crossley and Crossley, 2001; Estroff, 2004; Haghighat, 2008; Haghighat and Littlewood, 1995; McLean, 2000; Reaume, 2002; Speed, 2006, 2007; Sass, 2007; Simmons et al., 2010). The lesson I draw from this scholarship is that it is important never to lose sight of the historical specificity of the language and the semantic contexts associated with schizophrenia, especially when attempting to grasp the theoretical disagreements over 'dementia praecox', 'schizophrenia', 'paraphrenia', 'psychosis', 'madness', and 'mental illness' from the late nineteenth to the early twenty-first centuries. Eugen Bleuler simply did not treat 'mental health service users'; R.D. Laing did not study the existential phenomenology of 'consumers'; however, the commitment of both men to improving the lives of people they diagnosed as schizophrenic patients is beyond dispute. In analysing these and other theoretical texts, I am careful to avoid assigning the paradigms and terminology of past eras a contemporary currency, but equally, I refuse the loose historiography that would map contemporary understandings or terminologies back onto the 'unenlightened' past. My concern throughout this book is to preserve the scholarly integrity of cultural and historical analysis. Schizophrenia's validity as a category of mental illness may be publicly and routinely called into question (Ferns et al., 2010), but suspending acceptance of diagnostic categories does not detract from or cast doubt upon the reality of people's suffering. What is *not* in dispute is the reality of people's subjective experience, the power of this diagnosis in shaping that reality, and the fact that notions about schizophrenia have had cultural impacts in excess of those acknowledged at the clinical level. The term 'schizophrenia' is powerful in its effects—it has potency, meaning, and agency in the clinical and cultural realms, which it is the task of this book to investigate.

* * *

Part One of *The Sublime Object of Psychiatry* examines the status of schizo-phrenia in clinical theory, concentrating on classical psychiatry and psychoa-nalysis. In Chapter 1, I look in detail at key works by the earliest and most influential theorists of schizophrenia—Emil Kraepelin's 1907 *Clinical Psychiatry* (1981), Eugen Bleuler's 1911 *Dementia Praecox or The Group of Schizophrenias* (1950) and Karl Jaspers's 1913 *General Psychopathology* (1972). Steady advances in psychopharmacology, neuroimaging, and genetic profiling notwithstand-ing, the basic *clinical* conceptualizations of schizophrenia offered by Kraepelin, Bleuler, and Jaspers have changed little in over a century (Johnstone et al., 1999, p. 38). Changing focus from the psychiatric to the psychodynamic, Chapter 2 locates at the heart of psychoanalytic theories of schizophrenia an autobiographical account of psychosis: Daniel Paul Schreber's 1903 *Memoirs of My Nervous Illness* (1955). Schreber's text was the subject of Sigmund Freud's major account of schizophrenia, his 1911 'Psycho-Analytic Notes on an Autobiographical Account of a Case of Paranoia (Dementia Paranoides)' (1981) and, in turn, a central focus of Jacques Lacan's third seminar in 1955–1956 *The Psychoses* (1993). Although Freud and Lacan were by no means the most influ-ential psychoanalysts when it came to treating psychosis, their influence on cultural theory was and continues to be profound.

The five much shorter chapters of Part Two bring together under the broad category of cultural theory four conflicting but interrelated discourses: the antipsychiatry of R.D. Laing and Thomas Szasz, the early work of Gilles Deleuze and Félix Guattari, the oeuvre of phenomenological psychologist Louis A. Sass, and the writing of Fredric Jameson and Jean Baudrillard. All these theorists challenge psychiatric and psychoanalytic accounts of schizo-phrenia, and focus much of their attention on the relationship between this disorder and contemporary society and subjectivity. Concentrating on Laing's 1960 *The Divided Self* (1990) and *The Politics of Experience* (1967), and Szasz's *Schizophrenia: The Sacred Symbol of Psychiatry* (1976), Chapter 3 examines the vociferous critiques of clinical theory mounted by the antipsychiatry move-ments of the 1960s and 1970s, but looks as well at the alternative models of schizophrenia they proposed. Chapter 4 offers what is to my knowledge the first sustained close reading of schizophrenia in Deleuze and Guattari's icono-clastic *Anti-Oedipus: Capitalism and Schizophrenia* (1982). Chapter 5 discusses Sass's critique of clinical and antipsychiatric theory, his phenomenological model of schizophrenia, and his analysis of its relationship to modernism, focussing on his magnum opus *Madness and Modernism* (1992). Chapter 6 addresses the work of a group of postmodern cultural theorists, led by Jameson and Baudrillard, who have suggested that schizophrenia is the exemplary mode of subjectivity in postmodernity. Jameson's 'Postmodernism, or the Cultural

Logic of Late Capitalism' (1984b and 1991) and Baudrillard's *The Ecstasy of Communication* (1983 and 1988) are key texts here. Part Two concludes with a close reading of Bret Easton Ellis's *Glamorama* (2000), a novel which helps us to explore in more depth the phenomenological and symbolic dimensions of cultural theory's account of 'postmodern schizophrenia'.

This book is an analysis of how 'schizophrenia' came to acquire such potency in a wide range of critical and cultural discourses, of how a diagnostic category from clinical theory came to be transformed into a topos of cultural theory, and in that transformation, how 'schizophrenia' came to be associated with the everyday experience of post/modern life. My aim is not to arbitrate between competing accounts of schizophrenia, but to examine trends in the writing of those who have sought to do so. What meanings have *they* attributed to schizophrenia? How does *the concept function* within different discursive fields, and to what ends is it mobilized? Is it possible to identify a dominant vocabulary through which schizophrenia has been articulated?

Viewed collectively, these chapters chart the theoretical overlaps and divergences between disciplines. But this book makes a further argument regarding the metatheoretical relationship between competing clinical and cultural accounts of schizophrenia by using the aesthetic category of the sublime. In aesthetic theory, the sublime is defined as something that exceeds or exists beyond our capacity for comprehension and representation. Because it threatens to overwhelm our senses and unsettle our sense of self, the sublime initially inspires in its subjects feelings of awe and terror, but these, it is said, are then superseded by the sense of delight that comes from mastering the perceived threat. In Chapter 1, I use art historian Mark Cheetham's suggestion of a 'disciplinary sublime' (derived from a reading of the Kantian sublime) to develop a conceptual apparatus through which to understand the connections and hierarchies of influence between competing accounts of schizophrenia. In so doing, I identify four distinct representational modes, which together can be called the schizophrenic sublime: the elevation of schizophrenia to the status of sublime object (psychiatry), the framing of schizophrenia as a sublime text (psychoanalysis), the celebration of schizophrenia as an experience of the sublime (antipsychiatry and *Anti-Oedipus*), and the rendering of schizophrenia as paradoxically sublime (postmodern cultural theory). Sass's work engages but then refuses the logic of the sublime, and supports my analysis of it, whereas *Glamorama* returns to the heartland of psychiatry for its portrayal of a sublime 'postmodern schizophrenia'. Referring always to the 'schizophrenia' that appears in the texts of clinical and cultural theory, the 'schizophrenic sublime' is a concept located within orders of clinical and cultural representation, rather than unproblematically reflecting embodied experience.

* * *

To scholars working in the medical humanities, and particularly those who herald from literary and cultural studies backgrounds, I hope that this book can make accessible some important aspects of the clinical history of schizophrenia, and demonstrate its relevance to cultural theory. An understanding of the key concepts used in psychiatric and psychoanalytic theory is essential if we are to explain how and why schizophrenia became so 'awash with significance' over the course of the last century,[8] and I hope my close reading of major theoretical texts in these fields furthers both our understanding and our capacity for explanation. It has also been my aim to challenge the assumption that a literary and cultural studies approach to this topic would necessarily focus on literary representations of psychosis, on the textuality of 'schizophrenic' writing, or on the theme of madness in contemporary cultural productions.[9] The central texts of this book are not novels or films, but psychiatric textbooks and studies of schizophrenic experience; its contribution is to the history of ideas in theoretical, not fictional, writing; as such, its commitment is to traversing disciplinary boundaries.

Regular readers of the International Perspectives in Philosophy of Psychiatry series may likewise find that this book introduces material that might not otherwise be familiar. However, cultural theory—particularly the work of Michel Foucault, Gilles Deleuze, R.D. Laing, and Louis A. Sass—undoubtedly deserves to be thought of as philosophical, and, as I hope my close reading of key texts makes clear, as making important contributions to the broad, and intrinsically interdisciplinary, field of the philosophy of psychiatry. Cultural theory invites sustained analytic attention for its critique of clinical theory as well as for its radical, compelling, and puzzling appropriations of clinical accounts of schizophrenia to explain models of twentieth- and twenty-first-century selfhood. The phenomenology of schizophrenia, in the discourse of cultural theory, is used to interpret modern and postmodern existence, and rather than simply dismiss theorists' use of schizophrenia as illegitimate, insensitive, or inappropriate, we must instead ask why this might be the case.

----

[8] In his masterful book *The Weariness of the Self: Diagnosing the History of Depression in the Contemporary Age*, Alain Ehrenberg observes in passing that 'We do not have, to my knowledge, a social and cultural history of schizophrenia' (Ehrenberg, 2010, p. 249). *The Sublime Object of Psychiatry* is intended as a contribution to this long overdue project, and I hope that our respective analyses of the way schizophrenia and depression can illuminate structures of the self in the late twentieth century can be drawn in to fruitful discussion in the future.

[9] Although see *Madness in Post-1945 British and American Fiction* for an extended analysis of these themes, in particular a discussion of the 'psychoticisation of the text' in the postmodern fiction of William S. Burroughs and Kathy Acker (Baker et al., 2010, p. 165).

This is not a book about schizophrenia and everyday life. It does not discuss in detail contemporary clinical practice. And it is not an analysis of the way schizophrenia is portrayed in popular culture. But to people who have received a diagnosis of schizophrenia, psychiatrists, and others working or involved in the mental health system, I hope that this book offers some insights into why schizophrenia has been seen for so long as 'ununderstandable' and how this, in turn, has influenced the ongoing conflict between competing clinical accounts of the disorder. Whether cultural theory's use of some of these accounts to interpret aspects of postmodern culture is to be applauded or condemned is, I hope, a question that readers will feel better equipped to debate after reading this book.

Part 1

Clinical theory

Chapter 1

Psychiatry on schizophrenia: clinical pictures of a sublime object

Cats, mice, and modern psychiatry

Psychiatric studies of schizophrenia frequently begin by announcing the arrival of an 'exciting' new era in schizophrenia research. The typical introduction to an edited collection of essays goes like this:

> This costly, devastating, and puzzling disorder is beginning to yield up its long-held secrets to systematic scientific inquiry. We now have the capability to explore, understand, and eventually control the biological foundations of schizophrenia in its myriad forms. [. . .] The pessimism that once permeated both the scientific study of schizophrenia and its clinical treatment has been replaced by a new spirit of excitement and hope that schizophrenia can be understood and conquered within a reasonable time frame.

> (Judd, 1994, p. xii)

The tone and tenor of Lewis Judd's introduction to *Schizophrenia: From Mind to Molecule* are distinctive but by no means unusual. Schizophrenia is often introduced as a huge burden—a disorder whose significant costs must be measured in economic terms as well as at the level of individual psychic health (McDonald et al., 2004, p. xvii)—and is further presented as an intellectual puzzle that is on the verge of being solved thanks to rapid advances in medical technology (Andreasen, 2004, p. x). Optimism, it seems, is the order of the day: 'It is now *unequivocally* established that schizophrenia is a brain disorder', Judd continues, and we are but moments away from being able to 'pinpoint' its origins (Judd, 1994, p. xii, my italics).

Or are we? Ten years after the publication of *Schizophrenia: From Mind to Molecule*, Glenn Shean—in his bluntly titled *What is Schizophrenia and How Can We Fix It?*—argues with equal conviction that 'We do not presently know what causes schizophrenia, nor do we know that the term refers to a single disorder. We continue to use the term for lack of a better or widely acceptable alternative' (Shean, 2004, p. 95). Judd's 'unequivocal' assurances cannot disguise the fact that today, as in more 'pessimistic' eras, the psychiatric arena abounds with competing interpretations of this incurable disorder. Although there seems to be relative consensus among psychiatrists regarding key symptoms, there are no pathognomic signs unique to schizophrenia and hence no definitive way to test for its presence.[1] Further complicating this diagnostic indeterminacy is the lack of compelling evidence consistently implicating specific physical, genetic, neurological, psychological, or environmental factors, or combinations of factors, in the aetiology of schizophrenia (Editor, 2010). The research field is as varied as it is inconclusive: 'Could Schizophrenia Be a Viral Zoonosis Transmitted from House Cats?' (Torrey and Yolken, 1995; see also Torrey, 1988; Torrey and Miller, 2001; Torrey and Yolken, 2007). Or is it the case that genetically engineered mice will unlock its neurochemical and genetic secrets (see Kellendonk et al., 2006; Jaaro-Peled et al., 2010; O'Tuathaigh et al., 2010)? After over 100 years of intensive research the debates still rage (Chung et al., 2007, pp. 1–2). That schizophrenia refuses interpretive 'closure', however, does not mean that it is an empty or free-floating signifier: the 1% of any given population identified as suffering from schizophrenia attest if not to its existence then certainly to the consistency of its professional diagnosis and management.[2] What is the status, then, of a disorder for which there is no

[1] Although research continues into the diagnostic potential of blood testing (Noll, 2006; Tsuang et al., 2005) and electrovestibulography (Haghgooie et al., 2009).

[2] The figure of 1% is an approximation that is widely cited but heavily contested, especially as it says nothing about the severity or duration of suffering. Gender is a key variable, as it has been widely observed that more men than women are diagnosed with severe early-onset schizophrenia, whereas women outnumber men in later-onset cases (Castle, 2000). Meta-analytical studies suggest that 'psychotic outcomes are associated with growing up in an urbanized area, minority group position, cannabis use and developmental trauma' (van Os et al., 2010). In a recent review of research into the epidemiology of schizophrenia, Kinney et al. (2009) confirm findings of an up to ten-fold variance in the prevalence rates for schizophrenia in different geographic sites, increasing significantly with latitude and colder climate. Within these climatic zones, city dwellers are at greater risk than people living in the country, as are recent immigrants, particularly those living in ethnically mixed communities (Bentall, 2004, p. 475). For example, in the UK it has been consistently shown for 40 years that people of Afro-Caribbean descent are up to seven times more likely to be diagnosed with schizophrenia (Morgan and Hutchinson, 2009), a fact that continues to cause justifiable concern and outrage (Lewin, 2009; O'Hara, 2010). In the USA, Jonathan Metzl has argued convincingly that the figure of 1% is 'a delusion', as pernicious as it is persistent. Metzl cites a 1960s National Institute of Mental Health study (which found that '"blacks have a 65% higher rate of schizophrenia than whites"'), and a 2004 study of over 130,000 veterans diagnosed with schizophrenia (which identified a four-fold increase in the likelihood that African-American identified men would receive the diagnosis), as two of the many and varied pieces of evidence in analyzing 'how schizophrenia became a black disease' (Metzl, 2009, pp. x–xi, 187–8).Without ever losing sight

uncontested explanation, but which is itself used to 'explain' roughly one person in every hundred?

Schizophrenia's importance to modern psychiatry cannot be overestimated, as it is through the definition and clinical management of this disorder that psychiatry claimed, and continues to claim, its authority to legislate in the name of science between normal and abnormal, sane and insane, reason and unreason. However, schizophrenia is also a profoundly problematic psychiatric concept: to the extent that its aetiology remains impenetrable, it threatens to undermine the legitimacy of the discipline's claims to have conquered, or be on the verge of conquering, severe mental illness. As Arthur Kleinman succinctly states, 'Schizophrenia is *the* defining problem for psychiatry' (2004, p. xv, italics in the original); so '"to know schizophrenia is to know psychiatry"' (Roy Grinker, quoted in Grinker, 2010, p. 168). But if schizophrenia is '"the heartland of psychiatry"' (Kendall quoted in McGuffin, 2004, p. vi), then it has frequently been described as a heart of darkness. According to Michael Foster Green, this has two negative consequences:

> Schizophrenia is shrouded in an overpowering sense of mystery—which is a wonderful quality for a romance or a novel but not for an illness. When an illness is viewed as inexplicable and impenetrable, people tend to react to it with one of two extremes: either they *stigmatize* the illness or they *romanticize* it.
>
> (Green, 2003, p. 1, italics in the original)

There is, I will argue, a third response to the mystery of schizophrenia—clearly Green's own response—and that is to construe it as a professional challenge; to position it at the centre of psychiatric enquiry. My focus in this chapter is not on how 'people tend to react' to the mystery of schizophrenia, but on how psychiatrists very consciously write about it *as* a mystery. In doing so, psychiatry, I will argue, does not stigmatize or romanticize schizophrenia, but elevates it to the status of the sublime. Drawing primarily on the thinking of philosopher Immanuel Kant (1969) and art historian Mark Cheetham (1995), this chapter argues that schizophrenia becomes psychiatry's 'sublime object' by being perpetually invoked as its disciplinary limit point. Through its ongoing construction in psychiatric writing as opaque, bizarre, and resistant to analysis, schizophrenia at once attracts and frustrates ever more sophisticated

---

of these epidemiological differences and their impact, it will be more accurate to say that schizophrenia has been diagnosed in at least 0.5 to 1% of populations across the world since the introduction of standard WHO guidelines. Whether the guidelines themselves have led to 'The Globalization of the American Psyche' is a question taken up by Ethan Watters (Watters, 2010) in his aptly-titled book of the same name.

forms of scientific enquiry, exceeding and thus marking the limits of any given interpretive model.

This chapter, then, opens up a new perspective on the history of schizophrenia by analysing how it acquired and maintained its function as the sublime object of psychiatry. We begin with a controversial but crucial text in the interdisciplinary study of madness: Michel Foucault's *Madness and Civilization* (1993). Foucault's analysis of the shifting historical constructions of madness, the development of psychiatric practices, and the precariousness of psychiatry's assertion of scientificity inform my own work; however, it is his metatheoretical claims that are of most significance to this project. My analysis of *Madness and Civilization* leads to a discussion of the 'disciplinary sublime' and its relevance to understanding the status of schizophrenia in psychiatric discourse. The key psychiatric texts under consideration in the remainder of this chapter are those most influential in twentieth-century psychiatry: Emil Kraepelin's *Clinical Psychiatry* (1981), Eugen Bleuler's *Dementia Praecox, or The Group of Schizophrenias* (1950), and Karl Jaspers's *General Psychopathology* (1972). As my close reading of their work seeks to demonstrate, Kraepelin, Bleuler, and Jaspers among them not only laid the foundation for the way in which psychiatry would diagnose, treat, and perpetually re-theorize schizophrenia; their clinical pictures of the disorder have played a decisive role in constructing schizophrenia as sublime. The final part of the chapter traces the influence of these accounts in shaping competing contemporary representations of schizophrenia and generating the psychiatric controversies that mark schizophrenia's sublime status in this discipline.

Madness and Civilization: insanity and scientificity

Michel Foucault's *Folie et Déraison: Histoire de la Folie à l'Âge Classique* was published in 1961. Six years later, a translation of the abridged French edition appeared as *Madness and Civilization: A History of Insanity in the Age of Reason*. *Folie et Déraison* has a place of distinction in Foucault's oeuvre as the text that launched, to considerable acclaim, his career-long inquiry into the archaeology of the human sciences. Although it rankled—and occasionally outraged— some British historians of psychiatry,[3] there has been a grudging acknowledgement that this 'cavalier philosopher' has in many ways set the research agenda (Houston, 2000, p. 12). Foucault's work influenced scholars of madness from across the humanities by issuing a sophisticated challenge to psychiatry's

---

[3] Colin Gordon (1992) provides an overview and rebuttal of the debate, which centres principally on questions of the calibre of Foucault's historical records and the accuracy of their interpretation.

narrative of its own enlightened progression. It was a challenge that also reso-
nated powerfully with the 1960s counter-cultural antipsychiatry movement
spearheaded by R.D. Laing. Laing's reader's report, which praised Foucault's
'exceptional book' for advancing 'a thesis that thoroughly shakes the assumptions of traditional psychiatry' (Laing, quoted in Foucault 2009), guaranteed
that from the moment of its publication *Madness and Civilization* would enjoy
a political resonance and significance beyond the confines of the academic and
medical establishments.

Nearly 40 years later, Foucault's ongoing importance to the study of madness in the West is attested to by the publication of two new books: *Psychiatric
Power* (Foucault, 2008), which collates for the first time Foucault's lectures
around this theme held at the College dè France in 1973–1974, and *History of
Madness*, the first full English translation of *Folie et Déraison*. Although additional and extended chapters explore in greater depth competing seventeenth-
and eighteenth-century schemas of madness, *History of Madness* also returns
nearly 1000 footnotes to the text (and with them a scholarly apparatus that
appears to have reignited long-smouldering academic disputes[4]). These two
important texts reward close and sustained reading; however, as their publication has not significantly altered the ideas and subsequent debates that are the
focus of my analysis, my references throughout remain to the original *Madness
and Civilization* and to the little-known work that preceded it, *Mental Illness
and Psychology.*

The first part of *Mental Illness and Psychology* has received scant critical
attention, and yet only here does Foucault explicitly consider what madness
must be like for the mad themselves. Rejecting any parallel between organic

---

[4] Far from resolving debate about the quality of Foucault's archival and scholarly research,
the publication of *History of Madness* seems to have prompted Foucault's detractors and
defenders back in to the ring with renewed vigour. In a scathing review entitled 'The fictions of Foucault's scholarship: The frail foundations of the Foucaldian monument',
Andrew Scull (2007) suggests that the only lesson to be learned from *History of Madness* is
'the ease with which history can be distorted, facts ignored, the claims of human reason
disparaged and dismissed, by someone sufficiently cynical and shameless, and willing to
trust in the ignorance and the credulity of his customers'. In response the theory blogo-
sphere erupted with an increasingly impassioned series of posts, led by a long-standing
champion of Foucault, Colin Gordon. Wondering 'why Scull chooses to gamble his own
scholarly credibility on such an ill-founded and malevolently unbalanced polemic',
(Gordon, 2007a) he extols *History of Madness* as 'a work of masterful accomplishment and
prodigious and prodigal energy, grasp and daring', going so far as to claim that 'No richer,
more multidimensional work of cultural and intellectual history has been written – including
by Foucault himself' (Gordon, 2007b). A more balanced evaluation from the perspective
of psychiatry and political theory respectively can be found in the work of Bracken et al.
(2007) and Hooke (2009).

and mental pathology, Foucault examines specific forms of mental illness produced by theories of psychic evolution (psychology), individual history (psychoanalysis), and existence (phenomenology), in order to 'determine the conditions that have made possible this strange status of madness, a mental illness that cannot be reduced to any illness' (Foucault, 1976, p. 13). Although the teleological, normalizing narratives of psychology and psychoanalysis imply otherwise, for Foucault 'the pathological structure of the psyche is not a return to origins; it is strictly original' (Foucault, 1976, p. 26). Foucault's attempt to understand the experience of mental illness from the 'inside' is one of the most original and intriguing aspects of his work on madness, not least because it directly prefigures R.D. Laing's (1990) existential phenomenological model of schizophrenia. Tracing how each pathological condition distinctively alters the subjective experience of time, space, embodiment, and social relationships, Foucault finds none more radical in its effect than schizophrenia. Foucault's description of the texture of schizophrenic experience brings the reader tanta-lizingly close not to the object of professional analysis, scientific treatment, or juridical management, but to a subject engaged in a dynamic relation with the world:

> [In schizophrenia, the person] is submerged in the morbid world and aware of the fact; and, as far as one can guess from the accounts of cured patients, the impression remains ever present to the subject's consciousness that reality can be grasped only in a travestied, caricatured, and metamorphised, in the strict sense of the term, dream mode.
>
> (Foucault, 1976, p. 49)

Foucault then claims that psychology, psychoanalysis, and phenomenology can elucidate the forms that mental illnesses take, but are unable to provide satisfactory aetiological explanations:

> It would be a mistake to believe that organic evolution, psychological history, or the situation of man in the world may reveal these conditions [of appearance]. It is in these conditions, no doubt, that the illness manifests itself, that its modalities, its forms of expression, its style, are revealed. But the roots of the pathological deviation, as such, are to be found elsewhere.
>
> (Foucault, 1976, p. 56)

It is at this point in the text that Foucault abandons his focus on the experi-ences of different forms of mental illnesses. Collapsing this spectrum of difference to reinstate a simple opposition between aberrant and normal sub-jectivities enables Foucault to argue that mental illness is simply madness alienated in and by psychology. This argument, developed in the second part of *Mental Illness and Psychology*, lays the foundations for Foucault's later work on the history of madness.

Madness and Civilization is a genealogy of the shifting interpretation and management of the mad from the medieval period to the rise of the asylum in the nineteenth century; an investigation of the cultural mechanisms that opposed madness to reason, excluding it as an unreason with which there could be no exchange. Challenging dominant historical narratives that explain the evolving treatment of mad people as a humanistic progression away from the barbarity of Bedlam towards an informed and compassionate care for the sick (a progression largely determined by advances in medical knowledge of the 'reality' of mental illness) Foucault draws attention to other factors that were critical in defining madness, thereby instigating and/or legitimizing societal responses to it. For example, he argues that the Classical period's 'great confinement' of the mad as 'socially useless' was anchored in a moral injunction against idleness as the root of sin, such that in addition to its limited economic benefits, enforced labour in hospital workhouses had a significant ethical status. 'What made [confinement] necessary', Foucault writes, 'was the imperative of labour. Our philanthropy prefers to recognize the signs of a benevolence toward sickness where there is only a condemnation of idleness' (Foucault, 1993, p. 46). Madness was later transformed into a spectacle displaying 'a bestiality from which man had long since been suppressed', and the free and frenzied animality of the mad warranted control through discipline and brutalization (Foucault, 1993, pp. 70, 75). By the end of the eighteenth century, madness, according to Foucault, had become moral aberration, and the asylum both punished and organized the mad person's guilt:

> The asylum of the age of positivism . . . is not a free realm of observation, diagnosis, and therapeutics; it is a juridical space where one is accused, judged, and condemned, and from which one is never released except by the version of this trial in psychological depth—that is, by remorse. Madness will be punished in the asylum, even if it is innocent outside of it. For a long time to come, and until our own day at least, it is imprisoned in a moral world.

> (Foucault, 1993, p. 269)

Variously excluded and punished as idleness, animality, and moral fault, madness, as Foucault argues, is not an innate difference, disease, or dysfunction. Rather, under the more general rubric of 'unreason', its definition is determined by the governing ideology and medico-juridical apparatus of the period.

Madness and Civilization, as Rudi Visker argues, is more than a history of madness; it is a powerful critique of psychology's understanding of its own history as the discovery and progressive scientific conquest of mental illness. If psychology 'conceives its emergence literally as a discovery, as the exposure of an object which was already there before being discovered, not an object constituted by its discovery', Foucault's counter-history suggests that mental illness, the object of psychology's discovery, 'not only arose historically, but is also dependent on that discovery' (Visker, 1995, pp. 9, 19).[5] Psychology's selective interpretation of its history enables the construction of a positivist narrative through which psychology lays claim to its own scientificity. And this claim conceals a crisis:

> By [Foucault's] account, the positivistic forgetting in which psychology gradually loses itself, does not, as one might expect, to a crisis of psychology, but in fact covers up a crisis [. . .] Having arisen as a moral practice, it can only lay claim to being a science by forgetting the stigma of its conditions of emergence, a stigma which has never disappeared.

(Visker, 1995, p. 21)

Whereas other historians celebrate in Philippe Pinel's release of the mad from their chains the beginnings of humane and scientific asylum practice, Foucault suggests in *Mental Illness and Psychology* that psychology would not exist 'without the *moralizing sadism* in which the nineteenth-century "philanthropy" enclosed [madness], under the hypocritical appearances of "liberation"' (Foucault, 1976, p. 73, italics in the original). Psychology thus 'befalls madness', alienating it in mental illness and further subjecting it through the telling of its own 'inauthentic' or 'improper' history (Visker, 1995, p. 28). By radically destabilizing psychological metanarratives, constructed in part through histories of psychology's discovery, epistemological conquest, and progressively enlightened treatment of mental illness; by emphasizing the distinctions between each historical period's conceptualization of madness; and by focussing on the economic, legislative, religious, and ethical factors at play in the regulation of the mad, Foucault suggests that both the form and aetiology of modern madness must be sought not in the mad body or psyche, but in the history of their discursive construction.[6]

---

[5] In his recent work, acclaimed Foucauldian sociologist Nikolas Rose (Rose, 2006; Abi-Rached and Rose, 2010) extends this enquiry into the domains of neuroscience, biotechnology, genomics, and psychopharmacology.

[6] Recent critical inquiries into the validity of contemporary diagnostic categories have reached a similar conclusion by different means. Berrios, Luque and Villagrán, for example, in their analysis of the history of the concept of schizophrenia, have mounted a cogent critique of what they term the 'continuity hypothesis'. Their sarcastic tone speaks volumes about the esteem in which these authors hold one of the founding premises of psychiatry: 'According to this view: (a) "schizophrenia" has *always* existed (say, as a "rough diamond"), (b) 19th and 20th centuries alienists (Kraepelin, the Bleulers, the Schneiders, etc.) have polished away its blemishes and impurities, culminating in: (c) the DSM IV definition which can therefore be considered as a paragon (RRUS [*real, recognizable, unitary* and *stable* object of inquiry]), and (d) The end of history is nigh for it is only matter of months before the genetics and aetiology of schizophrenia is sorted out for good'

Foucault posits critical differences between mental illness and madness, emphasizing that madness is something inherently beyond the classificatory schema essential to the scientificity and self-proclaimed efficacy of modern psychiatry. At their most intimate, madness is only the 'lyrical halo of illness' (Foucault, 1996, p. 101). Whereas discussions of nosology, comparative symptomatologies, and specific forms of mental illness surface intermittently in *Madness and Civilization*, the term 'madness' retains its 'strange status', remaining difficult, opaque, and seemingly free from positive content. For philosopher Jacques Derrida, Foucault's use of an 'unverifiable . . . popular and equivocal notion of madness',

> . . . would not be serious if Foucault used the word in quotation marks, as if it were the language of others, of those who, during the period under study, used it as a historical instrument. But everything transpires as if Foucault *knew* what 'madness' means. Everything transpires as if, in a continuous and underlying way, an assured and rigorous precomprehension of the concept of madness, or at least of its nominal definition, were possible and acquired. In fact, however, it could be demonstrated that as Foucault intends it, if not as intended by the historical current he is studying, the concept of madness overlaps everything that can be put under the rubric of *negativity*. One can imagine the kind of problems posed by such a usage of the notion of madness.
>
> (Derrida, 1978, p. 41, italics in the original)

According to Foucault, madness was distinguished as a particular form of unreason only when other forms of social uselessness (poverty, licentiousness, blasphemy) were no longer locked in the asylum. Beyond these historically determined definitions of what madness is or was not, Derrida correctly points out that there are few explicit references to its positive content in the text. However, Foucault's thesis presupposes that there existed, and perhaps exists, an essential or tragic experience of madness. This structuring presupposition is explicit in *Mental Illness and Psychology*: 'Generally speaking, madness [prior to its confinement] was allowed free reign; it circulated throughout society, it formed part of the background and language of everyday life, it was for everyone an everyday experience that one sought neither to exalt nor to control' (Foucault, 1976, p. 65). The peculiar sentimentality of this portrait of quotidian madness underscores its loss and the impossibility of a cultural return to it. For in Foucault's account, by the beginning of the twentieth century, madness had become psychiatry's victim, at once tragic and noble as the inarticulate truth of unreason.

(Berrios et al., 2003, p.113). Writing in *Nature*, Thomas Insel (2010) rather courageously offers a view of what schizophrenia will look like in 2030 which resists the narrative just outlined.

How, then, can one speak of this madness? 'One day', Foucault writes in *Mental Illness and Psychology*, 'an attempt must be made to study madness as an overall structure—madness freed and disalienated, restored in some sense to its original language' (Foucault, 1976, p. 76). Some commentators claim Foucault has indeed sought and found 'the keys to the language of madness':

> From now on, we have to allow those whom we have not heard previously to speak, even if the substance of their words is madness. . . . During three centuries of misery, we have spoken of a mute; and here [in *Madness and Civilization*] he [*sic*] recovers his abolished language and begins to speak by himself, of himself.
>
> (Serres, 1994, p. 38)

In my view, this is a case of wishful thinking rather than close reading, as Foucault performs neither a gesture of semantic recuperation on behalf of the mad person nor an act of ventriloquism. In *Madness and Civilization*, Foucault positions the experience of madness, the mad, and mad speech, as analytically inaccessible to those living in the age of psychiatry:

> As for a common language [between modern 'man' and the 'madman'], there is no such thing; or rather, there is no such thing any longer; the constitution of madness as a mental illness, at the end of the eighteenth century, affords the evidence of a broken dialogue, posits the separation as already effected, and thrusts into oblivion all those stammered, imperfect words without fixed syntax in which the exchange between madness and reason was made. The language of psychiatry, which is a monologue of reason about madness, has been established only on the basis of such a silence.
>
> I have not tried to write the history of that language, but rather the archaeology of that silence.
>
> (Foucault, 1993, pp. xii–xiii)

The idea of an archaeology of silence evokes the sense of loss Foucault so strongly associates with madness, the sense that civilization has crushed the life out of a madness now fossilized in the rubble called scientific progress. But sifting through this debris is, as Derrida argues, an impossible project, for,

> . . . is not an archaeology, even of silence, a logic, that is, an organized language, a project, an order, a sentence, a syntax, a work? Would not the archaeology of silence be the most efficacious and subtle restoration, the *repetition*, in the most irreducibly ambiguous meaning of the word, of the act perpetrated against madness—and be so at the very moment when this act is denounced?
>
> (Derrida, 1978, p. 35)

Derrida further contests that '*Nothing* within this language, and *no one* among those who speak it, can escape the historical guilt . . . which Foucault apparently wishes to put on trial' (Derrida, 1978, p. 35). As reason cannot

speak unreason, so to speak of madness is thus to reiterate the crime perpe-
trated against it. It seems one must either remain silent about (but somehow
cognizant of) this silence, or 'follow the madman down the road of his exile'
(Derrida, 1978, p. 36). Through reference to the 1961 preface of *Folie et déraison*, Colin Gordon (1992, p. 35) argues that Foucault's awareness of this
impasse is already apparent in his description of the project as 'a structural
study of the historical ensemble—notions, institutions, juridical and police
measures, scientific concepts—which hold captive a madness whose wild state
can never in itself be restored' (Foucault, 2009, p. xxxiii). However, as Derrida
notes, this wildness that is supposedly beyond language 'must reverberate
within the language used to describe the history of madness', and therefore
Foucault 'acknowledges the necessity of maintaining his discourse . . . without
support from an absolute reason or logos' (Derrida, 1978, p. 36).

Following Derrida, Shoshana Felman argues that Foucault undertakes a
philosophical search 'for a *new status of discourse*, a discourse which would
undo both exclusion and inclusion, which would obliterate the line of demar-
cation and the opposition between Subject and Object, Inside and Outside,
Reason and Madness' (Felman, 1985, p. 42). Felman suggests that this new
discourse is essentially one of pathos and metaphor: 'On the idea that literature, fiction, is the only possible meeting-place between madness and philosophy, between delirium and thought, Foucault would doubtless agree with
Derrida' (Felman, 1985, p. 48). For Felman, madness can only, if elusively,
express itself through literary writing. Foucault's own valourization of writers
like Friedrich Nietzsche and Antonin Artaud (Foucault, 1993, p. 272) is ech-
oed in Felman's appraisal of Foucault, although it is unclear why for Felman
literature alone should enjoy privileged access to the truth of madness, as if
madness were inherently literary in form.[7] The search for a new literary
discourse of madness is motivated by Foucault's refusal to speak either as madness or its captor. His poetic archaeology of madness's silence effectively suggests a position, however tenuous, outside this reductive dualism; the
possibility of a witness who is neither the agent of oppression nor entirely
deranged, who might, as Derrida puts it, 'provide a reason without objectifying, or
even identifying, that is to say, without examining' (Derrida, 1998, p. 71). So, might
what Derrida interprets as pathos, and Felman as the literary, be re-conceptualized

---

[7] The pathos of Foucault's writing, and the relationship between madness and literature in
Madness and Civilization, has also received attention from more hostile quarters. So
Cutting (1994, p.65) makes the conservative claim that Foucault's analysis of madness in
fact 'lies outside of history . . . because it is ambiguous in a way appropriate to literature,
rather than an academic discipline'.

as a space somehow beyond the reason/unreason dichotomy? For Dominick LaCapra,

> Foucault at his most provocative writes neither from the side of the mad nor that of the sane but from the problematic margin that divides the two. Yet a liminal status on this margin, which allows or constrains a hybridized, internally divided voice, is particularly tenuous in the modern world as Foucault himself understands modernity, for modernity has been largely successful in reducing unreason to pathological madness if not at times to mere muteness. In some obscure fashion, Foucault would apparently like that torn and ragged margin to expand or even to explode in affirmatively changing society and culture.

(LaCapra, 1992, p. 83)

It may be that only by writing from this 'torn and ragged margin' suggested by Foucault that future theorists can avoid the further oppression of madness. But the question remains: what exactly is this object of oppression, this impossible and incomprehensible speaking position, this madness?

For Felman, as for Foucault, madness is simply 'nothing other than an irreducible resistance to interpretation' (Felman, 1985, p. 254). Ironically, considering their collective attentiveness to metatheoretical implications of writing (about) madness, Foucault, Felman, and to a lesser extent Derrida, fail to recognize that despite their claims to the contrary they have not resisted interpreting madness. Each implicitly positions madness not just as external to reason, but as an authentic, transgressive, and illuminating experience somehow lost to modernity.[8] For these authors madness cannot escape its transcendent status. The caution against perpetuating reason's unjust treatment of madness elevates it as a truth whose essence cannot, or must not, be subjugated in discourse. The origins of mental illness, as alienated madness, can be traced to the disciplinary regimes of psychiatry, but madness itself has no origin in Foucault's account, instead it is held to undergo a passage from the quotidian to the transcendent. Absent from *Madness and Civilization* is the sense, present in *Mental Illness and Psychology*, that there are particular forms of madness complicating and calling into question a simple opposition between madness and normalcy. In its place, there is the conviction that any attempt to speak directly of madness further violates an integrity guaranteed only by silence; a conviction which serves to sever madness from its relationship to the bodies and experience, to the sufferings and insights, of the mad themselves. Can madness be so easily

---

[8] In this, the speech of madness, as Michele Crossley and Nick Crossley note, is produced by Foucault as 'the ahistorical "other" of contemporary forms of medical power; a subjugated but authentic discourse which might be recovered and restored through progressive political measures' (Crossley and Crossley, 2001, p. 1477).

separated from its material incarnation in the mad person? Is madness a silent or an unspeakable experience for the mad as well as their spectators? Does not disconnecting madness from its referent in suffering potentially inflict a further injustice on the mad, paradoxically recapitulating the rhetorical gestures of psychiatrists at their most scientifically self-assuring?

In his analysis of the 'strange status of madness, a mental illness that cannot be reduced to any illness', Foucault himself assigns madness a strange status, one apparent also in the writing of Derrida and Felman. Already I have referred to this unacknowledged valuation of madness as some form of transcendence or transgression, as a form of unreason demanding to be reclaimed from reason's interminable colonization. In what follows, I suggest that the strange status of madness in *Madness and Civilization* can be understood as Foucault's association of madness with the sublime, and that this, moreover, points towards Foucault's elliptical recognition of associations already made between schizophrenia and the sublime in psychiatric discourse.

Approaching a disciplinary sublime

'The sublime' is a concept that appears deceptively easy to grasp. On the one hand it is a word we use almost casually to suggest something that is so awe-inspiring it defies description; on the other, we tend to be uncomfortably aware that the term comes laden with subtleties, contradictions, and a history that spans two millennia. The sublime takes us from the Roman oratory of Longinus through to eighteenth-century philosophy and politics, Romantic poetry and painting, Lacanian psychoanalysis, and the representation of post-modern technology. Supplying a definition suitable for such a wide sweep of experiences, historical periods, and discursive contexts is a challenge met by Philip Shaw in his book-length study of the sublime:

> In broad terms, whenever experience slips out of conventional understanding, whenever the power of an object or event is such that words fail and points of comparison disappear, *then* we resort to the feelings of the sublime. As such, the sublime marks the limits of reason and expression together with a sense of what might lie beyond these limits . . .

(Shaw, 2006, p. 2)

Floating far from its moorings in aesthetic theory, the sublime can call to mind a range of images: from the lone cliff-top figure gazing across a stormy sea, to the rousing multi-sensory spectacle of Wagnerian opera; from the shuttle's orbit through deep space to the elation of an electoral victory.

The relevance of the sublime to an inquiry into theoretical representations of schizophrenia may not be immediately obvious, so it is the task of the next two sections to elucidate this relationship more fully. The first step, then, is to highlight the features of the sublime that inform the development of this theoretical model, as well as the kinds of areas and relations that the sublime might be particularly well-suited to exploring. One of the chief virtues of the sublime is that it focusses our attention on an encounter between subject and object, and on the importance of context in giving meaning to that encounter. As we shall see, the object in this encounter has no fixed properties: it is produced (rather than simply perceived) as sublime through the interplay of temporal, spatial, and social factors. Unsettling and affirming, the dynamics of the encounter make the sublime a site of subjective transformation, ensuring the subject and object are not fixed or static but remain 'in process'. Despite appearances to the contrary, then, the sublime is not an endpoint or an outcome; its emphasis is on singularity, certainly, but of a kind that bears within it the capacity for repetition. For these reasons, as I hope to demonstrate, it can be developed into a compelling model for thinking about the relationship between and the development of subjects and objects of knowledge.

Published in 1757, Edmund Burke's *A Philosophical Enquiry into the Origin of Our Ideas of the Sublime and Beautiful* (1987) is the first philosophical work to offer a sustained exposition of these two aesthetic categories. Like the Romantic artists and thinkers he helped to inspire, Burke's fascination clearly lies not with the calm of beauty but with the tempest of the sublime and the terror which is its ruling principle:

> Whatever is fitted in any sort to excite the ideas of pain, and danger, that is to say, whatever is in any sort terrible, or is conversant about terrible objects, or operates in a manner analogous to terror, is a source of the *sublime*; that is, it is productive of the strongest emotion which the mind is capable of feeling.

> (Burke, 1987, p. 39)

The sublime swells in the subject prior to a process of reasoning; it is a moment of temporal suspension in which the object overwhelms psychic space. For Burke the objects of the sublime can be classified according to their sensory appeal on a schema that ranges from the concrete (stenches, serpents, and sudden noises) to the less tangible (the terrible privations of vacuity, darkness, solitude, and silence). Although danger as an immediate threat is 'simply terrible', 'at certain distances, and with certain modifications' these otherwise terrible objects can provoke delight in the subject, a sensation derived from the removal or negation of their threat (Burke, 1987, pp. 40, 45). Without discussing the form of this distance between subject and object (is it spatial? sensory? a function of power, or of mediated perception?), *A Philosophical Enquiry* figures distance as an essential condition of the sublime. Whereas anyone with an instinct for self-preservation is susceptible to being terrified by the immediate, obscenely proximate object, the sublime is exclusively the prerogative of the safe subject, one whose distance, however we may interpret it, affords a perception of the terrible as delightful.

Combining empiricism with 'homespun' psychology, Burke's sublime, as Terry Eagleton (1990, p. 54) correctly notes, is associated with 'enterprise, rivalry and individuation', a 'phallic swelling' fostered in aesthetic experience as a culturally permissible antidote to 'spiritual emasculation'. The sublime, for Burke, eclipses our capacity for meaning-making, plunging us into,

> . . . that state of the soul, in which all its motions are suspended, with some degree of horror. In this case the mind is so entirely filled with its object, that it cannot entertain any other, nor by consequence reason on that object which employs it. Hence arises the great power of the sublime, that far from being produced by them, it anticipates our reasonings, and hurries us on by an irresistible force.

(Burke, 1987, p. 57)

Burke's account of the sublime strongly influenced Romantic writers and thinkers who located the sublime with the spectacles of the natural world. Despite its endurance in the popular imaginary, this idea of the sublime as an 'irresistible force' in nature, arousing in us a tremendous depth of feeling, is precisely *not* the basis for the theoretical model I want to develop. For that we must turn to Kant's third critique and his discussion of the mathematical and dynamic sublime.

In his 1790 *Critique of Judgement* Kant does not concern himself with identifying a cornucopia of essentially unrepresentable objects indirectly presented in the sublime, for he argues that 'the sublime is to be found in an object even devoid of form, so far as it immediately involves, or else by its presence invokes, a representation of *limitlessness*, yet with a super-added thought of its totality' (Kant, 1969, p. 90). Formlessness, unboundedness, incomparable magnitude, powerfulness: whereas these might be the potentially terrifying qualities of such an object, the sublime 'cannot be contained in any sensuous form, but rather concerns ideas of reason' (Kant, 1969, p. 92), the faculty that is able to 'super-add' the thought of totality upon limitlessness. The sublime must therefore be understood as a process internal to the judging subject, occasioned by a conflict between the faculties of imagination and reason that is triggered by the perception of an object but is nonetheless distinct from it. The sublime is '*the mere capacity of thinking which evidences a faculty of mind transcending every standard of sense*' (Kant, 1969, p. 98, italics in the original). For example, in the idea of infinity, an instance of the mathematically sublime, we encounter the limits of our capacity for imaginative representation. However, this humbling recognition of the triumph of nature is immediately superseded by the feeling of delight produced by the rational faculty's mastery of the concept in its totality, a mastery at once demonstrating and securing our independence from nature. So, for Kant, sublimity 'does not reside in any of the things of nature, but only in our own mind, in so far as we may become conscious of our superiority over nature within, and thus also over nature without us (as exerting influence upon on us)' (Kant, 1969, p. 114).

Eagleton downplays the dimension of delight in his discussion of the Kantian sublime:

> [I]n the turbulent presence of the sublime we are forcibly reminded of the limits of our dwarfish imaginations and admonished that the world as infinite totality is not ours to know. It is as though in the sublime the 'real' itself—the eternal, ungraspable totality of things—inscribes itself as the cautionary limit of all mere ideology, of all complacent subject-centeredness, causing us to feel the pain of incompletion and unassuaged desire.
>
> (Eagleton, 1990, p. 89)

Evocative as it is, I would argue that Eagleton obscures the effect of the sublime in affirming the rational subject's ascendancy over nature and hence in actively re-centring the subject. Kant insists that the drama of the sublime spares our 'humanity' from 'humiliation', and is quick to reassure the reader that such an 'estimation of ourselves loses nothing by the fact that we must see ourselves safe in order to feel this soul-stirring delight' (Kant, 1969, p. 111). Rationality, it seems, exercises its supremacy only at a distance. Kant here, like Burke, emphasizes distance as a precondition of the sublime encounter's edifying transformation of self; however, he is more explicit in his assertion that moral development alone can secure safe access to the sublime, which 'merely strikes the untutored man as terrifying' (Kant, 1969, p. 115). Rationality as an index of the subject's humanity is affirmed through a sublime experience predicated upon one's already accomplished rational development. Burke's *Philosophical Enquiry* sidesteps the circularity of this logic by positioning the sublime as an emotive response preceding rational engagement with a necessarily terror-invoking object. By contrast, it could be argued that for Kant the aesthetic judgement of sublimity has a dimension of pleasurable performativity about it, being at once constitutive and indicative of the judging subject's reason as a transcendence of the natural realm. The Kantian sublime is 'edifying', as Mark Cheetham (1995, p. 353) notes, because 'it simultaneously reveal[s] and consists in our awareness of . . . the mind's ultimate intellectual control— through reference to morality—over anything it perceives'.

For this founding moment in the formation of modern subjectivity, the sublime object is clearly instrumental: 'we have no interest whatever in the Object, i.e. its real existence may be a matter of no concern to us', provided 'its mere greatness, regarded even as devoid of form, is able to convey a universally communicable delight' (Kant, 1969, p. 96). Kant's insistence upon the non-essential, almost incidental, form of the sublime object is, for my purposes, crucial. As Cheetham observes: 'The experience and pleasure of the sublime does not stem from the promise of something noumenal, outside a given frame, but rather from the perpetual, yet always provisional, activity of framing itself, from the parergon' (Cheetham, 1995, p. 354). Extending Derrida's (Derrida, 1987) reading of the Kantian sublime, Cheetham suggests that the judging subject's delight in parergonal activity can be utilized to interpret contemporary debates surrounding the limits of discourse:

> At different times and from different perspectives, even large and imprecisely defined constructs such as disciplines will have their own sublimes, those issues that are at once feared and desired and which, through the disciplinary attention they garner, work to mark the provisional limits and flash points of particular disciplines.
>
> (Cheetham, 1995, p. 360)

Cheetham's notion of the disciplinary sublime is central to my analysis of schizophrenia as the sublime object of psychiatry. Developing this analysis requires that we examine the relationship between schizophrenia and the (non)qualities of the sublime object, the theme of distance, and the question of subjective, or in this case, discursive, transformation that structures Kant's account of the sublime.

Schizophrenia and sublimity

As Ronald Paulson cautions: 'if the human sublime means the assumption of sublime qualities, then either the human has to be truly raised into a natural/supernatural force, as by a kind of possession, or we are dealing with at best a metaphorical and at worst a pseudo/sublime' (Paulson, 1985, p. 428). It would certainly be possible to press Burke's sublime into the service of such a metaphor, for, as Foucault demonstrates in *Madness and Civilization*, madness has indeed passed through a number of historical incarnations as wild animality and divine or satanic possession, and scientificity and secularization notwithstanding, early psychiatric representations of schizophrenia do bear the residue of these interpretations of madness. We could even go further, perhaps, and argue that mountain peaks and stormy seas (sublime objects par excellence) find their anthropomorphic echo in the mute immobility of catatonia and the violence of some delusional acts. Such analogies, however, are tenuous, dehumanising, and ultimately unproductive, depending as they do upon perceiving the person diagnosed with schizophrenia as a terrifying spectacle of calamity, misery, and privation.

Rather than search for a 'human sublime', then, Kant's analysis directs our attention away from the object in isolation, and on to the distance between object and subject in the sublime encounter. For an object to be judged sublime is, according to Kant, dependent not on its apprehension, a process that 'can be carried on ad infinitum', but on its ability to exceed the limits of our imaginative comprehension (Kant, 1969, p. 99). Recalling that sublimity is, for Kant, a property not of the object but the judging subject, the subject's position as regards the object is nonetheless crucial in staging reason's transcendence of imagination's limits. Kant uses the example of the pyramids to explore this in detail:

> [I]n order to get the full emotional effects of the size of the Pyramids we must avoid coming too near just as much as remaining too far away. For in the latter case the presentation of apprehended parts (the tiers of stones) is but obscure, and produces no effect upon the aesthetic judgement of the Subject. In the former, however, it takes the eye some time to complete the apprehension from the base to the summit; but in this interval the first tiers always in part disappear before the imagination has taken in the last, and so the comprehension is never complete. The same explanation may also sufficiently account for the bewilderment, or sort of perplexity, which, as is said, seizes the visitor on first entering St. Peter's in Rome. For here a feeling comes home to him of the inadequacy of his imagination for presenting the idea of a whole within which that imagination attains its maximum, and, in its fruitless efforts to extend this limit, recoils upon itself, but in so doing succumbs to an emotional delight.

> (Kant, 1969, pp. 99–100)

Where the sublime object appears within a disciplinary context the careful negotiation of proximity appears equally as necessary. Up close and personal, schizophrenia may be perceived as 'simply terrifying'; too far removed, and apprehension itself becomes strained.

Rather than theorize distance solely in terms of a spatial separation between actors (the psychiatrist and patient), I suggest that the distance between subject and object that is an essential precondition of the sublime encounter can be best conceptualized as an ensemble of discursive practices. It is the development of a *professional* position from which to view (label, probe, and manage) schizophrenia that produces it as a sublime object; instigating and legitimizing a mediated gaze focussed on, but not jeopardized by, this disorder. Foucault writes persuasively on this point, observing that the regimen of the early psychiatric asylum was,

> ... necessary for the very constitution of medical knowledge, since exact observation is not possible without this discipline, without this order, without this prescriptive schema of regularities. The condition of the medical gaze (*regard médicale*), of its neutrality, and the possibility of it gaining access to the object, in short, the effective condition of possibility of the relationship of objectivity, which is constitutive of

medical knowledge and the criterion of its validity, is a relationship of order, a distribution of time, space, and individuals.

(Foucault, 2008, pp. 2–3)[9]

Once it has been confined in the asylum—brought into spatial proximity with the professional subject, but subjected to various distancing measures that make it a suitable object of study, while containing and organizing its threat to the social order—can schizophrenia become capable of producing 'delight'? For Kant, the answer must surely be yes, if we consider that the sublime object's role is to function as a site through which judging subject can exercise the power of their (professional) reasoning. As the sublime 'must in every case have reference to our *way of thinking*' (Kant, 1969, p. 127, italics in the original), in this instance schizophrenia's status as an object of the sublime is dependent on discursively mediated distance, but is simultaneously an incitement to extend discursive limits, to capture the disorder in its totality.

To argue that schizophrenia acquires the status of sublime object for psychiatry, then, is not to imply similarities between the disorder and the qualities of the sublime object. It is, more significantly, to suggest that schizophrenia functions as a limit point for this discipline, a potentially daunting unknown, which perpetually spurs greater efforts at analytic conquest. I am not suggesting that the logic of sublimity is the only means by which psychiatry has shored up the rationality of its discourse. On the contrary, the sublime 'unsettles every locus of power'; destabilizing the very discursive structures whose expansion it enables. The sublime is not 'an end in itself but the power to make every end seem preliminary . . . [it] spontaneously surpasses every designation intended to locate it' (Pease, 1984). Eliding reason's colonization and existing beyond conclusive analytic explanation, schizophrenia serves both as an exemplary site of unreason upon which psychiatry can exercise an ongoing claim to scientificity, *and* as a challenge to the scientificity of those very claims. The unceasing

---

[9] Writing of Foucault's work on medicine more generally, Alan Bleakley and John Bligh question whether Foucault's analysis of the disciplinary medical gaze needs to be reconceptualized in an era when simulation, diffusion, and fragmentation have superseded the physical encounter between doctor and patient: 'the future of medical diagnostics is in the technology of imaging and the art of reading such images, which effectively scatters or distributes the diagnostic gaze as it draws in mediating instruments and a variety of specialist practitioners. Also, Foucault does not address the issue of how the clinical gaze is further shaped by the development and sophistication of tests – of sputum, blood, urine, biopsies – where, as with imaging, the diagnostic gaze is now splintered, distributed across a variety of specialty and subspecialty practitioners preserving their boundaries, and no longer holds that original intensity of the *coup d'oeil*, the penetrating glance of the individual doctor' (Bleakley and Bligh, 2009, pp. 376–7).

proliferation of theories and treatments of schizophrenia testifies to its capacity to produce a delightful confirmation of ever more sophisticated reasoning, whereas the marked inability of these theories and treatments to comprehend or cure schizophrenia can be seen as symptomatic of its sublimity, its capacity to exceed comprehension. Here, schizophrenia also fulfils Burke's condition of sublime obscurity: it remains hidden from the psychiatric gaze while being constantly under the scientific spotlight (Burke, 1987, pp. 58–9).

Before turning to consider in more detail how the logic of sublimity illuminates specific accounts of psychiatry's framing of schizophrenia, the 'strange status' of madness in Foucault's writing warrants re-examination. Although my analysis of the importance of discursively produced distance in the establishment of schizophrenia's sublimity owes much to Foucault's reading of the psychiatric confinement of madness, it also suggests a way of interpreting his indebtedness to the discourses he so robustly critiques. Foucault, and Derrida and Felman after him, identify a crisis of representation when it comes to speaking (about) madness, a crisis which I think is only partially resolved through recourse to a literary mode of writing. The 'lyrical halo of illness' is extinguished in the language of reason, just as madness has endured disfigurement in its transformation from the quotidian to the sublime via the discourse and practices of psychology. Foucault's historical dramatization of the confinement of the insane could therefore be re-read as an allegory for madness's elevation to the status of the sublime, and it is *as* an inherently unrepresentable, sublime object that Foucault politicizes madness, imparting to it a transgressive potential as a freedom outside reason.[10] Put simply, his valourization of madness depends on its confinement, on its sublime status in psychiatry. If, as I have suggested, these disciplines have a Kantian turn about them (that is, the sublime encounter reveals the supreme agency of reason) it is one Foucault radically rejects. Pursuing a liberatory ideal, Foucault is in fact closer to Burke in implicitly hinting at madness's obscurity, power, and unintelligibility; its capacity to elicit pre-rational astonishment rather than the delight of self-contained superiority. Foucault's anamorphic recognition of the sublimity of madness since the great confinement therefore suggests that his hostility towards psychiatry conceals his complicity with the creators of mental illness.

What, then, does this tell us about schizophrenia, specifically? Although Foucault strategically uses the all-encompassing term 'madness' to distance his analysis from psychiatry and its classificatory schema, and to distinguish madness from mental illness, it is clear that by 'madness' Foucault means

---

[10] This is also the case for other antipsychiatric thinkers, as we shall see in Chapters 3 and 4.

something very close to 'schizophrenia'. Indeed, in *The Order of Things* he goes so far as to describe 'madness *par excellence*' as that 'which psychiatrists term schizophrenia' (Foucault, 1970, p. 375). However, as it is my intention throughout this book to insist on the specificity of schizophrenia—on the clinical and cultural significance of the concept, as well as the particular set of experiences it describes—we must resist the temptation to pursue an easy equivalence between the terms 'madness' and 'schizophrenia' in Foucault's work or indeed my analysis of it.

Madness and Civilization charts a history of madness from the middle ages to the birth of modern psychiatry in the nineteenth century, a history that stops short of schizophrenia's identification as a discrete clinical entity in 1896. Although it is commonly assumed that schizophrenia is as old as humanity itself, a significant number of scholars argue strongly that it first appeared in the West during the industrial revolution. Edward Hare, a psychiatrist and advocate of the 'recency hypothesis', claims that 'few if any adequate descriptions of schizophrenia were written before the year 1800' (1988, pp. 153, 521). Notwithstanding the methodological problems of retrospective diagnosis (Fraguas and Breathnach, 2009), Louis Sass also dates the first comprehensive case study of schizophrenia to 1810 (1992, p. 325), and neuropsychologist Christopher Frith and psychiatrist Eve Johnstone to 1809 (2003, p. 7). Hare, advancing a less than popular viral hypothesis, suggests that 'some change of a biological kind occurred about 1800, such that a particular type of schizophrenia thereafter became much commoner [*sic*]' (1988, p. 521), gradually spreading throughout the industrialized world in a slow epidemic. Analysing asylum records and evaluating the relationship between social factors and burgeoning asylum populations, Hare concludes that the spread of schizophrenia provides the best explanation for the stark increase in admissions over the nineteenth century (Hare, 1983). This notion of a substantive increase in insanity, whatever the suggested cause, has been fiercely debated,[11] but the idea that schizophrenia has a special relationship with modernity remains fruitful, as the second half of this book attests.

----

[11] *The invisible plague* (Torrey and Miller, 2001) offers a comprehensive – if ultimately unconvincing – case for the existence of an epidemic of insanity, as well as a survey of competing views. Challenging the viral hypothesis, sociologist Andrew Scull (1984) draws attention to shifts in lunacy legislation, asylum management practices, and cultural attitudes to poverty that significantly affected asylum admissions in the nineteenth century, arguing that definitions of insanity have always been contingent, historically determined, and governed by the ideological interests of those in positions of psychiatric and legal authority.

My point, then, is to suggest that the foregoing analysis of madness in Foucault's influential work provides an important foundation for the current study of schizophrenia in multiple ways. Schizophrenia clearly inherits the fraught legacy of an alienated madness analysed by Foucault, but its appearance in the last years of the nineteenth century prompts us to examine its status as the discovery of a new era of psychiatry. It is this discovery that constitutes the focus of the rest of this chapter.

Clinical psychiatry and dementia praecox

Schizophrenia's status in psychiatric discourse cannot be understood without reference to the writings and practices of one nineteenth-century north German clinician, Emil Kraepelin. A contemporary of Freud, and one-time colleague of Paul Flechsig (who we will meet as Daniel Paul Schreber's 'soul-murderer' in Chapter 2), Kraepelin presented in his 1896 textbook of *Clinical Psychiatry* the first detailed descriptions of dementia praecox. Although dementia praecox was swiftly renamed schizophrenia by Eugen Bleuler, Kraepelin's account of this major form of psychosis has endured without radical alteration for over 100 years: the hebephrenic, catatonic, and paranoid forms of Kraepelin's dementia praecox have become, in the most recent American Psychiatric Association *Diagnostic and Statistical Manual* (DSM-IV-TR) (2000), disorganized, catatonic, and paranoid schizophrenia (complemented by 'undifferentiated' and 'residual' types).[12] As a more detailed examination will make evident, it is not just the psychotic symptoms described by Kraepelin, theoretically reconfigured by Bleuler, and ranked by Kurt Schneider that have been established as diagnostic gospel by today's DSM-IV-TR; an entire conceptual apparatus has survived a century of psychiatric practice. Indeed,

----

[12] At the time of writing, one of the most significant areas of contention in schizophrenia research is the simultaneous contraction and expansion of definitions of schizophrenia proposed for the fifth edition of the American Psychiatric Association's *Diagnostic and Statistical Manual*. DSM-5, as it is known, is due to be published in mid-2013, and there is little doubt that the fifth 'bible' of American psychiatry will continue to exert a huge influence worldwide. Overturning a century of nosological convention, the current draft aims to 'streamline' schizophrenia by replacing its five subtypes with a simple scale for assessing the severity of specific symptoms. At the same time, however, it adds the new diagnostic category of 'psychosis risk syndrome'. Although its proponents hope the diagnostic category will facilitate early and effective intervention for those in the prodromal phase of schizophrenia (Carpenter, 2009; Woods et al., 2009), critics argue that psychosis risk syndrome risks exposing tens of thousands of people with false positive diagnoses to stigma, unwelcome clinical attention, and the debilitating side effects of antipsychotic drugs (Dobbs, 2010; Frances, 2010). If *DSM-V* has begun a 'civil war' in psychiatry (Aldhous, 2009), psychosis risk syndrome is surely among its most conflict-ridden arenas (Aldhous, 2010).

the psychiatrist whose analysis of dementia praecox met with, at best, 'lively resistance' (Kraepelin quoted in McKenna, 1994, p. v) from his peers now occupies a position of almost imperial authority in orthodox psychiatry. As Berrios and Hauser note: 'The Kraepelinian classification of the psychoses *governs* twentieth-century psychiatric thinking and neurobiological research' (Berrios and Hauser, 1995, p. 280, my italics). Through a close reading of Kraepelin's treatment of dementia praecox in *Clinical Psychiatry*, I aim to demonstrate that schizophrenia's sublime status in psychiatry—its paradoxical legitimization and destabilization of psychiatry's scientificity, its construction as other to the centred modern subject—is already clearly established in the first and most influential clinical picture of this disorder. So multifaceted is the influence of this text that a detailed analysis of its account of dementia praecox is indispensable to understanding the status of schizophrenia in contemporary psychiatric discourse.

It is possible that dementia praecox might not have been identified by Kraepelin at all if it were not for two idiosyncrasies: his bad eyesight and his meticulous record keeping. German psychiatry, by the end of the nineteenth century, had become almost exclusively focussed on the somatic aetiology of psychiatric disease. The microscope was the privileged tool of the alienist's trade, and the goal of biological analysis was to identify post-mortem areas in the cerebral cortex responsible for various psychotic symptoms (Shorter, 1997, pp. 79–80). As a consequence, any interest in the effect of psychosis upon the patient and their behaviour was considerably diminished. Kraepelin's poor eyesight, however, meant that he was unable to pursue his career through the microscope (Shorter, 1997, pp. 100–1). Instead, he followed his then rather unfashionable interest in psychology and focussed his investigations on the family and personal history of the patient and the course of their illness. Recording this information alongside clinical observations on his famous patient cards, Kraepelin was able to track patients as they moved from university clinics to asylums, relapsed, or recovered (Engstrom, 1995, pp. 294, 297). He therefore acquired enough statistical data on patient populations to pursue a longitudinal approach to the study of psychiatric illness and its nosology, an approach that proved instrumental to his formulation of dementia praecox.

In 1860 the French alienist Bénédict-Augustin Morel, famous for introducing to asylum science the notion of degeneration, first used the term *démence précoce* to describe a chronic insanity predominantly affecting young men (Healy, 2002, p. 18).[13] Morel filled a taxonomic gap—psychosis with adolescent

---

[13] German Berrios and colleagues note that 'Because Morel did not propose "*démence précoce*" as an official clinical category but as a mere description, it had already sunk into oblivion by the time Kraepelin had decided to use the term "dementia praecox"', and was

onset had joined the ranks of other age-specific psychoses and absorbed the earlier diagnosis of masturbatory insanity (Gilman, 1988, p. 205). But it was Emil Kraepelin who used the term to reconfigure fundamentally the psychiatric approach to mental illness, interpreting all psychotic behaviour not shown to have been caused by intoxication or direct damage to the brain as the product of one of two natural disease entities: manic–depressive psychosis or dementia praecox. Kraepelin distinguished dementia praecox from manic–depressive psychosis primarily by the course of the illness: although there was some overlap in symptoms, the outcome of manic–depressive psychosis was favourable, whereas dementia praecox, as the name suggests, was characterized 'by a pronounced tendency to mental deterioration of varying grades' (Kraepelin, 1981, p. 219). It was the tendency towards significant deterioration, which Kraepelin identified in hebephrenia, catatonia, and paranoia, that led him to reconceptualize these previously distinct psychoses as the three forms of one illness. In Kraepelin's longitudinal analysis, dementia praecox was one 'disease entity with a tangible underlying morbid process' (Johnstone et al., 1999, p. ix). Unable to define this entity or demonstrate its process, however, Kraepelin could only speculate about dementia praecox's probable causes. Conceding that 'the disease process in dementia praecox is not known', he nevertheless believed there was 'a definite disease process in the brain', perhaps triggered by an 'autointoxication . . . related to processes in the sexual organs', and that a large percentage of patients were made vulnerable to the disease by their 'defective heredity' (Kraepelin, 1981, pp. 221–2).[14]

These unsubstantiated aetiological conjectures did not prevent Kraepelin from writing at length and with conviction about the hallmark symptoms of this new disease entity. Upon admission to the asylum, sufferers of dementia praecox could be identified by their lack of attention, volition, judgement, appropriate emotional responsiveness, and, of course, by the 'silliness' of intermittent hebephrenic delusions and hallucinations, the rigid immobility of catatonic stupor, and the complexities of the fantastical delusions characteristic of paranoia. Significantly, the symbolic content of the bizarre delusions, hallucinations, or immobile postures of the dementia praecox patient was deemed by Kraepelin to be inconsequential, a position in sharp contrast to the hermeneutical analyses of the psychoses advanced by psychoanalysts. It was not the probing analysis of individuals and their symptoms, but the 'majesty of

most probably not known to him (Berrios et al., 2003, p. 117). However, as Rob Barrett (1998a) observes, the *concept* of degeneration remained profoundly important to Kraepelin's account of dementia praecox.

14 Richard Noll (2007) offers a comprehensive contemporary reappraisal of Kraepelin's theories of autointoxication.

Kraepelin's overall structure' that, in the estimation of neoapologist historian Edward Shorter, 'transfixed the psychiatric world' (Shorter, 1997, p. 108).

Although Kraepelin's work was viewed as controversial by his contemporaries, it swiftly grew in status throughout the twentieth century, 'eclipsing' Jean Esquirol's (1965) earlier taxonomies of insanity, Carl Wernicke's study of brain localization,[15] and finally the psychodynamic and psychoanalytic approaches to mental illness that dominated American psychiatry until the late 1970s. As Paul Hoff notes:

> Kraepelin's psychiatry became so influential, because it offered a pragmatical, clinically and prognostically oriented nosology, developed by a self-confident author who focussed on rather straight-forward quantitative and naturalistic research methods and claimed to abandon speculative aspects from psychiatry as much as possible.

> (Hoff, 1995, p. 273)

Kraepelin has been viewed less as a visionary or revolutionary thinker than as the natural product of a positivist movement in the late nineteenth century, a movement that privileged empiricism over metaphysics and evinced a 'profound confidence in the ideas of development and progress' (Hoff, 1995, p. 263). Although the empirical analysis of symptomatology and longitudinal analysis of the course of illness enabled Kraepelin to draw together several approaches to psychosis under the umbrella concept of dementia praecox, only a confidence in the authoritative scientificity of psychiatry justified his assertion that the different forms of dementia praecox were the result of a single but as yet indeterminate disease process.

Kraepelin's methodological approach to dementia praecox can be interpreted as the decisive factor in explaining how schizophrenia is at once the bedrock of psychiatry's claim to scientificity and the source of its seismic tremors. The genius of Kraepelin's concept of dementia praecox lies in his rejection of the primacy of aetiology and brain localization in the identification of this disease entity, in favour of describing and cataloguing its symptoms and tracing their development in each patient. The 'clinical picture' of dementia praecox, distilled from the observation of presumably hundreds of patients, was detailed enough to be of diagnostic and hence prognostic use to clinicians both in the identification of patients for treatment and of patient populations for research purposes. However, what further guaranteed its efficacy and longevity was its extreme flexibility. This clinical picture could, and would, be broken down into its constitutive elements and redrawn under new principles; it did not rely upon or advance any specific treatment of the whole disease, ensuring

---

[15] There is still no English translation of Wernicke's most comprehensive publication – *Outlines of Psychiatry*. See Wernicke (1900).

it would become a site for the development of new methods; finally, and most importantly, by subordinating and deferring the question of aetiology, Kraepelin's concept of dementia praecox not only stimulated further research but itself provided no grounds upon which to discriminate between theoretical analyses, thus ensuring their ongoing proliferation in and beyond the field of biological psychiatry. Twenty years after identifying dementia praecox, Kraepelin wrote that the causes of the illness were 'still mapped in impenetrable darkness' (Kraepelin, quoted in Johnstone et al., 1999, p. 4). Fifty years later, with its aetiology still the subject of psychiatric debate, and its treatment confined for the most part to ECT, insulin therapy, and the new and serendipitously discovered antipsychotic drugs, Kraepelin's clinical picture could even be compatible with *anti*psychiatric models of socially constructed schizophrenia. With this in mind, we can consider how those aspects of Kraepelin's clinical picture of dementia praecox, which have been intensely productive, if not pivotal, for psychiatry's project of scientificity, can be simultaneously interpreted as undermining, if not undoing, that project.

In her book, *Schizophrenia: A Scientific Delusion*, Mary Boyle claims to 'make understandable some of the reasons for the chaos and controversy which have so often surrounded the concept [of schizophrenia], for its persistence in spite of these, and to make clear why no amount of tinkering with it will bestow scientific respectability' (Boyle, 1990, p. vii). Kraepelin is again invoked as the founding father of schizophrenia, but here he bequeaths not order, scientificity, or 'majesty' to psychiatry but an unstable, unsubstantiated, and deeply flawed concept developed, Boyle argues, as a last resort to impose order upon the bizarre behaviour of asylum patients (Boyle, 1990, p. 45). Boyle's attack on Kraepelin's methodology is multilayered and unremitting. Drawing attention to the inadequacy of his patient card system, his failure to quantify his findings, and his recourse to a rhetoric of authority when faced with a distinct lack of empirical evidence, she lays her most severe charge:

> Instead of *concluding* by inferring his construct, having presented evidence in support, Kraepelin *began* with the construct and proceeded to describe what he called cases of dementia praecox. [. . .] Kraepelin's descriptions are in the form, 'one often notices'; 'it is occasionally observed'; 'in some cases', and so on. Thus, Kraepelin wrote as if by some independent and valid criteria, established by past research, dementia praecox had already been inferred in this sample and he was merely engaged in recording his impressions of the group. He wrote, that is, as if data supporting the introduction of his concept had already been presented when in fact they had not.
>
> (Boyle, 1990, p. 46)

What Boyle finds so striking about Kraepelin's work on dementia praecox is that despite purporting to emerge from a scientific framework, it is supported not by data but purely by belief (Boyle, 1990, p. 75). In this account, the elasticity of Kraepelin's clinical picture of dementia praecox stretches to breaking point; scientificity is performative, an effect of masterful rhetoric rather than 'properly' scientific practice.

Boyle's call to de-centre and dismantle the psychiatric delusion of schizophrenia goes to the core of the discipline's claims to scientificity. And she is not alone. 'The Kraepelinian dichotomy: the twin pillars crumbling?' asks one historian of psychiatry (Greene, 2007). 'The Kraepelinian dichotomy—going, going . . . but still not gone' molecular geneticists lament (Craddock and Owen, 2010b; see also Crow, 1985, 1995; Craddock and Owen, 2005, 2007; Craddock et al., 2009; Craddock, 2010; Craddock and Owen, 2010a). If progress is to be made in schizophrenia research, it is claimed, clinical, neuroscientific, genetic, and phenomenological data must be gathered and analysed without regard to diagnostic labels (Cuthbert and Insel, 2010; Heckers, 2008). More daringly, Richard Bentall, another clinical psychologist, has consistently called for the abandonment of the concept of schizophrenia altogether (see Bentall et al., 1988a; Bentall et al., 1988b; Bentall, 1990), and in *Madness Explained* (Bentall, 2004) mounts a comprehensive argument in favour of dismantling the entire nosological structure of Kraepelinian psychiatry. Kraepelin's failings, for Bentall, are many, but stem primarily from his claim that psychosis can be explained by two distinct underlying disease processes, and that there is an unambiguous separation between psychotic and 'normal' experiences. Bentall concludes from his review of the scientific literature that 'Studies of patients' symptoms, of the role of genes, of the course and outcome of illnesses over time, and of the response of symptoms to treatment, all point to similarities between schizophrenia and bipolar disorder rather than to differences' (Bentall, 2004, p. 94). He then advances the continuity principle, which argues for a continuum in the frequency, severity, and phenomenology of abnormal and normal experiences and behaviours (Bentall, 2004, p. 115). Although his call to '*abandon psychiatric diagnoses altogether and instead try to explain and understand the actual experiences and behaviours of psychotic people*' (Bentall, 2004, p. 141, italics in the original) remains a minority and contested view (Lawrie et al., 2010), it is supported by a growing number of researchers (Greene, 2007; Romme and Morris, 2007).

Kraepelin's work emerged from a positivistic scientific framework even if it did not, upon closer analysis, conform to contemporary understandings of a properly scientific methodology. Boyle acknowledges that the limitations of Kraepelin's clinical picture of dementia praecox were in part dictated by the status of scientific research in the late nineteenth century; what emerges as particularly problematic for her, as for Bentall, is the enormous and enduring influence of Kraepelin's ideas into the twentieth and early twenty-first century. Stephan Heckers, who agrees that the differentiation of schizophrenia and bipolar disorder is arbitrary and unhelpful, provides a succinct reminder of the value of Kraepelin's underlying disease entities:

> While not perfect, they have predictive power. They simplify complex human behavior and provide a framework for communication among affected individuals, relatives, caregivers, and the society at large. They also justify research efforts that pledge to uncover the basis of mental illness (eg the gene or brain region for schizophrenia). Kraepelin's vision of progress in psychiatric research gives hope to those who struggle to make sense of mental illness. Any research agenda that challenges the Kraepelinian model will have to provide the same kind of inspiration.

(Heckers, 2008, p. 592)

In an editorial introduction to a special issue of *History of Psychiatry* on Kraepelin's legacy, Eric Engstrom and Matthias Weber further note that in dominant psychiatric discourse 'Kraepelin has become a touchstone of professional loyalties and that he is put to use in the strategic organization and apportionment of disciplinary resources, power and knowledge' (Engstrom and Weber, 2007, p. 268). It seems clear that for psychiatry to recognize the central object of its scientific enquiry as the beliefs—not the discovery—of one nineteenth-century clinician would be to risk much, including, perhaps, its own undoing.

We will return to these issues later in the chapter. What I want to do first, however, is to look at the extent to which in 'resurrecting' Kraepelin's clinical picture of dementia praecox 'to reimpose an order on world psychiatry' (Healy, 2002, p. 174), psychiatry imported not only an unscientific concept, but also a concept embedded in and dependent on a grand narrative of modern Western selfhood.[16] Attending closely to a number of tropes deployed repeatedly in *Clinical Psychiatry*, we can see how dementia praecox is primarily figured by Kraepelin as a disruption in the capacity of the patient to engage in a specific type of labour, figured, that is, as a disorder of the modern labouring individual.

----

[16] The relationship between schizophrenia and notions of the self has been widely studied (see for example Fabrega, 1989; Estroff, 1989, 2004; Jenkins and Barrett, 2004a, b; Lysaker and Lysaker, 2010), and is one of the central problematics explored in this book. I agree with Barrett that 'psychiatric formulations of schizophrenia have emerged from the background of Western cultural formulations of the person', and see the ensuing analysis of the centrality of labour in Kraepelin's account of dementia praecox as confirmation of Barrett's observation that in a culture oriented towards development and progress, 'The person with schizophrenia, at least in the West, becomes the antithesis of the idealised person' (Barrett, 1998a, p. 618).

For the secular, rational, self-determining subject—the modern self—progress 'becomes part of the imperative of selfhood', conceptually underpinning the project of organized, disciplined self-development in the pursuit of 'a state of grace' (Jervis, 1998, p. 189). Psychiatry has been pivotal in shaping, managing, and promulgating the regulatory ideal that Nikolas Rose (1996, p. 2) calls the 'regime of the self', an ideal which, in the modern West, 'embodied the social norms and values of a middle class' (Goldberg, 1999, p. 185). Kraepelin's writings on dementia praecox clearly construct the disease entity as antithetical to this ideal of a bourgeois selfhood capable of and committed to the perpetual labour of self-improvement. By articulating dementia praecox as the dramatic collapse or rupture of the rationality and volition that define the modern self and underpin its capacity for this edifying labour, Kraepelin locates the patient not only symbolically outside the teleological narrative of modern selfhood, but also as actively resistant to the imperatives of that narrative. In this, Kraepelin's clinical picture of dementia praecox, as a modern form of madness, exemplifies trends in the asylum psychiatry of his era. Foucault argues that the great confinement was an effect of the classical period's ethical injunction against idleness; labour was 'an infallible panacea' for the sinful sloth of the poor and the insane (Foucault, 1993, p. 56). Early asylum administrators reconfigured the meaning of labour but retained it as a central form of treatment, creating a scenario in which 'work is deprived of any productive value; it is imposed only as a moral rule; a limitation of liberty, a submission to order, an engagement of responsibility' (Foucault, 1993, p. 248). I would suggest that the psychiatry of Kraepelin's era—claiming its authority primarily on medical and not religious grounds—is nonetheless reliant upon these earlier 'unscientific' beliefs in the moral value of labour and the importance of labour to the definition and maintenance of the modern self. Nowhere is this more in evidence than the portrait of that self's psychotic Other.

In his inventory of the symptomatology of dementia praecox, the first 'fundamental symptoms' Kraepelin identifies are 'a pronounced impairment of voluntary *attention*', profound disturbance of the train of thought, a failing of judgement resulting in 'irrational' actions, and 'disturbance in the emotional field' (Kraepelin, 1981, pp. 223–6, italics in the original). These symptoms appear to culminate or crystallize in,

> ... disturbances of *conduct*, of which the most fundamental is the progressive *disappearance of voluntary activity*. One of the first symptoms of the disease may be the loss of that activity which is peculiar to the patient. He may neglect his duties and sit unoccupied for the greater part of the day, though capable of doing good work if persistently encouraged.
>
> (Kraepelin, 1981, p. 227, italics in the original)

Inactivity—not only a lack of productivity, but also an implicit rejection of the imperative to be productive—is a hallmark characteristic of sufferers of dementia praecox prior to their institutional confinement (Kraepelin, 1981, p. 231). The situation deteriorates following admission to the asylum: by now the patient's '*capacity for employment* is seriously impaired', and three-quarters of those admitted become 'dull, indolent, apathetic, anergic, sluggish', 'slovenly', 'unproductive and mute', in short, unfit for work (Kraepelin, 1981, pp. 228, 238, italics in the original).[17] Eventually, the patient no longer has the desire or the ability to perform mental and manual labour, and as an 'unproductive vegetative organism' is no longer a self as such (Kraepelin, 1981, p. 239). A minority of 'apparently recovered' patients might regain their capacity to labour, but 'fail to employ themselves profitably' for their work does not reflect an appropriate commitment to the ideals of productivity, rationality, and ambition (Kraepelin, 1981, p. 240). Either 'they spend much time in reading, evolving impractical schemes, and pondering over abstract and useless questions', or they 'show a lack of interest, are unbalanced, and unable to advance in their profession or occupation' (Kraepelin, 1981, p. 240). Finally, the question of employment reveals that there can be no complete recovery in Kraepelin's model: even those well-educated patients who exhibit no symptoms find themselves unable to realize their professional ambitions and instead must seek situations with few or no intellectual demands (Kraepelin, 1981, p. 241).

Kraepelin's comparative analysis of dementia praecox among the population of Java is noteworthy here. While asserting the universal validity of his diagnosis (the 'overall familiarity' of the phenomenon in Java 'far outweighed the deviant features') he does repeatedly remark on the 'much less florid, less distinctively marked' and less severe symptoms exhibited by the Javanese, which he suggests can be explained by their 'lower stage of intellectual development' (Kraepelin, 2000, p. 40). Europeans, possessed of what Kraepelin considered to be a greater intellectual capacity and commitment to higher forms of labour, would seem to be more at risk of devastation by dementia praecox as a disease process that isolates and opposes them to modern Western selfhood. The resistance to labour, present at every stage in the course of dementia praecox and even in its wake, is not simply a perceived neglect of or disinterest in a particular type of employment; it incorporates a resistance to the labour of self-improvement and recovery, and thus becomes the central problem of the disease entity and a marker of its strangeness.

---

[17] Reading these descriptions immediately brings to mind Goffman's (1973) classic study of the role of the asylum, or 'total institution', in producing this 'symptomatic' behaviour.

For Kraepelin, then, the most significant measure of a patient's wellbeing is not how they communicate with others, or express themselves, but their capacity for work performance. 'Performance turns into "work"', writes Karl Jaspers, 'when it is carried out as a steady effort for a practical purpose, absorbs the person as a whole, depends on his getting tired and refreshed, and is generally subject to quantitative measurement' (Jaspers, 1972, p. 205). Kraepelin pioneered experimental methods for measuring work performance in relation to subjective variables, and 'called the characteristics obtained from his "working-curve" (fatiguability, capacity for recovery, drive, etc.) "*basic personality characteristics*"' (Jaspers, 1972, p. 622, italics in the original). The concepts of functionality and productivity thus are essential to the Kraepelinian view of the self; indeed, it is through work performance and the attendant labour of self-improvement that selfhood is guaranteed in health and ultimately jeopardized in psychosis. It is of little surprise, then, that in the case of dementia praecox, Kraepelin insists that an 'essential feature of the care of these mental shipwrecks is healthful employment, preferably out of doors' (Kraepelin, 1981, p. 275). What *is* surprising is that the centrality of labour—employment and self-improvement—to Kraepelin's system should have been largely overlooked in the many analyses of his hugely influential work on dementia praecox.[18]

Returning to the matter at hand, we must now consider how, by positioning dementia praecox as outside and fundamentally resistant to modern, autonomous, secular selfhood, Kraepelin elevates this disease entity to the status of the sublime. Twice in *Clinical Psychiatry* (Kraepelin, 1981, pp. 241, 275), Kraepelin uses the striking image of a 'mental shipwreck' to describe patients afflicted by dementia praecox. A seafaring vessel broken by unrepresentable meteorological forces; a psyche blown off the narrow course of self-improving progress, ravaged by an unrelenting and unknown disease process: in a sudden rupture of his own scientific discourse, Kraepelin records his perception of the catastrophe of dementia praecox through a staple image of the sublime. The ship is a convenient metaphor for Kraepelin's view of normal/ideal selfhood: progressing through the vicissitudes of life to the destination of psychic maturity, it is autonomous, imperial, and can be both rationally explained and repaired by mechanically minded men of science. As a spectacle of privation, recalling Burke's term, the 'mental shipwreck' of dementia praecox suggests it is other to the modern self because of the stark visibility of its dysfunction rather than for any inherently supernatural qualities. Burke further argued

---

[18] Although see 'Labours of Schizophrenia' in Peter Barham's *Schizophrenia and Human Value* (1993).

that obscurity, in terms of mental as well as sensory apprehension, was a vital part of the sublime, for 'When we know the full extent of any danger . . . a great deal of the apprehension vanishes' (Burke, 1987, pp. 58–9). In the case of Kraepelin's dementia praecox, a clear presentation of the disease entity (comprising a detailed inventory of symptoms, illuminating descriptions of the vivid psychotic delusions, and statistical analysis of patient populations) belies the essential obscurity surrounding the aetiology and treatment of the disease process.

Clearly the psychiatrist is not merely the witness of dementia praecox, but from the moment of diagnosis engages with psychosis through the hierarchical structures of the asylum and the culturally mediated roles of clinician and patient, professional and inmate, rational explicator and irrational victim of the disease process. Distance, as I have already indicated, is of supreme importance in the apprehension of an object as sublime, and, in addition to the physical and disciplinary boundaries of the asylum, Kraepelin's methodology, his longitudinal approach to mental illness, depends upon further maintaining the patient object at a particular and predetermined distance. The intimacy of a psychoanalytic encounter—the guided exploration of the latent content of symptoms, the repetition of sessions building an analytic relationship— although not inconceivable in an asylum context, was neither sought after nor valued by Kraepelin. Instead, his patient card system kept *people* suffering from specific psychic disturbances at a distance, but ensured a certain proximity to each *patient* (or 'symptom-carrier' (Porter, 2002, p. 184)) as their illness progressed under statistical scrutiny.[19] As a clinician, not a laboratory practitioner, Kraepelin was close enough to the patient populations of the clinics and asylums in which he worked to be confronted daily with the spectacle of insanity; armed with the undertaking of a comprehensive longitudinal analysis of all psychiatric disorders, and rising quickly in the professional ranks, it appears that he was seldom if ever engaged with psychotic people in any long-term or individually meaningful way. Kraepelin's position can be juxtaposed with that of his contemporaries, Wernicke and Kahlbaum, whose 'brain-localizing' fondness for the microscope paradoxically separated them from dementia praecox as they attempted to capture and conquer it in the cerebral cortex. Kant's lengthy description of the best place from which to apprehend the pyramids as sublime (rather than as triangles on the horizon or as mere slabs of rough-hewn stone) finds a strong if strange equivalence in the precision of Kraepelin's physical and discursive positioning of the object of his analysis.

---

[19] Kraepelin (2010) gives a fascinating insight into the structure and operation of the surveillance wards he established for this purpose.

The qualities attributed to dementia praecox and the institutionally medi-ated modes of identifying and categorizing those qualities contributed to the production of dementia praecox, and in turn schizophrenia, as a sublime object of early psychiatry. However, it is the third aspect of the sublime encoun-ter, its 'delightful' (re)affirmation of the subject's rationality, that I would argue is the most significant factor in twentieth-century psychiatry's elevation of schizophrenia to the status of sublime object. It is not the isolated encounter between mad doctor and the mad person that is at stake here, but rather the cumulative effect that the theoretical framing of these encounters has in per-petually extending the parameters of psychiatry. Recall, once again, Mark Cheetham's constructive observation:

> At different times and from different perspectives, even large and imprecisely defined constructs such as disciplines will have their own sublimes, those issues that are at once feared and desired and which, through the disciplinary attention they garner, work to mark the provisional limits and flash points of particular disciplines.

(Cheetham, 1995, p. 360)

Kraepelin's clinical picture of dementia praecox has been framed and reframed countless times; it is the capacity of that picture to fit almost any scientific frame drawn around it that has secured schizophrenia unparalleled and ongoing disciplinary attention. Underscoring that clinical picture is Kraepelin's belief that human behaviour can be measured, quantified, and ultimately rendered transparent by psychiatry; as Jaspers observes, Kraepelin's 'basic conceptual world remained a somatic one', his discussions of psychology regarded 'as temporary stopgaps until experiment, microscope and test-tube permitted objective investigation' (Jaspers, 1972, p. 852). In his own erudite writing on the subject, Jaspers makes clear that no such totalizing 'objective investigation' into human behaviour is possible:

> *Psychopathology is limited* in that there can be no final analysis of human beings as such, since the more we reduce them to what is typical and normative, the more we realise there is something hidden in every human individual which defies recognition. We have to be content with partial knowledge of an infinity which we cannot exhaust.

(Jaspers, 1972, p. 1, italics in the original)

Jaspers locates the disorder in relation to the unknowable dimensions of *all* human experience, not as radically other to a normative model of bourgeois selfhood. Although the spectacle of an individual's psychosis may be a sublime moment for any psychiatrist (a moment, that is, in which a sense of terror is swiftly mitigated by the diagnosis of that behaviour as a symptom of the disease process dementia praecox), dementia praecox is a sublime object for orthodox psychiatry because it is visible (as a clinical picture) but fundamentally obscure (as a disease process of unknown origins) and so a perpetual site of contestation in a discipline that would demystify, rationalize, and render transparent every dimension of human behaviour.

If a pivotal tension in psychiatry arises from the conflict over the aetiology of mental illness—namely, is it of somatic, environmental, psychic, or intersubjective origin—schizophrenia has been the prime site for what psychiatrist David Healy describes as a series of ongoing 'turf wars' (2002, p. 145). Kraepelin was a leader of the eugenic biological psychiatry that developed from the middle of the nineteenth century only to be disgraced by its association with and appropriation by Nazi psychiatry.[20] A strong psychoanalytic focus guided American, and in turn global, psychiatry from the Second World War until the 1970s when, in the triumphant words of Edward Shorter, 'biological psychiatry came roaring back on stage, displacing psychoanalysis as the dominant paradigm and returning psychiatry to the fold of other medical specialities' (Shorter, 1997, p. 239). If Kraepelin, the first to identify dementia praecox, is the intellectual ancestor of the biological psychiatry once again dominating the management of mental illness today, Eugen Bleuler is the psychiatrist who psychologized dementia praecox, renaming it schizophrenia and broadening the analytic possibilities for its diagnosis and treatment. In the following section of this chapter, I will discuss the detail and significance of Bleuler's reconceptualization of dementia praecox as schizophrenia, and suggest that even in its departure from Kraepelinian orthodoxy it serves to reinforce the validity and scientificity of Kraepelin's claims.

From dementia praecox to schizophrenia

Eugen Bleuler's 1911 text, *Dementia Praecox, or The Group of Schizophrenias*, is most frequently cited simply for introducing the term schizophrenia to modern psychiatry.[21] A cynical explanation of this change in nomenclature would note that Bleuler's departure from the Latin phrase brought psychiatric taxonomies in line with the fashion for Greek neoclassicism (Gilman, 1988,

---

[20] For an accessible account of the Nazi's psychiatric genocide see Torrey and Yolken (2009). This horrific chapter in psychiatric and medical history has not received the attention it has deserved. However, as Rael Strous notes, 'That it has taken close to 60 years to confront this dark period in the history of psychiatry does not diminish the importance of finally dealing with it. It is painfully shameful that close to 300 000 individuals with schizophrenia were either sterilized or killed at the behest of members of our profession' (Strous, 2010).

[21] In fact, he first used the term 3 years earlier in a lecture at the German Psychiatric Association in Berlin (Fusar-Poli and Politi, 2008).

p. 203). However, the arguments Bleuler advances in favour of abandoning the cumbersome 'dementia praecox' reveal that the shift is more than superficial. First, Bleuler notes that as dementia praecox 'designates the disease, not the diseased', the term is not only awkward but limited in its application (Bleuler, 1950, p. 7).[22] Secondly, he draws attention to a fact that Kraepelin, too, was forced to acknowledge: dementia praecox does not, as the name suggests, always have early onset, nor does it always result in dementia. Such were the problems seemingly resolved by the rejection of 'dementia praecox', but 'schizophrenia' was in no way an innocent or unassuming replacement. Although he writes that 'it is really quite impossible to find a perfect name for a concept which is still developing and changing', Bleuler advocates the term schizophrenia, meaning 'split mind', because in his view 'the "splitting" of the different psychic functions is one of its most important characteristics' (Bleuler, 1950, p. 8). Schizophrenia rapidly replaced dementia praecox as the preferred term of psychiatric discourse, but proceeded to acquire a life of its own in the non-psychiatric imaginary:

> The rise of the term 'schizophrenia' was probably due, in part, to the simultaneously exotic and familiar sound of the word itself, with its echoes of 'schism' and 'frenzy' and 'frenetic', but also, less superficially, to the meaning commonly attributed to the word: not so much 'split mind', as 'split personality'. . . . Although this has had a regrettably powerful influence on what most people understand schizophrenia to be, it bears virtually no resemblance to schizophrenia as currently diagnosed.

> (Crichton, 2000, p. 14)[23]

Bleuler's understanding of the disease—'a specific type of alteration of thinking, feeling, and relation to the external world which appears nowhere else in this particular fashion' (Bleuler, 1950, p. 9)—has been less than uniformly accepted, its perceived validity dependent on whether psychological or biological models of psychosis dominate psychiatric enquiry.[24]

----

[22] Although Bleuler's positive view of using schizophrenic as a noun no doubt appears scandalous today (the mental health sector strenuously rejects such terminology as stereotyping and stigmatizing), it is worth noting that he in no way intended for this to be dehumanizing. On the contrary, Bleuler's interest in and attachment to his patients has been well documented (see, for example, the second chapter of Bentall, 2004).

[23] In an interesting analysis of the history of this informal usage, Kieran McNally takes a different view: 'Schizophrenia as split personality was not then a result of misinterpretation by the general public. It was generated, maintained, and reinforced from within the culture of the psychological professions until it was no longer useful' (McNally, 2007, p. 78).

[24] Thus Eve Johnstone (Johnstone et al., 1999, p. 30) writes: 'Although Kraepelin's view retained their popularity in Europe until the 1960s and 1970s, Bleuler's ideas held sway in the United States. His concept of schizophrenia as an essentially psychological

The key distinction between Bleuler's account of schizophrenia and Kraepelin's clinical picture of dementia praecox has been isolated by Healy: 'whereas Kraepelin's dementia praecox was simply descriptive, Bleuler offered a model that made sense of the descriptions' (Healy, 2002, p. 265). Bleuler did not significantly extend, narrow, or otherwise dispute Kraepelin's inventory of symptoms of dementia praecox so much as offer a different rationale for their appearance. His account of schizophrenia hinges upon the idea that the normal mind works by unifying psychic functions, drives, and processes. In schizophrenia, these become 'split off' from each other, and the psyche is fragmented by the dominance or impotence of various incomplete psychic processes. Utilizing this dynamic model, Bleuler divides Kraepelin's inventory of schizophrenic symptoms into two dichotomies: fundamental and accessory, and primary and secondary symptoms. Summarized as the Four As—Autism, Ambivalence, Affective disturbance, and impaired Associations—the fundamental symptoms are, according to Bleuler, present in all cases and at all stages of the illness (Bleuler, 1950, p. 13). The symptoms traditionally identified as 'properly' psychotic—hallucinations, delusions, and catatonic stupor—are deemed accessory, as they are less consistent in presentation and duration. The primary/secondary dichotomy appears to extend the relationship between fundamental and accessory symptoms.[25] In the dynamic disease process of schizophrenic splitting, the psychiatrist must 'distinguish the symptoms stemming directly from the disease process itself from those secondary symptoms which only begin to operate when the sick psyche reacts to some internal or external process' (Bleuler, 1950, p. 348). For example, hallucinations (accessory and secondary symptoms) would be interpreted as a reaction or adaptation to psychic malfunctioning precipitated by the fundamental and primary symptoms of the disease process. Directly influenced by Jung and others of the Zurich School, Bleuler believed that such symptoms could be meaningfully interpreted, no matter how incomprehensible they appeared to be (Bleuler, 1950, p. 96). For Jaspers this is essentially 'a *translation to schizophrenia of concepts which have been arrived at during the analysis of hysteria*' (Jaspers, 1972, p. 410, italics in the original); hence, as we shall see in the next chapter, it is an approach that overlooks the specific structure of symptom formation in

---

disorder, possibly with a psychogenic basis, rather than a pathological condition of the nervous system, was compatible with the psychoanalytic orientation prevailing in the USA at that time'.

[25] Although as Boyle (1990, pp. 60–1) observes, 'Bleuler's writings give no indication that he meant this to be the case . . . some behaviours called fundamental symptoms appear later as secondary, while behaviours called accessory symptoms were later labelled primary'.

schizophrenia. In any event, the enduring effect of psychologizing Kraepelin's dementia praecox and foregrounding the importance of the least bizarre symptoms of psychosis (such as ambivalence and a lack of affect) was to broaden further both the concept and the diagnostic criteria of schizophrenia (Crichton, 2000, p. 14).

For all their differences, Bleuler's account of schizophrenia is the first and perhaps the strongest testament to the flexibility of the clinical picture of dementia praecox advanced by Kraepelin. As I have already discussed, Kraepelin described dementia praecox as a disease process with three forms (hebephrenic, catatonic, and paranoid), each of which could be distinguished from manic–depressive psychosis by a pronounced tendency to deterioration. The title of Bleuler's work, *Dementia Praecox or The Group of Schizophrenias*, thus appears to contradict Kraepelin fundamentally: if deterioration is no longer the defining feature of schizophrenia, of which there are not three forms but potentially many, how can the two terms designate the same disease process? The simple answer is because the question of what that disease process actually is remains unanswered in both texts. For Kraepelin, a belief in the neurobiological origin of psychosis was enough to justify his unsubstantiated claim that dementia praecox was a disease of the brain. This belief propels him from the uncertain to the definitive in a single sentence:

> The nature of the disease process in dementia praecox is not known, but it seems probable, judging from the clinical course, and especially in those cases where there has been rapid deterioration, that there is a definite disease process in the brain, involving the cortical neurones.

> (Kraepelin, 1981, p. 221)

Bleuler evinces no such unshakable faith in somatic aetiology, but his opening caveat similarly betrays an uncertainty regarding the nature of the disease process:

> Our knowledge of the disease group which Kraepelin established under the name of Dementia Praecox is too recent to warrant a complete description. The whole complex is still too fluid, incomplete, tentative. Since it would be rather tedious to draw attention to all the reservations implied by this fact, I hope I am justified in assuming that the reader will bear this in mind.

> (Bleuler, 1950, p. 1)

Here, the reader must be complicit with an author who states that producing a 'complete' description of schizophrenia is virtually impossible, yet who presents his work, following Kraepelin, as a comprehensive if not definitive account of the disease. Like the author, the reader must (but only in the interests of avoiding boredom) effectively repress questions as to the scientific validity of his claims.

Bleuler's systematic presentation and psychological subtlety cannot disguise the fact that the symptomatological dichotomies constitutive of his depth model of schizophrenia derive from a phantom origin: he confesses towards the end of the book '*We do not know what the schizophrenic process actually is*' (Bleuler, 1950, p. 466, italics in the original). Kraepelin's clinical picture of dementia praecox is therefore reframed and re-theorized in Bleuler's account of schizophrenia, but it is not rendered invalid or obsolete. Although introducing a non-biological theory of psychic splitting to Kraepelin's clinical picture appears to reconfigure it quite radically, in doing so Bleuler repeated and so confirmed Kraepelin's most basic assertion, that there was a consistently identifiable asylum population suffering from a particular form of psychosis. (Indeed, Bleuler's addition of 'simple' and 'latent' schizophrenia to the hebephrenic, catatonic, and paranoid forms further supported this assertion, as if the illness could manifest itself now in essential or not yet wholly perceptible forms.) Bleuler's account further clarified the symptomatology of schizophrenia, but left the disease process itself shrouded in obscurity, and so reinforced the sublime status of the disorder. Furthermore, by positing a qualitative difference in groups of symptoms, Bleuler opened up new possibilities for (re) framing the clinical picture of this disorder, so extending schizophrenia as a point around which psychiatry could assert and reassert its scientific conquest of mental illness. Before addressing competing models of schizophrenia that reconfigure a Bleulerian split in symptom groups, we must turn to the work of his contemporary, Karl Jaspers, whose phenomenological analysis distinguishes itself from both the Kraepelinian and Bleulerian accounts of schizophrenia in its examination of the sheer 'ununderstandability' of schizophrenia.

Although Jaspers retained the term schizophrenia to designate a particular constellation of symptoms, his critique of the philosophical and methodological assumptions underlying both Kraepelin's and Bleuler's accounts of the disorder is a powerful one. Commending Kraepelin both for his vivid descriptions of mental illness and his methodological emphasis on the patient's life history (Jaspers, 1972, pp. 849, 852), Jaspers nonetheless remained sharply critical of what he calls the inherently unscientific 'somatic prejudice' underlying Kraepelin's analytic project, and the 'brain mythologies' promulgated by other biological psychiatrists (Jaspers, 1972, p. 18). Clearly unconvinced by the rhetorical posturing and lack of aetiological analysis or evidence in Kraepelin's account of dementia praecox, he anticipated the arguments of Boyle and Bentall in writing '*No real disease entity has been discovered* by this method of approach' (Jaspers, 1972, p. 567, italics in the original). Jaspers's critique of the Bleulerian model of schizophrenic splitting is less explicit; however, in advocating the empathetic analysis of psychopathological phenomenon (the patients' communication, behaviours, and gestures), Jaspers aimed to ensure that '*the psyche* itself does *not* become *an object*' (Jaspers, 1972, p. 9, italics in the original), which arguably it is for Bleuler. Jaspers argued that by identifying with patients, psychiatrists could achieve an empathetic understanding of how mental events and mental disorders arise: the phenomenological analysis of patients' behaviour would produce insight into the experience of psychopathology. Schizophrenia is unique in Jaspers's account because it is a psychic experience that frustrates genetic understanding. 'The most profound distinction in psychic life', Jaspers writes, 'seems to be that between what is meaningful and *allows empathy* and what in its particular way is *ununderstandable*, "mad" in the literal sense, schizophrenic psychic life (even though there may be no delusions)' (Jaspers, 1972, p. 577, italics in the original).

Schizophrenia in Jaspers's *General Psychopathology* is described as a compelling spectacle of sublimity—it is 'particularly fascinating and psychologically interesting', its changes to the individual's psychic '"machinery"' are 'remarkable and alarming', and 'in certain cases the very manner of it, its contents and all that it represents can in itself create quite another kind of interest; we find ourselves astounded and shaken in the presence of alien secrets' (Jaspers, 1972, pp. 608, 577). Unlike Kraepelin and Bleuler, Jaspers advances neither a comprehensive clinical picture nor psychodynamic model of schizophrenia. Echoing Kant's analysis of the sublime encounter as essentially an intrasubjective event, Jaspers insists:

> It is easier to describe the common factor [among schizophrenic patients] in subjective terms, that is, in terms of the effect on the observer, rather than try to do so objectively. All these personalities have something baffling about them, which baffles our understanding in a peculiar way; there is something queer, cold, inaccessible, rigid, and petrified there, even when the patients are quite sensible and can be addressed and even when they are eager to talk about themselves. We may think we can understand dispositions furthest from our own but when faced with such people we feel a gulf which defies description.
>
> (Jaspers, 1972, p. 447)

The immediately perceptible collapse of the *psychiatrist*'s empathetic structures of understanding is pathognomonic of a disorder unequivocally construed as sublime. If the 'nuclear symptom of schizophrenia' is this 'praecox feeling', as Dutch psychiatrist H. C. Rümke also suggests (Hoenig, 1995, p. 345), it is a symptom latent in but not absent from more orthodox accounts of the disorder. Jaspers's frank account of the fundamental 'ununderstandability' of the psychic experience that appears as schizophrenia is already implicit in Kraepelin's description of 'mental shipwrecks' and Bleuler's anxiety regarding the obscurity of the schizophrenic disease process. The feeling of a 'gulf which defies description' is not here dependent on the perception of any particular fundamental and accessory symptoms; it is produced in the overall apprehension of the person. Foregrounding the emotional dimension of the clinical encounter, non-phenomenological psychiatry also incorporated an account of the uniquely ununderstandable, or quintessentially bizarre, dimension of schizophrenia but attributed it exclusively to the presence of florid, or what Bleuler called the accessory, symptoms. Effectively ignoring their theoretical and methodological specificity, mainstream psychiatry ended up synthesizing Jaspers's notion of a 'praecox feeling' with Bleuler's separation of non-bizarre from bizarre symptoms.

Bleuler inaugurated an approach to mapping schizophrenic symptomatology that persisted throughout the twentieth century. However, whereas his division of symptoms into distinctive groups endured, Bleuler's hierarchized dichotomies of fundamental and accessory, primary and secondary symptoms were uniformly inverted such that the most 'bizarre' accessory symptoms came to be seen as the most distinctively schizophrenic. An early and hugely influential reconfiguration of Bleuler's symptom division was made in the late 1950s by Kurt Schneider, who produced a list of so-called first-rank symptoms of schizophrenia displayed in acute episodes of the disorder. Striking for its detail, the list includes the experience of thought insertion and thought broadcasting, the presence of hallucinatory voices in dialogue, delusional perception and experiences of extreme passivity, and victimization in the fields of drive and willpower (see Smith, 1982, p. 36). Schneider claimed no particular theoretical significance for his hierarchical division of symptoms (Johnstone et al., 1999, p. 24); he advanced them merely as an aid to cross-sectional (as distinct from longitudinal) diagnosis (McKenna, 1994, p. 46). However, it is no coincidence, given their close professional relationship, that Schneider's list was constituted exclusively of symptoms that Jaspers believed were beyond genetic understanding (Farmer et al., 1988, p. 38). More surprising is the distillation of Jaspers's phenomenological analysis into an easy-reference list, when Jaspers himself was vehemently opposed to the (over)simplification of psychiatric concepts:

> Those who teach should compel their students to rise to a scientific level. But this is made impossible if 'compendia' are used, which give students fragmentary, superficial pseudo-knowledge 'for practical purposes', and which sometimes is more subversive for practice than total ignorance. One should not allow a façade of science. There is a decline in culture and intellectual effort in our day and it is the duty of everyone not to compromise.

(Jaspers, 1972, p. xi)

Twentieth-century psychiatry, in its quest to conquer if not mental illness then certainly the burgeoning market for mental illness management, has made many such 'compromises' in the form of internationally standardized and disseminated diagnostic manuals. Schneider's symptom ranking was clearly an instance in which this 'façade of science' was put to strategic ends. By highlighting 'key' elements of Kraepelin's clinical picture of dementia praecox in order to facilitate faster, more 'objective', and therefore more consistent diagnoses, Schneider shifted the diagnostic emphasis from the apprehension of the person to the identification of specific and isolated behaviours. After Bleuler had significantly broadened the concept of schizophrenia, Schneider tightened and delimited it, but still did not address the question of aetiology.

Thus ranked, the symptom groups Bleuler identified as fundamental and accessory have also been qualitatively differentiated as negative and positive symptoms of schizophrenia. This differentiation draws upon the much earlier work of English neurologist Hughlings Jackson. In 1860, Jackson hypothesized that the symptoms of both neurological and psychiatric disorders were caused by anatomical lesions, lesions that could cause the loss of a function and pro-duce so-called negative symptoms, or disinhibit excessive behaviour and so generate positive symptoms (Johnstone et al., 1999, p. 22). Divesting itself of Jackson's theoretical framework, modern psychiatry deploys the terms more simplistically: a negative symptom designates the absence of a certain function, whereas the presence of a behaviour deemed pathological, such as a delusion, is a positive symptom (Johnstone et al., 1999, p. 22). Temporality and causal-ity are noteworthy points of distinction between the three symptom-dividing models so far discussed. Clearly for Bleuler the fundamental and primary symptoms (the 'four As') not only precede but also produce the secondary, accessory symptoms. Schneider, by contrast, ranks symptoms according to whether or not they manifest at the temporal apex of psychosis, the acute epi-sode. Finally, the positive/negative symptom grouping of modern psychiatry merely subdivides a static clinical picture, offering no account of the causal relationship between or sequential development of symptoms. Like Kraepelin's clinical picture of dementia praecox, the Jackson/Bleuler-inspired differentia-tion of positive from negative symptoms was advanced as a disinterested description of ways in which schizophrenic behaviour could be demarcated from other forms of pathological and normal behaviour, and retained regard-less of the scientific veracity of its assumptions (Jackson's anatomical lesions, Bleuler's vague biological origin). It was, in short, highly flexible and proved to be adaptable to wildly divergent accounts of schizophrenia: epidemiological researchers utilize the symptom division to explain gender differences in schizophrenia (Goldstein and Lewine, 2000, p. 115); 'institutional neurosis' theories attributed personality-flattening negative symptoms to hospitali-zation or asylum incarceration; 'defective filter theories' held that positive

symptoms arose from the schizophrenic inability to screen stimuli and negative symptoms were a strategy of withdrawal from this overwhelming state;
and Tim Crow's theory of two types of schizophrenia saw the second, negative
type as a form of degenerative brain damage, possibly triggered by a virus, that
affected some patients already suffering from the first, positive type (Crow,
1985; see also Healy, 2002, p. 266).

Schizophrenia today

Although theoretical divergences of this magnitude exert a certain fascination,
especially when they underpin the diagnosis of on average 1% of the population, we cannot here chart the rise and fall of every theory of schizophrenia
developed by twentieth-century psychiatry.[26] Kraepelin's clinical picture of
dementia praecox and Bleuler's model of schizophrenia are the foundational
accounts of schizophrenia; balancing symptomatological clarity and aetiological obscurity, they have ensured that schizophrenia is perceived as a definite
disease entity but one that attracts ongoing analysis in order to prove this is so.
If a demonstrable organic lesion or an underlying disease process had been
discovered, schizophrenia, like the tertiary form of syphilis (general paralysis,
or paresis, of the insane), might well have faded from view as a somatic madness curable with something as simple as penicillin. In the absence of such a
discovery or even such a treatment, new theories continue to be developed and
frustrated within the conceptual frameworks of early psychiatry, theories that
are not only substantively indebted to but metatheoretically complicit with
these early presentations. In the rest of this chapter, I argue that schizophrenia
continues to function as the sublime object of psychiatric discourse by focussing upon three things: the influence Kraepelin's *Clinical Psychiatry* exerts on
modern psychiatry, schizophrenia's position at the cutting edge of psychiatric
treatments, and the indeterminacy that still characterizes the discursive representations of the disorder.

The clinical picture of schizophrenia in the pre-eminent contemporary cata-
logue of mental disorders, the revised fourth edition of the American Psychiatric
Association's (APA's) *Diagnostic and Statistical Manual* (DSM-IV-TR), is a
detailed inventory of schizophrenic symptoms unhampered by any overtly
theoretical account of the disorder.[27] Since the publication of DSM III in 1980,
the APA's taxonomic enterprise has 'attempted to be neutral with respect to
theories of etiology' (American Psychiatric Association, 2000, p. xxvi), and its

---

[26] For a comprehensive overview of current international research, see Hirsch and
Weinberger (2003); MacDonald and Schulz (2009); Mueser and Jeste (2008).

[27] For a discussion of DSM-V, due to be published in 2013, please see footnote 12.

striving for impartiality is evident in the shifting definitions of the term 'psychotic' in successive editions of the manual. Previously defined as a 'loss of ego boundaries', a 'gross impairment of reality testing', and a gross interference 'with the capacity to meet the ordinary demands of life', in DSM-IV-TR 'psychotic' simply 'refers to the presence of certain symptoms', namely, positive schizophrenic symptoms (American Psychiatric Association, 2000, p. 297). DSM-IV-TR lists five subtypes of schizophrenia distinguished by the non/appearance of certain symptoms. Of these, the first three—paranoid, disorganized (hebephrenic), and catatonic—reproduce Kraepelin's three forms of dementia praecox; undifferentiated and residual schizophrenia correspond to Bleuler's addition of simple and latent subtypes. The APA's general diagnostic criteria are worth reproducing in full for despite their many flaws (Cooper, 2004, 2005; Kirk and Kutchins, 1992), they comprise the single most influential contemporary clinical picture of schizophrenia:[28]

Diagnostic criteria for schizophrenia

A *Characteristic symptoms*: Two (or more) of the following, each present for a significant portion of time during a 1-month period (or less if successfully treated):

(1) delusions

(2) hallucinations

(3) disorganized speech (e.g. frequent derailment or incoherence)

(4) grossly disorganized or catatonic behavior

(5) negative symptoms, i.e. affective flattening, alogia, or avolition

Note: Only one Criterion A symptom is required if delusions are bizarre or hallucinations consist of a voice keeping up a running commentary on the person's behavior or thoughts, or two or more voices conversing with each other.

B *Social/occupational dysfunction*: For a significant portion of the time since the onset of the disturbance, one or more major areas of functioning such as work, interpersonal relations, or self-care are markedly below the level achieved prior to the onset (or when the onset is in childhood or adolescence, failure to achieve expected level of interpersonal, academic, or occupational achievement).

---

[28] The World Health Organisation's *International Classification of Diseases* (ICD) *10* (2007) is also widely used. One of the key differences between the diagnostic schemas is that ICD only requires that symptoms to be present for 1 month.

C *Duration*: Continuous signs of the disturbance persist for at least 6 months. This 6-month period must include at least 1 month of symptoms (or less if successfully treated) that meet Criterion A (i.e. active-phase symptoms) and may include periods of prodromal or residual symptoms. During these prodromal or residual periods, the signs of the disturbance may be manifested by only negative symptoms or two or more symptoms listed in Criterion A present in an attenuated form (e.g. odd beliefs, unusual perceptual experiences).

D *Schizoaffective and Mood Disorder exclusion*: Schizoaffective Disorder and Mood Disorder with Psychotic Features have been ruled out because either (1) no Major Depressive, Manic, or Mixed Episodes have occurred concurrently with the active-phase symptoms; or (2) if mood episodes have occurred during active-phase symptoms, their total duration has been brief relative to the duration of the active and residual periods.

E *Substance/general medical condition exclusion*: The disturbance is not due to the direct physiological effects of a substance (e.g. a drug of abuse, a medication) or a general medical condition.

F *Relationship to a Pervasive Developmental Disorder*: If there is a history of Autistic Disorder or another Pervasive Developmental Disorder, the additional diagnosis of Schizophrenia is made only if prominent delusions or hallucinations are also present for at least a month (or less if successfully treated). (American Psychiatric Association, 2000, p. 312, italics in the original)

This is Kraepelin's clinical picture of dementia praecox reframed in late-twentieth-century psychiatric terminology, incorporating the Bleulerian distinction between symptoms for ease of identification, and recoding Jaspers's hallmark 'ununderstandability' of schizophrenic behaviour as distinctively 'bizarre' positive symptoms. It is a disorder marked by an inability to labour (where labour signifies paid employment as well as social interaction), identified through longitudinal analysis, and explicitly differentiated from manic–depressive psychosis and substance-induced psychosis. DSM-IV-TR's rhetoric of scientificity and its strategic silence on the fiercely debated question of aetiology facilitate global consistency in the diagnosis of mental illness, but legitimize the tendency to ignore the very vexed issue of whether schizophrenia is indeed a disease entity. The clinical picture offered here, like Kraepelin's before it, stimulates an already prolific research interest in this indeterminate disorder by itself being impotent to discriminate between findings. So it is precisely in being a dry, detached description of this modern madness that the DSM reinforces schizophrenia's status as the sublime object of psychiatry.

The *Diagnostic and Statistical Manual* itself does little to explain or resolve the seemingly inexhaustible and irresolvable challenges posed by Kraepelin's elusive disease entity. It also does not give a strong indication of the specific importance of schizophrenia to the disciplinary development of psychiatry, nor the psychiatric representation of schizophrenia as a fundamentally indeterminate or unknowable disorder, both of which contribute, I argue, to schizophrenia's sublime status in psychiatric discourse. Whereas some forms of major mental illnesses have been forgotten (for example, governess psychosis (Bleuler, 1950, p. 342)), subsumed by subsequent taxonomies (masturbatory psychosis (Gilman, 1988, p. 205)), abandoned as a result of political protest (homosexuality (Shorter, 1997, p. 301)), and vehemently contested even within orthodox psychiatry (multiple personality disorder (Goldberg, 1999, pp. 183–4)), schizophrenia has, since its identification, been consistently viewed as the proper object of a scientific psychiatry anxious to alleviate one of the most severe forms of human suffering, as well as secure and maintain its position as pre-eminent authority on mental health. Still comprising a significant percentage, if not the majority, of long-term psychiatric cases, people diagnosed as suffering from schizophrenia are also at the 'core of psychiatric business' (Healy, 2002, p. 329).

Psychiatrists, like most medical practitioners, did not delay the treatment of severe disorders until outstanding theoretical issues had been resolved but pursued a number of different therapeutic pathways simultaneously. Modern psychiatry's most notorious interventions in mental illness have been made in the name of 'curing' schizophrenia. As Thomas Szasz wryly observed in 1976 (pp. 112–9), people diagnosed with schizophrenia have been subjected to a plethora of largely ill-conceived 'cures', from mega-vitamins to fasting, religious instruction to regular beating. More common and widely known treatments such as insulin coma therapy and electro-convulsive treatment, although credited with alleviating certain psychotic symptoms, are not necessarily better theoretically substantiated than their more bizarre predecessors (Shorter and Healy, 2007). The practice of treating schizophrenia by performing frontal lobe lobotomy—also developed without significant theoretical justification—is unquestionably the most infamous of all psychiatry's strategies of symptom management.

It was, however, the use of antipsychotic drugs to control the positive symptoms of schizophrenia that revolutionized psychiatric practice, forging new and powerful connections between psychiatry and the pharmaceutical industry. In *The Creation of Psychopharmacology*, David Healy describes the discovery of chloropromazine as no less than 'one of the seminal events of human history' (2002, p. 4), and makes clear that schizophrenia's importance to the development of psychopharmacology and the pharmaceutical management of all mental illness cannot be overemphasized. The efficacy of neuroleptic drugs in relieving certain florid psychotic symptoms was the first great success story of psychopharmacology, but a success not without negative side-effects. Early antipsychotics caused the extremely debilitating tardive dyskinesia, failed to affect the so-called negative and cognitive symptoms of schizophrenia, and qualitatively and quantitatively diminished the communication between patient and psychiatrist (Healy, 2002, pp. 245–85). Second-generation, or 'atypical' antipsychotics have been successful in reducing the appearance of extrapyramidal symptoms, but do not necessarily improve upon earlier anti-psychotics (Abbott, 2010; Geddes et al., 2000; Lieberman et al., 2005), particu-larly in their propensity to cause diabetes, loss of libido, and considerable weight gain (Nasrallah, 2003, 2008).[29]

The acknowledgement or realization that schizophrenic symptoms could be modified if not abolished signalled a significant shift in psychiatric thinking. Early twentieth-century psychiatrists regarded schizophrenia as a hereditary, endogenous disease, and as such any response to treatment would have been evidence that the diagnosis itself was incorrect (Healy, 2002, p. 72). The con-troversial treatments of schizophrenia that arose throughout the twentieth century, and those now endorsed in the twenty-first,[30] exist in such numbers

---

[29] Psychiatry's dependence on neuroleptic drugs in the treatment of schizophrenia has been widely criticized by certain antipsychiatrists, as I discuss in Chapter 3, and has also attracted passionate criticism from those within its own ranks. Peter Breggin, for exam-ple, argues that antipsychotic drugs are the pharmacological equivalent for surgical lobotomy: by placing a 'chemical clamp on the higher brain' they 'can have no specifi-cally beneficial effect on any particular human problem' regardless of whether or not they modify the appearance of schizophrenic symptoms (Breggin, 1991, pp. 55–7). Recent books by Joanna Moncrieff (2009) and Richard Bentall (2009) similarly argue for a radi-cal reappraisal of received wisdoms about the efficacy of psychopharmacological inter-ventions, and the UK-based critical psychiatry network (http://www.critpsynet.freeuk. com/) has as one of its main goals 'the development of a critique of the influence of the pharmaceutical industry on the theory and practice of psychiatry' (Bracken and Thomas, 2010a, p. 226).

[30] Although the exploration of off-beat therapies persists (see Mitchell and Michalczuk, 2010; Xia and Grant, 2009), the evidence base is building for a range of psychosocial (Dixon et al., 2010; Tai and Turkington, 2009; Velligan, 2009) as well as psycho-pharmacological treatments (Buchanan et al., 2010). The latest report from the Patient Outcomes Research Team (PORT) identifies '24 treatment areas that have strong empir-ical evidence for improving outcomes and which should comprise the basic menu of treatments and services available to all people with schizophrenia' (Kreyenbuhl et al., 2010, p. 100). Frustrated by the pace of evidence-based research in this area, and the lack of any significant breakthroughs, the PORT authors are careful to note that 'These treat-ments do not "cure" schizophrenia or fully ameliorate symptoms and problems for the

in part because of divergences in psychiatric opinion regarding the aetiology of schizophrenia. In some cases, new treatments have not simply relied upon but have directly spawned new theories of the disorder—the dopamine hypothesis of schizophrenia being a case in point.[31] Genetic theories of schizophrenia have continued to be influential since Kraepelin and Bleuler advanced their beliefs that the disease was inherited, although the search for schizophrenia's genetic origins remains elusive (Crow, 2008; Kendler, 2005; Williamson, 2007) and still criticized (Bentall, 2009). But thanks in part to the influence of antipsychotic drugs, developments in neuroscience, and the re-emergence of a Kraepelinian account of schizophrenia in DSM-III and IV, the idea that schizophrenia is caused by an as-yet-unknown brain disease still dominates contemporary psychiatry.[32]

The recent *Diagnosis: Schizophrenia: A Comprehensive Guide for Patients, Families and Helping Professionals* disseminates this received wisdom to a lay reader:

> Schizophrenia is a disease of the brain that affects about one percent of the population. [. . .] A number of researchers are investigating different possible causes of schizophrenia, but for now the exact cause is unknown. . . . But no matter how this disease develops, it is important to remember that schizophrenia is an illness of the brain, and it's no one's fault.
>
> (Miller and Mason, 2002, p. 35)[33]

---

majority of affected individuals; such objectives remain for future generations of research' (Kreyenbuhl et al., 2010, pp. 101–2).

[31] Writing in 2002, Healy suggests that 'The dopamine hypothesis of schizophrenia . . . argued backward from the efficacy of the treatment to what might be the cause of the disorder. That made little more sense that arguing that because aspirin was useful in treating rheumatoid arthritis there must be some kind of aspirin deficiency implicated in rheumatoid arthritis. Yet, despite its weakness, the dopamine hypothesis of schizophrenia was successfully used by the pharmaceutical industry to sell drugs' (p. 191). The current status of the dopamine hypothesis is usefully summarized in Howes and Kapur (2009).

[32] This point finds support in the fascinating research conducted by Harland and colleagues (2009) into the attitudes of trainee psychiatrists. Measuring the trainee's attitudes towards eight models of mental illness as applied to four psychiatric disorders, the researchers found that attitudes towards schizophrenia were expressed with the greatest conviction and that of the 32 possible models the biological model of schizophrenia enjoyed the strongest support. As the authors point out, a more comprehensive understanding of the attitudes with which mental health professionals approach mental illness, perhaps especially schizophrenia, has the potential to improve multi-disciplinary communication and ultimately patient care.

[33] Jeffrey Poland suggests that the public education campaigns around the biology of schizophrenia have been 'aggressive' 'partly in an attempt to offset widespread stigma associated with the label and partly to reinforce the existing practices centred around the

Even expert opinion reproduces Kraepelin's authoritative rhetoric as well as his neural preferentialism: 'Eventually, there will be some highly specific physical method for detecting schizophrenia, as well as the predisposition to it. We know that something goes wrong chemically and/or physically in the brain of the schizophrenic, but we do not yet know what' (Gottesman, 1991, p. 19). Others are more candid about psychiatry's failure to prove conclusively Kraepelin's beliefs:

> As far as defining the clinical boundaries of schizophrenia/dementia praecox is concerned, we have not moved very far in the last 100 years. We still have the same difficulty that Kraepelin had; we believe we are defining an entity which will be shown to have a tangible underlying morbid process, but we cannot demonstrate that process. Things are better for us than they were for Kraepelin . . . the darkness does not seem so impenetrable any more, but the dawn will have to break more fully before we can be clear about the central cluster of clinical features which mean that someone should be diagnosed as having schizophrenia.
>
> (Johnstone et al., 1999, p. 38)

In 1913, Jaspers attacked the perception that 'brain research' should be 'not only one task among many but *the* task of psychiatry', and urged his colleagues to 'guard against *any one viewpoint becoming an absolute* even if such a viewpoint proves fruitful for research and might now and then even be decisive for radical therapy' (Jaspers, 1972, p. 577, italics in the original). It is the inability to produce conclusive evidence of schizophrenia's aetiology (Fatemi and Folsom, 2009; Stephan et al., 2009) that prevents 'brain research' from curtailing the investigation of schizophrenia. Eluding psychiatry at both the macro and molecular levels, schizophrenia has yet to be shot down either by 'magic bullet' treatments or by aetiological explanation.

Although neuroscientific accounts of schizophrenia remain dominant, new approaches to the study and treatment of schizophrenia are emerging as part of broader shifts in clinical practice and policy. We are, according to Patrick Bracken and Philip Thomas, entering an era of 'postpsychiatry' characterized by a diversity of clinical perspectives, an attentiveness to social and cultural difference, a robust questioning of the dominance of the biomedical model and of psychopharmacological interventions, and a profound commitment to increasing the involvement of service users in reforming, researching, and delivering mental health services (Bracken and Thomas, 2005, 2010a, b; Gawith and Abrams, 2006). There is also increasing recognition that culture is

concept' (Poland, 2007, p. 168). However, recent studies have shown that such programmes of education in mental health literacy can have the unwanted and unanticipated effect of *increasing* stigma and the desire for social distance (Angermeyera et al., 2009; Sartorius, 2010).

critical to understanding every aspect of schizophrenia (Jenkins and Barrett, 2004a, p. 6), and thus that experiences of schizophrenia will vary from region to region as well as from person to person. Where once schizophrenia was synonymous with long-stay hospitalization and an expectation of permanent disability, today the 'recovery' approach is rapidly growing in influence (Craig, 2008; Davidson, 2010; Ramon et al., 2007).[34] Although there is great hope among many that an emphasis on recovery, on valuing individual experience, and on a service-user-led approach to psychiatric research and therapeutic support will significantly improve the experience of people diagnosed with severe mental illness (Hornstein, 2009), challenges to the concept of schizophrenia itself have yet to reach a tipping point.

'Is it possible to summarise these themes and variations, or is the notion of schizophrenia too diffuse to clarify?' asks Trevor Turner (1995, p. 355). For Healy, lack of clarity has been integral to schizophrenia's status in the big business of psychopharmacology: 'The emergence and survival of concepts in both the business and academic marketplaces is often determined by the "slogan" value of the concept [and] terms like schizophrenia . . . worked because they carried just the right level of ambiguity' (2002, p. 254). The stark presentation of diagnostic criteria in DSM-IV-TR disguises the inherent indeterminacy of the concept, and it is this balance between Kraepelinian clarity and conceptual indeterminacy that has been crucial to psychiatry's disciplinary legitimization and expansion. Books on schizophrenia endlessly reiterate the professional fascination with this disorder, poetically describing the disciplinary pursuit of this distinct but unknowable 'essence of madness' as if it were indeed the mapping of the sublime:

> Albeit the heartland of psychiatry, schizophrenia remains a will o' the wisp landscape, full of shadows and chimeras. Explorers here have laboured hard to define the territory, establish landmarks, and to discover the cause and meaning underlying what they have seen. Alas, this journey of discovery has been painstakingly slow . . . [However] the inadequacy always apparent in our theories is gradually giving rise to new appraisals of a more radical kind. These reappraisals enshrine what we have always known, that schizophrenia is a most subtle and challenging disorder, but, in addition, they are accompanied by a new determination to meet the challenge with a whole range of sophisticated techniques.
>
> (Bebbington and McGuffin, 1988, p. 1)

---

[34] In the UK, for example, *New Horizons* was the first cross-government strategy to foreground well-being, health, and recovery in the treatment of schizophrenia (Mental Health Division, 2009), and the multi-million pound *Time to Change* campaign has explicitly challenged misconceptions about schizophrenia as part of its effort to end mental health discrimination.

No matter how great their determination, or how sophisticated their techniques, psychiatrists have so far been unable to reduce schizophrenia to the comfortable status of something like a substance-abuse psychosis—aetiologically and symptomatologically explicable, and routinely cured. But although this observation may apply to a range of psychiatric disorders, schizophrenia is frequently assigned a special status: 'Among all the maladies and disorders that challenge our species, there is, quite simply, nothing else like it' (Green, 2003, p. xii). Szasz's claim that like '"divine" and "demonic", "schizophrenic" is a concept wonderfully vague in its content and terrifyingly awesome in its implications' (Szasz, 1976, p. xiv) still resonates over 30 years later.

This chapter has presented an account of psychiatry's ongoing Kraepelinian conviction that schizophrenic symptoms result from an underlying disease process.[35] I have described a psychiatry confident in its potential to manage schizophrenia in theory and in practice but unable to explain or treat it conclusively. These claims need now to be understood in relation to clinical theory more broadly. The disciplinary domination of biological psychiatry was brought to an end by the Nazis' genocidal eugenics programme, and it took the publication of DSM-III in 1980 to bring Kraepelin's clinical picture of dementia praecox back to the centre of psychiatric thinking, where it now dominates the research agenda. To provide a more comprehensive account of schizophrenia in twentieth-century clinical theory, it is vital to consider the ways in which psychoanalysis not only challenged psychiatric models of schizophrenia but also advanced competing accounts of this disorder. The following chapter, then, extends my analysis of the status of schizophrenia to the key texts of psychoanalysis. Whereas psychiatry pursues schizophrenia primarily through its symptomatology and cannot, even by its own estimation, provide an adequate aetiological explanation for the disorder, psychoanalysis investigates the meaning of schizophrenic experience and offers vivid accounts of its psychic origins. Despite the significant theoretical differences between these disciplines, I will argue that in the case of schizophrenia they converge at the level of metatheory: for psychoanalysts, psychiatry's sublime object refuses the conventional parameters of the analytic encounter only to be interpreted as a sublime text.

---

[35] Indeed, despite the fact that 'accumulating genomic evidence indicates that there may be scores or hundreds of lesions contributing to [a] final common syndrome', and that the 'clinical evidence supports the possibility that what we have labelled schizophrenia for the past century may be many different disorders with different outcomes' (Insel, 2010, p. 191), the sense that 'it' is and will still be a meaningful concept seems doggedly to persist.

Chapter 2

Schizophrenia: the sublime text of psychoanalysis

The schizophrenic symptom and its secret

As we have seen, schizophrenia occupies a central position in psychiatric discourse: framed as an opaque and bizarre disorder of unknown or unknowable aetiology, it exceeds and thus marks disciplinary limits as a form of unreason which can be neither adequately represented nor analytically mastered. Although psychiatry is unquestionably the dominant clinical discourse on schizophrenia today, the influence of psychoanalytic accounts of schizophrenia on the critical and popular imaginaries is indisputable, even though dementia praecox, paranoia, paraphrenia, and psychosis are the terms privileged in psychoanalysis.[1] So, what is the status of schizophrenia in key psychoanalytic texts? Do psychoanalytic accounts of psychosis relate schizophrenia to the sublime; and if so, how? And how can an analysis of schizophrenia and sublimity in psychoanalytic writing better equip us to identify and interpret the subsequent appropriation, adaptation, and rejection of psychoanalytic concepts in cultural theory?

It is not the aim of this chapter to provide a comprehensive chronological survey of a century of psychoanalytic writing on schizophrenia. Nor is it to provide a detailed comparative study of psychiatric and psychoanalytic clinical practice. My concern is rather with the broad theoretical and methodological differences between the disciplines that centre on questions of the aetiology and content of schizophrenic symptoms. Extending my inquiry into the status of schizophrenia in clinical theory along these axes, in this chapter I consider how the 'disciplinary sublime' of psychiatry is reconfigured as what I call a 'textual sublime' by psychoanalysis. Privileging the analysis of psychotic speech over somatic symptom or genetic make-up, psychoanalysis, I will argue,

---

[1] Whereas Freud and Lacan prefer to retain paranoia (or paraphrenia) as a separate diagnostic category, I follow Louis Sass (1994b, p. ix) in identifying their object of analysis as paranoid schizophrenia, hence, schizophrenia. I also consider Lacan's use of the term psychosis to encompass schizophrenia.

approaches schizophrenia as a disorder of signification, and the schizophrenic patient as a text. The goal of the psychoanalytic treatment of hysteria is to uncover and translate the repressed psychosexual origin of neurotic symptoms, effectively relieving them. In the case of schizophrenia, however, there is no intrinsic connection between the hermeneutic reading of the schizophrenic symptom and the therapeutic treatment of the patient. It is through a process of 'textualization', an implicit division between speech and patient, that psychoanalysis simultaneously dispels and perpetuates the aura of sublimity around schizophrenia. Schizophrenic signification can be rendered intelligible and analytically mastered; however, the person diagnosed with schizophrenia is deemed, at least for Freud, to be beyond dialogue, incapable of transference, and hence inaccessible to psychoanalytic treatment. The double, paradoxical gesture of the textual sublime is to tackle that which is bizarre or unknowable about schizophrenia—to 'rescue' through interpretation schizophrenic signification—while at the same time preserving the essential enigma of the disorder itself. Like psychiatry's disciplinary sublime, the ongoing operation of the textual sublime is ensured by the fact that no limit can be imposed on (re) interpretations of the schizophrenic text because no criteria of therapeutic success can be mobilized to arbitrate between them. As this chapter endeavours to demonstrate, the psychoanalytic construction of schizophrenia as a sublime text is nowhere more apparent than in the case of Daniel Paul Schreber's *Memoirs of My Nervous Illness* (1955), an autobiographical account of paranoid schizophrenia central to the accounts of psychosis advanced by Freud (1981), Lacan (1993), and innumerable psychoanalytic, or psychoanalytically engaged, commentators.

A detailed discussion of the work of Freud and Lacan is indispensable for analysing the influence of psychoanalysis on the portrayal of schizophrenia in the theoretical texts under consideration in Part Two of this book. Furthermore, as Freud and Lacan's respective interests in schizophrenia are primarily theoretical and textual, rather than psychotherapeutic or even clinical, it is in their work on psychosis, and the work they inspired, that the textual sublime of psychoanalysis most clearly operates. By contrast, the psychoanalytic accounts of schizophrenia that dominated American psychiatry from the 1950s to the 1970s, and introduced the infamous schizophrenogenic mother to the popular imaginary, advance a different metatheoretical framework and so negotiate the sublime status of schizophrenia in diverse ways. Defining schizophrenia as a 'loss of ego boundaries' and a 'gross impairment of reality testing' (American Psychiatric Association, 2000, p. 297), ego psychologists and object-relations theorists reconceptualized schizophrenia as the regression to an earlier, infantile phase of psychosexual development. The effect of this 'regressive model of schizophrenia', as it has been called by Louis Sass (1992, p. 20), is essentially the diffusion of the sublime status schizophrenia acquires in psychiatric discourse. If schizophrenia is a stage through which everyone must pass, if it is marked by a return to infantile modes of behaviour, if it is caused by the 'transmission of irrationality' in a person's family (Fine, 1979, p. 288), if it should be located on a continuum with other mental disturbances, or indeed is seen to underlie all forms of 'mental morbidity' (Jones, 1948, p. 373), then it is not surprising that one famous American psychoanalyst should have claimed that half the adult population was affected by it to some degree (Harry S. Sullivan quoted in Fine, 1979, p. 497). It is also unremarkable that a contemporary ego psychologist would unequivocally state that 'There is perhaps no better example of a psychoanalytic theory that has turned out to be incorrect than the once prevalent theory regarding the etiology of schizophrenia' (Willick, 2001, p. 28). Clearly, this diffusion of the schizophrenic sublime is substantively different from the perpetuation of a textual sublime, and as it is the latter which has been most influential in cultural theory, I do not consider these 'regressive' psychoanalytic models of schizophrenia in detail here.[2]

Tempting as it would be to proceed straight to Freud's and Lacan's foundational psychoanalytic studies of schizophrenia, it is necessary first to examine the context in which they developed. At issue is the psychoanalytic distinction between the psychic structure and mechanisms of neurosis and those of psychosis, and the first part of this chapter addresses the problems dementia praecox initially posed for the emerging discipline. Carl Jung and Karl Abraham published the first sustained psychoanalytic accounts of dementia praecox while working with Bleuler at the University Clinic in Zurich. Directly influenced by Freud, they in turn contributed to Freud's seminal analysis of Schreber's *Memoirs*. Working at the intersection of psychiatry and psychoanalysis, Jung and Abraham sought to extend psychoanalytic concepts developed through the study of the neuroses to the analysis of dementia praecox, and did so by highlighting the disorders' structural and symptomatological similarities. In *The Psychology of Dementia Praecox* (1944), Jung argued that the psychological mechanisms of dementia praecox and hysteria are similar but that the former is triggered by a much deeper and more central disturbance, probably by the release of 'toxin', as Bleuler also hypothesized. Abraham's 'The Psycho-Sexual Differences between Hysteria and Dementia Praecox' (Abraham, 1972) adheres to Kraepelinian diagnostic criteria and

---

[2] For a useful overview of these models, see 'What's it like? Psychoanalytic theories of schizophrenia' in *Suffering Psychosis: Psychoanalytic Essays on Psychosis* (Hinshelwood, 2004).

orthodox Freudian concepts in its suggestion that dementia praecox is marked by the display of auto-eroticism and a diminished capacity for sublimation and transference. My analysis of these texts, including Jung's case study, foregrounds the way in which psychoanalysis distinguished itself methodologically and theoretically from psychiatry through its attentiveness to the content of schizophrenic symptoms. Although dementia praecox also played an important part in the politics of the psychoanalytic movement at that time (Jung's rejection of the primary role of the sexual libido in its aetiology was a central issue in his split from Freud (Steele, 1982)) Abraham's and Jung's accounts of the disorder are most significant, I will argue, for inaugurating the psychoanalytic approach to schizophrenia as a text, and privileging paranoid schizophrenia as the text most amenable to psychoanalytic interpretation.

Freud's definitive analysis of psychosis, his 'Psycho-Analytical Notes' on the Schreber case, crystallized this approach to schizophrenia as psychoanalytic orthodoxy. The choice of a self-published autobiography as the exemplary psychotic text allowed Freud to treat schizophrenia as an abstract interpretive problem quite detached from the incarcerated, bellowing Schreber himself. Furthermore, *Memoirs* provided Freud with an in-depth description of a delusional schema developed and refined over many years, a seductive illusion, I would suggest, of coherence and consistency from which a psychoanalytic account of paranoia could be derived. My reading of Freud's 'Psycho-Analytical Notes' concentrates on Freud's selective interpretation of Schreber's schizophrenic symptoms (in particular the hallucinations and delusions most clearly related to sexuality) to refine his hypothesis about paranoia. Strategically blurring diagnostic criteria in a manner Kraepelin would have abhorred, Freud theoretically distinguished psychotic and neurotic symptom formation but nonetheless treated insanity as a coded narrative of psychosexual trauma that could, like its hysteric counterpart, be psychoanalytically deciphered. This is most clearly reflected in Freud's emphasis on Schreber's 'unmanning' fantasy, which, without disputing the sophistication of Freud's interpretation of Schreber's transvestism, I argue entirely overlooks Schreber's more urgent and consistent efforts to prove his rationality to God.

Freud's 'Psycho-Analytic Notes' elevated *Memoirs* to the status of a psychoanalytic classic. It also inspired a proliferation of interdisciplinary interpretations of Schreber's text which continue the practice of selectively interpreting Schreber's symptoms in order to establish a coherent narrative of or beneath his madness. Each of the major accounts of Schreber's *Memoirs* purports to decipher, decisively, the 'textualized' sublimity of schizophrenia, to have found the interpretive master key that will reconcile the text's contradictions and its connection to the embodied reality of psychosis. My analysis of the interdisciplinary field of 'Schreber studies' argues that it is here that the operation of the textual sublime is most starkly revealed. If psychiatry's disciplinary sublime entailed the constant reframing of the general clinical picture of schizophrenia, here it is the specific content of a single symptomatological profile that is perpetually reinterpreted. As an intervention in the field, my analysis of Schreber's *Memoirs of My Nervous Illness* takes as its point of departure something omitted from Freud's analysis, namely, the centrality of the collapse and restitution of reason in Schreber's account of his symptomatology. The text of *Memoirs*, I will argue, can be persuasively interpreted as an articulation of the sublimity of his psychosis: it both records and continues a fight to establish critical distance from the sudden, direct, and unmediated revelation of the beyond-human; from the apprehension of a terrifying and magnificent cosmology. Recalling the importance of distance in facilitating the sublime encounter and affirming the rational faculty, I will argue that *Memoirs* is part of Schreber's ongoing project of detaching from, describing, and stabilizing his experience, constructing it as sublime as opposed to 'simply terrifying'. Schreber's undertaking in *Memoirs* therefore has multiple and hitherto unrecognized parallels with the psychoanalytic approach to psychosis. Freud and subsequent psychoanalytic commentators, like Schreber, maintain schizophrenia at a theoretical distance by treating the person as a text, downplaying the importance of somatic and cognitive symptoms, and privileging the pseudo-neurotic paranoid narrative.

The final part of this chapter will return us to the principal question of the relationship between schizophrenia, sublimity, and textuality in psychoanalysis, and specifically to the work of Jacques Lacan. In his account of psychosis, Lacan takes up directly the idea of schizophrenia as an experience of the sublime marked by a failure of symbolic representation. The psychotic exists, and, according to Lacan, has always existed, outside the symbolic realm, barred from access to it by the foreclosure of its grounding signifier, the Name-of-the-Father. In drawing out some of the fundamental differences between Freudian and Lacanian theories of psychosis, my aim is to illustrate ways in which Lacan nonetheless follows Freud in distancing the psychotic patient from psychoanalytic technique (insisting that people diagnosed with schizophrenia are beyond cure or even therapy, Lacan transforms the patient into a purely interpretive problem) while simultaneously suggesting that psychoanalysis provides the master theory of schizophrenia's aetiology, structure, and symptomatology.

Tackling dementia praecox: Jung and Abraham

In any study of psychoanalysis, especially one that involves the exchange between Freud and Jung, it is easy to be swept away by the politics of the psychoanalytic movement, the relationships of its key players, and the constellation of theoretical innovations that underpinned its development.[3] Although the significance of theoretical disputes cannot be overlooked, succumbing to these academic seductions is a temptation this chapter will resist; my aim here is to analyse the challenges early psychoanalytic theorists of dementia praecox faced, and the ways in which they attempted to resolve them. As a private practitioner for Vienna's middle classes, Freud did not treat psychotic patients; he had no direct access to asylum populations, nor did he particularly desire it (Shorter, 1997, p. 100). Furthermore, as is well known, hysteria and not psychosis is the privileged psychic disorder of psychoanalysis, and therefore it is unsurprising that Freud, at the outset, evinced little theoretical interest in the three forms of dementia praecox identified by Kraepelin. All but ignoring hebephrenia and catatonia, Freud did ponder the subject of paranoia in his letters to Wilhelm Fliess from 1895 to 1899, but viewed it alongside hysteria and obsessional neurosis as a 'sexual psychoneurosis' (Freud, 1985a, p. 209). By exploring connections between paranoia, autoeroticism, and sexual trauma (discussed in more detail later in this chapter) he defined paranoia in an 1896 paper as the 'neurosis of defense par excellence' (Freud, 1985b, p. 188), a statement which unequivocally demonstrates key nosological differences between psychoanalysis and the biological psychiatry of the day. These early speculations on the psychosexual origins of paranoia form the foundation of Freud's 1911 analysis of Schreber's *Memoirs*. However, it is Jung and Abraham, as practising psychiatrists, who are credited with the first major psychoanalytic incursions into the territory of dementia praecox.

By the early twentieth century, Eugen Bleuler's Burghölzli clinic was one of the Meccas of world psychiatry. Bleuler took a 'lively interest' (Freud, 1995, p. 32) in Freud's work, and Freud in turn courted the Swiss psychiatrists as they were in a unique position to test and legitimize psychoanalytic theory and practice through their work with asylum patients (Theweleit, 1990, p. 60). In sharp contrast to Jaspers's later account of the unbreachable gulf of understanding between clinician and schizophrenic patient, Jung's and Abraham's analyses, in their reliance on Freud's insights into the treatment of hysteric patients, pursued a strategy of equivalence rather than radical difference.[4] If structural and symptomatological similarities between dementia praecox and

---

[3] For an account in this vein, see Chapter 8 'Schizophrenia' of Lisa Appignanesi's book *Mad, Bad and Sad* (2008).

[4] Indeed, Jung (1944, pp. 16–17) states: 'In general we know by far too little about the psychology of the normal and the hysteric to dare accept in such an untransparent disease as dementia praecox, a totally new mechanism unknown to all psychology. One should be economical with new principles of interpretation'.

neurosis could be demonstrated, not only could psychosis be brought into the psychoanalytic fold, but the tenets of psychoanalysis would also win scientific legitimacy. Most striking about their work, however, is its complete departure from the modes of inquiry dominating biological psychiatry. Shunning the microscope, Kraepelin's longitudinal approach, and any concrete search for the somatic origins of dementia praecox, Jung and Abraham, with Bleuler's encouragement, focussed their attentions on the substance of symptoms. The most contentious issue between Jung and Abraham, and in turn Freud, was the role that infantile sexuality and the libido would play in their appearance.

The publication of Jung's *The Psychology of Dementia Praecox* followed Freud's *The Interpretation of Dreams* (of which Jung was an avid reader) and *Three Essays on the Theory of Sexuality*, but it preceded personal contact between the two men. Jung begins his study by hailing Bleuler as his respected superior and clarifying his position regarding the as yet relatively unknown science of psychoanalysis. His preface is worth quoting at length as it gives an indication of the status of psychoanalysis at the time and anticipates the major issues of contention between Jung and Freud:

> Even a superficial glance at my work will show how indebted I am to the ingenious conceptions of Freud [who] . . . has not yet attained fair recognition and appreciation . . . I can assure you that in the beginning I naturally entertained all the objections which are advanced in the literature against Freud. But, I said to myself Freud could only be refuted by one who himself had made much use of the psychoanalytic method . . . Fairness to Freud does not, however, signify, as many may fear, a conditionless surrender to dogma; indeed, independent judgment can very well be maintained beside it. If I, for instance, recognize the complex mechanisms of dreams and hysteria, it by no means signifies that I ascribe to the infantile sexual trauma the exclusive importance seemingly attributed to it by Freud. Still less does it mean that I place sexuality so preponderantly in the foreground, or that I even ascribe to it the psychological universality which Freud apparently postulates under the impression of the very powerful role which sexuality plays in the psyche . . . Nevertheless, all these are quite incidental and completely vanish beside the psychological principles, the discovery of which is Freud's greatest merit . . .
>
> (Jung, 1944, pp. iii–iv)

Jung's text struggles between guarded qualifications and praise of Freud as an 'ingenious' if 'as yet hardly recognized investigator' (Jung, 1944, pp. 29, 21). After reviewing the relevant contemporary literature, he takes as the starting point for his analysis Freud's hypothesis that paranoia arises *'from the repression of painful memories, and that the form of the symptoms is determined by the content of the repression'* (Freud (1896) quoted in Jung, 1944, p. 26, italics in the original). However, if the psychic mechanisms of hysteria can be discerned in the paranoid form of dementia praecox, what accounts for the greater rigidity of psychotic symptoms, and, moreover, what explains the appearance of one disorder rather than another? Pronouncing Freud's analysis insufficiently complex, Jung argues that 'we must therefore postulate that in the case of dementia praecox there is a specific resultant of the affects (toxine?), which causes the definite fixation of the complex by injuring the sum total of the psychic functions' (Jung, 1944, p. 32). The conceptual apparatus from which Jung develops his own account of dementia praecox is loosely psychoanalytic and yet decidedly opposed to Freud's analysis of paranoid symptom forma-tion: with the aetiological role of childhood sexuality explicitly rejected, and an unknown somatic origin repeatedly postulated, Jung integrates the received wisdom of *fin-de-siècle* psychiatry with Freudian concepts and methodologies and the Burghölzli's own brand of psychology.

Chief among the experimental techniques favoured by Bleuler and Jung was the word-association test, which resembles what we now think of as free asso-ciation.[5] According to Jung, the psyche is composed of many interconnected 'feeling-toned complexes', each of which has a sensory, affective, and intellec-tual component (Jung, 1944, p. 32). The word-association test revealed to him that '*every association belongs . . . to some complex*', that is, every word triggers already existing complexes within the psyche (Jung, 1944, p. 35, italics in the original). Although the ego complex is the 'highest psychic force' (ibid.), it exists in dynamic relation with other idiosyncratic complexes.[6] In order to theorize the aberrant functioning of complexes in dementia praecox as indi-cated by the word-association test, Jung investigated parallels between demen-tia praecox, dreams, and hysteria. Dreams, on his Freud-inspired model, appear as 'symbolic expressions of repressed complexes', which 'contain the characteristic features of mythological thinking' and are identical to those of dementia praecox: 'Let the dreamer walk about and act like one awakened and we have the clinical picture of dementia praecox' (Jung, 1944, pp. 51, 56, 79). Hysteria, like dementia praecox, is for Jung the result of a particularly pernicious (but not necessarily sexual) complex expressed in all areas of psychic activity, and in drawing elaborate parallels between the disorders on the levels of 'char-acterlogical abnormality', stereotypy, emotional and intellectual disturbance, Jung consistently implies that differences between them are a matter of degree.

---

5   Interestingly, it was from Kraepelin's clinic in Munich that Bleuler and Jung first learned of this psychological experiment, and in turn demonstrated its capacity to provide empir-ical evidence for the presence of unconscious patterns of association (Kerr, 1993, pp. 44–5).

6   Jung's junior colleague Ludwig Binswager identified 11 complexes in his superior, among them, Goethe and Siegfried complexes and the wish to have a son (Kerr, 1993).

Compelled, however, to account for the distinctive splitting, disintegration, and dissociation of psychic functions in dementia praecox, Jung hypothesized that a pathogenic complex produces 'an anomalous metabolism (toxine?), which injures the brain' and prevents the acquisition or development of new complexes (Jung, 1944, pp. 31–2). 'At best', the patient 'escapes with a psychic mutilation', but as they stand 'under the ban of an invincible complex' the 'separation of the schizophrenic from reality [and] the loss of interest in objective happenings' cannot really be remedied (Jung, 1944, p. 32). By attributing a single affective cluster of sensations and memories such devastating agency within the psyche, Jung was effectively saying 'that certain thoughts, or at least certain feelings, were metabolically dangerous' (Kerr, 1993, p. 180).

Following the publication of *The Psychology of Dementia Praecox*, Jung presented his toxin theory of dementia praecox at the First International Congress for Psychoanalysis, held in Salzburg in 1908. It was a prestigious and political occasion, and, thanks to the participation of the Burghölzli psychiatrists, it marked a turning point in the psychoanalytic understanding of dementia praecox. However, it was Karl Abraham, and not his erstwhile colleague Jung, whose paper was commended for its psychoanalytic innovations. The title of Abraham's paper, 'The Psycho-Sexual Differences between Hysteria and Dementia Praecox', succinctly states his principal assertion, namely that neurosis and psychosis could be substantively distinguished without recourse to either a Kraepelinian model of inevitable dementia or a toxic X-factor, but instead through a Freudian theory of psychosexual aetiology. Jung brought psychosis into the psychoanalytic fold methodologically by demonstrating that 'meaning' could be discerned behind the 'madness' of individual patients, but he refused to concede that a sexual complex was the decisive factor in all cases. By contrast, Abraham, in theoretically differentiating dementia praecox from hysteria, actually succeeded in forging the crucial (because psychosexual and therefore 'properly' psychoanalytic) connection between the two.

In his paper, Abraham spoke with clinical authority about all forms of dementia praecox and referred to a significant number of individual cases. He began by asserting that as the symptoms of both hysteria and dementia praecox 'originate in the repressed sexual complexes', the difference between them can therefore be understood in terms of the psychosexual development of the child, or, specifically, its capacity to transfer its libido onto the external world (Abraham, 1972, pp. 64–5). Noting the flatness of affect and tendency to hostility in dementia praecox, and having 'traced back all the transference of feeling of sexuality', the analyst must, according to Abraham, 'come to the conclusion that dementia praecox destroys the person's capacity for sexual transference, i.e. for object love' (Abraham, 1972, p. 69). In a striking early example of the psychoanalytic regressive hypothesis in action, Abraham urged his audience towards another conclusion:

> Only one similar sexual condition is known to us, namely, that of early childhood; we term it, with Freud, 'auto-eroticism'. In this period, too, interest in objects and sublimation is lacking. The psychosexual characteristic of dementia praecox is the return of the patient to auto-eroticism, and the symptoms of his illness are a form of autoerotic sexual activity.

(Abraham, 1972, pp. 73–4)

In lieu of supplying empirical evidence for his hypothesis, or any clear indication that an understanding of infantile auto-eroticism could aid in the treatment of dementia praecox, Abraham offers reassuring optimism:

> A great part of the pathological manifestations of dementia praecox would, it seems to me, be explicable if we assumed that the patient has an abnormal psychosexual constitution in the direction of auto-eroticism. Such an assumption would render the recently discussed toxin theory unnecessary.

(Abraham, 1972, p. 78)

Not only did Abraham supply precisely the theory that Freud had been trying to 'plant' with Jung and Abraham since the courtship with the Burghölzli psychiatrists began, he also succeeded in taking a direct swipe at the toxin theories of his rival, Jung. Salzburg was, as John Kerr wryly observes, Abraham's 'coming-out party' as a tactical psychoanalyst (Kerr, 1993, pp. 181–2).

Although its origins lay in Freud's unpublished thinking on paranoia, Abraham's presentation served the strategic function of linking a theory of auto-eroticism with clinical observations of dementia praecox patients from the highly respected Burghölzli.[7] 'The Psycho-Sexual Differences between Hysteria and Dementia Praecox' was proof that psychoanalysis had something to say about the *psychic origins* of dementia praecox. By contrast, Jung's toxin theory proved decidedly unpopular in psychoanalytic circles at the time, and, although he was still championing it as late as 1958 (Samuels, 1997, p. 6), it has consistently failed to win many non-Jungian supporters. Jung's bitter split from Freud, his development of an analytic psychology principally concerned with the archetypes of a collective unconscious, and allegations that he was a Nazi sympathizer have all but extinguished academic interest in his first major

---

[7] In later publications, Freud is careful to reference Abraham's paper in such a way that it is clear he assumes ultimate responsibility for its accuracy. Citing Abraham, Freud (1981, p. 41) states in a footnote: 'In the course of this paper its author, referring to a correspondence between us, scrupulously attributes to myself an influence upon the development of his views' (see also Freud, 1963a, p. 415).

publication. However, setting aside the subsequent career of its author, I would argue that *The Psychology of Dementia Praecox* is most significant not for the validity or influence of Jung's toxin theory of dementia praecox, but for the extremely detailed analysis of one of his patients, Babette S. This case study highlights Jung's principal contribution to the psychoanalytic investigation of dementia praecox, namely that:

> Unlike the majority of psychiatrists before or since, he gave serious attention to what his schizophrenic patients actually said and did, and was able to demonstrate that their delusions, hallucinations, and gestures were not simply 'mad' but full of psychological meaning.

> (Stevens, 1994, p. 12)

While Jung did not supply the kind of comprehensive, linear narrative Freud would produce from Schreber's *Memoirs*, he analytically untangled Babette's frequently bizarre word associations and succeeded in interpreting seemingly disconnected, disparate, impenetrable signifiers as elements of particular complexes. It is this impulse—this process—that most distinguishes the psychoanalytic approach to schizophrenia from its psychiatric counterpart.

Babette S., an impoverished seamstress, had been institutionalized for over 15 years before commencing analysis with Jung. She suffered from paranoid delusions of physical mutilation and grandeur, severe hallucinations and affectless, disconnected speech, but sought to explain herself as clearly as possible to Jung in the vain hope that he might secure her release from the Burghölzli. The case study includes list after list of Babette's word associations. Drawing attention to her 'extraordinarily long reaction times', her neologisms, and her bizarre and sometimes embellished responses, Jung concluded that his patient was psychically dominated by numerous complexes, so much so that 'she speaks, acts, and dreams of nothing else but what the complex inspires' (Jung, 1944, p. 101). Each neologism or stereotype connected to one of three interrelated complexes—wish-fulfillment (delusions of grandeur), ideas of injury (delusions of persecution), or an erotic complex. As part of his experiment, Jung repeated Babette's neologisms (what she calls her 'power-words') to her as stimulus words. Her response to the grandiose stereotype, 'I am the finest professorship', begins like this:

> This is again the highest activity—double—twenty-five francs—I am double polytechnic irretrievable—professorship includes in itself the fine learned world—the finest world of art—I am also these titles—snail museum clothing, am I, that emanates from me—to cut no thread, to choose the best samples, those representing much, and consuming little cloth—I created that—that concerns me—the fine art world is, to apply the trimming where it can best be seen—plum cake on an Indian meal layer . . . .

> (Jung, 1944, p. 106)

Where Jung proves masterful in his analysis of her 'word salad' (a term coined by Jung) is through a rigorous, meticulous reading of seemingly impenetrable neologisms as symptomatic of specific complexes. Reluctant to speculate on *why* these complexes developed, he aims to show 'how the patient, brought up under sad domestic conditions, amid distress and hard labor, creates in her psychosis an enormously complicated, and seemingly altogether confused fantastic structure' (Jung, 1944, p. 135).

It is difficult when reading Babette's responses not to be struck by the literary quality of her fantastic structure. Jung treats them as a code to be deciphered or a poem to be interpreted, and also remarks frequently on their resemblance to dreams:

> Like a poet impelled by his inner impulses, the patient pictures to us in the symptoms the hopes and disappointments of her life. [. . .] [She] speaks as if in dreams—I know of no better expression. [. . .] [T]his uneducated and scantily endowed patient thinks without any directing idea, in obscure dreamlike pictures and amid indistinct expressions. All this contributes to make her stream of thought as incomprehensible as possible. [. . .] [Unlike the dreams of normal people, here] we have long and extensively elaborated fancies, which on the one hand are comparable to a great poem and on the other to the romances and fantastic pictures of somnambulists.

> (Jung, 1944, pp. 135–6)

Although the comparison is seductive, Avital Ronnell challenges the move to equate dreams with dementia praecox, arguing that 'while the dream was thought to have latent content, a retrievable unconscious narrativity, the schizophrenic utterance remains a pistol shot in the dark of metaphysics, shattered, fragmented' (Ronell, 1989, p. 137). By 'making sense' of a number of Babette's more opaque phrases, what Jung ultimately delivers is only a series of discrete interpretations of elements of his patient's disturbed psyche rather than a narrative that would draw these together. Fragmentary understanding, then, comes to displace and replace any discussion of cure or the alleviation of symptoms and operates independently of a theory of aetiology, toxin-related or otherwise.

Through his analysis of Babette, Jung sought to establish the paranoid form of dementia praecox as the disorder most amenable to psychoanalytic investigation, demonstrating, albeit tenuously, how the idiosyncratic content of a patient's symptoms followed previously identified narrative patterns (delusions of grandeur and persecution). For Jung, the domain of dementia praecox was 'too extensive and yet too obscure' for his work on paranoia to be conclusive; promising to extend his inquiry into catatonic and hebephrenic schizophrenia at a future date, his final statement is at once apologetic, defensive, and self-aggrandizing: 'Somebody finally had to take it upon himself to set the stone rolling' (Jung, 1944, pp. 135–6). And roll it did—inexorably on towards

Freud's analysis of a text introduced to him by Jung, *Memoirs of My Nervous Illness*. Although many critics would prefer not to call attention to the influence of Jung's case study on 'Psycho-Analytic Notes', its importance should not be underestimated. What Jung presented was an analysis of an acutely psychotic *patient*—an analysis based upon psychological experiments in real time, conducted in an asylum, and involving a range of non-verbal and emotional communications which could not be captured adequately on the page. Babette did not provide him with a cogent or compelling narrative of her illness but with disconnected speech and 'difficult' behaviour. It is unsurprising, then, that Jung's text deals in fragments and cannot attempt a complete psychological picture of his patient, especially as he suggests that the disorder has a metabolic—not psychological—origin. Despite uncanny similarities between the delusional schema of Babette and Schreber,[8] the case history of this poor and uneducated woman could not match the analytic possibilities presented by the autobiography of an esteemed male jurist. Equally, when it came to the weaving of linear narratives, Jung's theory of co-existent complexes was no match for the capacity of libido theory to trace all symptoms and psychic dysfunctions back to a primary psychosexual disturbance. What Jung *did* establish was the possibility of penetrating the supposedly impenetrable symptoms of dementia praecox by subjecting them to psychoanalytic investigation. This, together with Abraham's authoritative account of the psychosexual origins of dementia praecox, constitutes a foundation for Freud's work on paranoia.

Before moving on to a detailed analysis of 'Psycho-Analytic Notes', it is worth recalling Karl Jaspers's comments on the work of Freud and the Zurich school on dementia praecox. Although Jaspers acknowledged that the psychoanalytic scrutiny of the 'delusional contents of dementia praecox' can be seen as an improvement on psychiatry's efforts to classify the chaos of schizophrenia, he remained justifiably suspicious of psychoanalytic methodology:

> They have thus come to 'understand' almost all the contents of these psychoses by applying a procedure which as the results show only leads on into endlessness. In the most literary sense they have rediscovered the 'meaning of madness' or at least they believe they have.

> The whole interpretation is a *translation to schizophrenia of concepts which have been arrived at during the analysis of hysteria*. We should, however, never forget the radical differences which exist between hysteria and a schizophrenic process . . .

> (Jaspers, 1972, pp. 539, 410, italics in the original)

....

[8] For example, Babette believes that her actions are continuously monitored by telephones, just as Schreber is consistently scrutinized by God's 'rays'. Both also suffer the presence of 'little men', literally, tiny figures emerging from or molesting their bodies (see Jung, 1944, pp. 140, 91; Schreber, 1955, pp. 112, 157).

Jaspers's observations from 1913 inform the primary argument of this chapter, that psychoanalysis approaches schizophrenia as a sublime text that reveals the collapse of psychic functioning if only it is properly deciphered. Jung's *The Psychology of Dementia Praecox* is, I suggest, the founding text in this psychoanalytic tradition. As he showed, the analyst's interpretive mastery over dementia praecox, secured through a potentially inexhaustible process, does not deliver the analysand from their schizophrenic symptoms as it might with neurosis. It is simply an end in itself, and, if Jaspers is correct, one that actually obfuscates the fundamental inaccessibility—or sublimity—of schizophrenia. Jung could only point to how Babette's speech revealed her complexes; the question of why she became psychotic, when others who experience 'distress and hardship' among 'sad domestic conditions' do not, is unanswered, and it is clear that his analysis did little to mitigate her distress. Although treating schizophrenia as a disorder of signification allows the analyst to restore or attribute meaning to schizophrenic speech, the analyst's narrative (like the psychiatrist's clinical picture) fails to address the structure of schizophrenic experience, or to explain *why* schizophrenia arises and cannot be 'cured'. The clinical picture of schizophrenia is recast as a text in which the 'meaning of madness' is rediscovered, but in revealing and exceeding the limits of interpretation or textualization, the person herself is assigned a sublime status in psychoanalytic discourse.

Freud on Schreber

Freud's 'Psycho-Analytical Notes on an Autobiographical Account of a Case of Paranoia (Dementia Paranoides)' has been described by one historian of psychoanalysis as 'the first time anyone had ever penetrated so deeply into the mental life of a psychotic' (Fine, 1979, p. 54). The same observation applies equally to the autobiographical account in question, the memoirs of psychiatry's most quoted and certainly most famous schizophrenic patient, Daniel Paul Schreber. Schreber was a distinguished jurist who suffered three distinct periods of what he called 'nervous illness' (Macalpine and Hunter, 1955b, p. 3). In 1884, he was admitted to the University Clinic of Leipzig and successfully treated by Paul Emil Flechsig for severe hypochondria. In 1893, soon after his appointment to the high office of *Senatspräsident* (President of the Court of Appeal) in Dresden, he was again admitted to Flechsig's clinic with psychotic symptoms, and was subsequently transferred to the Sonnenstein Asylum. *Memoirs of My Nervous Illness* is Schreber's account of his eight-year incarceration; written while he was still a patient at Sonnenstein, it was a key document in his legal appeal to be recognized as fit to manage his own affairs. Schreber's tutelage was eventually rescinded by the courts in 1902, and the following year he discharged himself and published his *Memoirs*. Unbeknown to Freud, Schreber's wife Sabine suffered a stroke in 1907, and immediately afterwards he was again admitted to an asylum with acute psychosis. He died there in 1911, months after Freud published 'Psycho-Analytic Notes'. Despite his painstaking efforts to elucidate for the reader the detail and significance of his religious revelations, Schreber's autobiographical account of his psychotic experiences is as byzantine as it is bizarre. At times daunting in its intricacy, *Memoirs* defies summary, so wherever possible we will let Schreber speak for himself.

The textual sources upon which Freud based his analysis of Schreber were both addressed, at least in part, to the legal question of Schreber's tutelage. The official medical reports submitted to the courts by the Sonnenstein Superintendent, Dr Weber, were published as appendices to *Memoirs*, and thus Freud had to reconcile conflicting accounts of Schreber's illness in his own presentation of the case history. Drawing a clear distinction between the psychiatric approach to psychotic behaviour and the psychoanalytic 'wish to go more deeply into the details of the delusion and into the history of its development' (Freud, 1981, p. 18), Freud begins by challenging Weber's description of Schreber's delusional system. In his report, Weber noted that Schreber's early delusions of bodily persecution eventually gave way to a fixed structure of 'pathological ideas':

> The patient's delusional system amounts to this: he is called to redeem the world and to bring back to mankind the lost state or Blessedness. He maintains he has been given this task by direct divine inspiration . . . The most essential part of his mission to redeem the world is that it is necessary for him first of all to be *transformed into a woman*. Not, however, that he *wishes* to be transformed into a woman, it is much more a 'must' according to the Order of the World, which he simply cannot escape, even though he would personally very much prefer to remain in his honourable manly position in life.

> (Weber, 1955, p. 268, italics in the original)

The 'natural' conclusion to draw from this, according to Freud, is that Schreber's emasculation fantasy was motivated by the original redeemer delusion; becoming a woman was, for Schreber, a secondary requirement of his messianic role. Freud points out, however, that *Memoirs* tells a very different story: the partial sexual transformation happened first, for the purposes of sexual abuse by God, and only later came to be related to the redeemer delusion. Assigning autobiography priority over psychiatric evaluation, he concludes:

> The position may be formulated by saying that a sexual delusion of persecution was later on converted in the patient's mind into a religious delusion of grandeur. The part

of the prosecutor was at first assigned to Professor Flechsig, the physician in whose charge he was; later, his place was taken by God Himself.

(Freud, 1981, p. 18)

Although presented as a statement of fact rather than the audacious analysis it is, this is the interpretive move upon which Freud's subsequent analysis of Schreber, and of paranoia more generally, hinges. Ignoring almost completely Weber's report of Schreber's complex symptomatology—severe hyperaesthesia, suicidal tendencies, periodic bellowing, and catatonic intervals being only some of the more striking—Freud focuses exclusively on the delusional structure, and assigns one aspect of it, namely the sexual one, unparalleled aetiological importance.[9] Significantly, delusional beliefs remain the sole focus of Freud's analysis, and by establishing a delusion of sexual persecution as primary, Freud attributes to Schreber's entire cosmology a sexual significance. This paranoid schizophrenia is not the '"negative case" which has so long been sought for—a case in which sexuality plays only a very minor part'; on the contrary, it is positively perfect for psychoanalysis: 'Schreber himself speaks again and again as though he shared our prejudice. He is constantly talking in the same breath of "nervous disorder" and erotic lapses, as though the two were inseparable' (Freud, 1981, p. 34).

Section two of Freud's essay, 'Attempts at Interpretation', begins by sketching two possibilities for the psychoanalytic investigation of psychosis as pioneered by Jung and Abraham: 'We might start either from the patient's own delusional utterances or from the exciting causes of his illness' (Freud, 1981, p. 35). Freud clearly sees little challenge in analysing the delusional utterance, but to prove the ease of the undertaking offers an interpretation of Schreber's 'miracled birds' as representing young girls (Freud, 1981, pp. 356).[10] However, it is clearly the 'exciting cause' that most excites Freud; psychoanalysis would have to answer the question of aetiology if it were to produce a theory of paranoia that explained delusional systems rather than mere utterances. Thus, having already established the primacy of the sexual persecution delusion, Freud turns to an analysis of Schreber's initial persecutor: the 'soul-murderer' Professor Flechsig. Freud offers his own 'simple formula' for explaining the delusion of persecution: the patient's intense emotional attachment to a particular person becomes unacceptable to the ego, so it is projected outwards

---

[9] Freud is unequivocal on this point: 'The idea of being transformed into a woman was the salient feature and earliest germ of his delusional system' (Freud, 1981, p. 21).

[10] Although clearly seeking to impress the reader through this 'easy' reading, it is ultimately isolated and ineffectual, as Freud fails to relate his findings here to the father-complex thesis subsequently developed.

onto that person and its affective content is transformed (Freud, 1981, pp. 40–1). In Freud's reading, Schreber denied his love for Flechsig and consequently imagined that Flechsig was his persecutor:

> The exciting cause of his illness, then, was an outburst of homosexual libido; the object of this libido was probably from the very first his doctor, Flechsig; and his struggles against the libidinal impulse produced the conflict which gave rise to the symptoms.

> (Freud, 1981, p. 43)[11]

The delusion of persecution is therefore a defence against what Freud calls a 'feminine (that is, a passive homosexual) wishful fantasy' (Freud, 1981, pp. 46–7). When Schreber believes that he is persecuted not just by Flechsig, but by God himself, the delusion appears to indicate psychic conflict on an even greater scale; however, its inflation instead provides the means by which the ego can accept the unconscious fantasy. Freud had hypothesized earlier that the redeemer delusion served to legitimate Schreber's fantasy of emasculation—becoming Flechsig's whore was intolerable, but if Schreber was chosen by God to redeem humankind then it was his duty to enjoy his transformation into a woman. If God is, in Schreber's cosmology, a symbol for the father, then the explanation for his longing for transsexual metamorphosis is easily identified: 'The feminine phantasy, which aroused such violent opposition in the patient, thus had its roots in a longing, intensified to an erotic pitch, for his father and brother' (Freud, 1981, p. 50). Freud explains Schreber's entire delusional structure—communication with rays and nerves, upper and lower Gods, the forecourts of heaven, and feelings of soul-voluptuousness—as derivative of a father complex wherein he assumes a 'feminine' attitude towards God-as-the-father.

Schreber's bizarre psychotic schema is effectively remoulded by Freud into a cogent neurotic narrative of psychosexual origins. Recognizing that 'in all this there is nothing characteristic of the form of disease known as paranoia, nothing that might not be found (and that has not in fact been found) in other kinds of neuroses', Freud turns to address psychic mechanisms particular to paranoia (Freud, 1981, p. 59). Projection is singled out as a process integral to paranoid symptom formation,[12] but it is the analysis of the particular mechanism of repression in paranoia that establishes a vital link to libido theory.

---

[11] And continues with dramatic flair: 'I will pause here for a moment to meet a storm of remonstrances and objections. Any one acquainted with the present state of psychiatry must be prepared to face trouble'.

[12] Freud (1981, p. 66) offers the following definition of projection: 'An internal perception is suppressed, and, instead, its content, after undergoing a certain kind of distortion, enters consciousness in the form of an external perception'.

Paranoia, according to Freud, is characterized by 'the failure of repression, of *irruption*, of *return of the repressed*' originating from a point of fixation, or a point of arrested development, in the libido (Freud, 1981, p. 68, italics in the original). One of the strongest and most persuasive passages in 'Psycho-Analytic Notes' is the interpretation of Schreber's 'world-catastrophe' delusion as one such irruption:[13]

> The patient has withdrawn from the people in his environment and from the external world generally the libidinal cathexis which he had hitherto directed on to them. Thus everything has become indifferent and irrelevant to him, and has to be explained by means of a secondary rationalization as being 'miracled up, cursorily improvised'. The end of the world is the projection of this internal catastrophe; his subjective world has come to an end since his withdrawal of his love from it.
>
> (Freud, 1981, p. 70)

The 'delusional formation' of a profoundly changed world is therefore not in itself the pathological product, rather it 'is in reality an attempt at recovery, a process of restitution'; it 'undoes the work of repression' by redirecting the libido on to the external world through a kind of radical projection, where 'what was abolished internally returns from without' (Freud, 1981, p. 71). Freud speculates that the withdrawal of libido from the world is in fact a regular feature of normal life and other less severe disorders; what is distinctive about paranoia is that the withdrawn libido is put to a 'special use', that it is, as the megalomaniac tendencies of paranoiacs indicate, redirected onto the ego (Freud, 1981, p. 72). Abraham had already argued that dementia praecox could be understood as regression to the auto-erotic (primary) stage of libidinal development; here, Freud suggests that in paranoia the libido is fixated at the second, narcissistic stage, and so associated with homosexuality.

Crystallized delusional structures, megalomania, passive homosexual fantasies—libido theory offers its own relatively comprehensive explanation for these elements of paranoia, but what of the more acutely psychotic, inaccessible dementia praecox? As I suggested earlier, Freud elided discussion of Schreber's panoply of schizophrenic symptoms, concentrating instead on his complex delusional formations. It becomes clear towards the end of 'Psycho-Analytic Notes' that the success of Freud's libido-theory analysis of paranoia depends upon grouping it among the neuroses, effectively rejecting Kraepelin's and Bleuler's clinical picture of paranoia as a type of dementia praecox or schizophrenia. 'What seems to me most essential', Freud writes, 'is that paranoia

---

[13] Schreber (1955, p. 86) reports that he had 'innumerable visions . . . in connection with the idea that the world had perished' and that these 'were partly of a gruesome nature, partly of an indescribable sublimity'.

should be maintained as an independent clinical type, however frequently the picture it offers may be complicated by the presence of schizophrenic features' (Freud, 1981, p. 76). Suggesting that dementia praecox be renamed 'paraphrenia', Freud proposes two key differences between dementia praecox and paranoia: first, dementia praecox does not involve projection but an unspecified 'hallucinatory (hysterical) mechanism'; secondly, the point of fixation is 'further back' at the stage of auto-eroticism (Freud, 1981, p. 77). If paranoia cannot, as Freud acknowledges, be definitively distinguished from other neuroses, and the more markedly psychotic aspects of paraphrenia similarly fail to warrant a significant innovation in psychoanalytic theory, then a continuum between neurosis, paranoia, and paraphrenia is implicitly established. Despite calling for distinct nosological categories, Freud only further confuses the issue: 'Our hypotheses as to the dispositional fixations in paranoia and paraphrenia make it easy to see that a case may begin with paranoiac symptoms and may yet develop into a dementia praecox, and that paranoid and schizophrenic phenomena may be combined in any proportion' (Freud, 1981, p. 77). Schreber's translators, psychoanalysts Ida Macalpine and Richard Hunter, note that in spite of Freud's equivocations, his theoretical formulations on paranoia 'were nevertheless imperceptibly extended in psychoanalysis to schizophrenia and the psychoses in general; as such they entered psychiatric literature as "the psychoanalytic theory of psychosis"'(Macalpine and Hunter, 1955b, pp. 10–11). Ultimately, as Lacan observes, Freud's analysis of paranoia/paraphrenia 'leaves the fields of the psychoses and the neuroses both on the same level' (Lacan, 1993, pp. 10–11), and, I would argue, establishes the translation of psychosis into a neurotic narrative a defining feature of the psychoanalytic approach to schizophrenia.

The key concepts introduced by Freud in his analysis of Schreber's *Memoirs*—homosexuality, narcissism, the return of the repressed, and the restitutive function of the symptom—became integral to subsequent psychoanalytic accounts of schizophrenia. However, 'Psycho-Analytic Notes' was arguably as influential in inaugurating a particular way of reading psychosis as it was for presenting a theory of paranoid symptom formation. I want to turn now to the significance of 'Psycho-Analytic Notes' in establishing a methodology for the analysis of psychosis, one that is summarized by Lacan's comment: '[Freud] deciphers [*Memoirs*] in the way hieroglyphics are deciphered' (Lacan, 1993, p. 10).

Two distinguishing features of the psychoanalytic approach to schizophrenia are made apparent in Freud's work: the presentation of schizophrenia as a textual puzzle, and the interrelated negotiation of intimacy and distance (close contact with the hieroglyphic, but spatial, temporal, and even psychic separation from its creator).[14] Freud makes it clear from the outset that people with psychosis pose specific difficulties for the analytic investigator: 'We cannot accept patients suffering from this complaint, or, at all events, we cannot keep them for long since we cannot offer treatment unless there is some prospect of therapeutic success' (Freud, 1981, p. 9). Any inquiry into paranoia is therefore frustrated by a lack of first-hand experience, a distance from the patients themselves. Freud overcomes this apparently insurmountable obstacle by arguing that such patients 'possess the peculiarity of betraying (in a distorted form, it is true) precisely those things which other neurotics keep hidden as a secret'; and by virtue of these flagrant displays of unconscious material, 'it follows that this is precisely a disorder in which a written report or a printed case history can take the place of personal acquaintance with the patient' (Freud, 1981, p. 9). Here it is a text, namely Schreber's *Memoirs*, that bridges the distance between psychoanalyst and patient, but in so doing calls into question the very nature of psychoanalytic technique.[15] The text is a substitute for not only the patient but also the analytic relationship; the hermeneutic enterprise has no therapeutic effects, and what would otherwise have been inaccessible to Freud is, by virtue of being laid bare on the page, ripe for pseudo-literary analysis.[16] Although Freud remarks no further on the significance of basing his remarks about paranoia on Schreber's *Memoirs*, rather than on a patient whose behaviour might disturb, undermine, confirm, or distract from the analytic process, it is clear that this text predetermines to some extent the scope of his inquiry. Unlike Babette's word associations, Schreber's story is both a memoir (a retelling of the history of his religious revelations, written during a period of relative

---

[14] Michel de Certeau (1983, p. 21) also notes that Freud 'preferred what was distant, as if a separation created the analytic space'.

[15] In a later paper, Freud resolved this by (re)defining paranoia as a 'narcissistic neurosis', which could not be cured by psychoanalysis due to the absence of transference. The paranoid person's indifference to the analyst means that 'the mechanism of cure which we carry through with other people—the revival of the pathogenic conflict and the overcoming of the resistance due to repression—cannot be operated with them. They remain as they are. Often they have already undertaken attempts at recovery on their own which have led to pathological results [i.e. delusions]. We cannot alter this in any way. [...] They manifest no transference and for that reason are inaccessible to our efforts and cannot be cured by us' (Freud, 1963b, p. 447). Establishing the impossibility of an analytic relationship as a cardinal feature of psychosis bears striking resemblance to Jaspers's thesis of an unbreachable gulf between the psychiatrist and schizophrenic patient. However, for Jaspers, unlike Freud, the gulf is structural to the definition of schizophrenia.

[16] As Pamela Thurschwell (2000, p. 62) observes, 'The Schreber case is . . . a psychoanalytic reading of a text, rather than an analysis of a person. In some ways it has more in common with Freud's reading of other literary and artistic works than it does with the other case histories'.

psychic stability) and an appeal (to have the validity of these revelations acknowledged, and his tutelage rescinded). Its form and function therefore allow for the presentation of a comparatively cogent narrative which charts the onset and development of Schreber's schizophrenic symptoms. Freud re-presents this narrative in order to give a psychoanalytic account of its origins.

The analytic distance imposed by the substitution of text for patient proved enormously productive for Freud and, paradoxically, it is this separation which allowed him to form an intimate identification with Schreber. Indeed, by consistently praising Schreber's intelligence, his professional accomplishments, and his powers of communication, Freud seems to align himself so closely with Schreber that by the end of 'Psycho-Analytic Notes' he feels compelled to assert his theoretical rigour and originality:

> [So many] details of Schreber's delusional structure sound almost like endopsychic perceptions of the processes whose existence I have assumed in these pages as the basis of our explanation of paranoia. I can nevertheless call a friend and fellow-specialist to witness that I had developed my theory of paranoia before I became acquainted with the contents of Schreber's book. It remains for the future to decide where there is more delusion in my theory than I should like to admit, or whether there is more truth in Schreber's delusion than other people are as yet prepared to believe.

> (Freud, 1981, p. 79)

Here, Freud echoes Schreber's own appeal to be believed:

> Even now I would count it a great triumph for my dialectical dexterity if through the present essay, which seems to be growing to the size of a scientific work, I should achieve only *the one* result, to make the physicians shake their heads in doubt as to whether after all there was some truth in my so-called delusions and hallucinations.

> (Schreber, 1955, p. 123, italics in the original)

So strong was his identification with Schreber that Freud used his neologisms to develop a private discourse with Jung, referred to him as 'the wonderful Schreber, who ought to have been made a professor of psychiatry and director of a mental hospital' (Freud, in Freud and Jung, 1974, p. 311), and, as John Farrell discusses at length, came to understand many of his own relationships through Schreber's paranoia (Farrell, 1996, pp. 188–94). Freud even attempted to insulate Schreber from any suspicion that he might be an average psychotic patient by disclaiming any similarity between Babette and Schreber: her 'dementia praecox' was apparently 'far severer than this one' and 'exhibited symptoms far more remote from the normal' (Freud, 1981, p. 35). These claims to know Schreber intimately, made in and beyond 'Psycho-Analytic Notes', serve, I would argue, a double function. First, they create the impression that psychoanalysis has privileged access to the secrets of psychosis, uncovering meaning in what psychiatry takes to be of diagnostic interest only. However, although it would appear that scrutinizing the symbolic content of delusions and hallucinations for the psychosexual origins of psychosis promotes a type of understanding unimaginable in an asylum, the idea of an intimacy between Freud and Schreber himself is utterly illusory as it is the schizophrenic text, and not the analytic relationship, in which Freud invests. Whereas Kraepelin routinely conceded that the behaviour of his dementia praecox patients was simply beyond comprehension, Freud's 'Psycho-Analytic Notes', in 'penetrat[ing] the dynamics of psychosis' (Fine, 1979, p. 83), can be read as a complex attempt to negotiate a safe distance from schizophrenia by treating it as a textual puzzle, and to mitigate the inscrutability of madness by solving that puzzle.

We have already seen that the careful control of distance was a determining factor in Kant's account of the sublime encounter, and that psychiatry's elevation of schizophrenia to the status of sublime object likewise depended upon a distance carefully controlled through an ensemble of discursive and clinical practices. The psychoanalytic approach to psychosis is in some sense similar to this process: the analyst purports to 'penetrate' the otherwise opaque internal dynamics of the patient through a pseudo-literary analysis made possible by a spatial and temporal gulf. But rather than inquiring into schizophrenia as disease, psychoanalysis frames schizophrenia as a sublime text, a series of signs that starkly expose the sublime 'secrets' of the unconscious, and challenge the analyst to assert their hermeneutic mastery by deciphering them.[17] What allows for the operation of a disciplinary sublime in psychiatry is the fact that schizophrenia retains its status as somehow 'unknowable'; psychoanalysis, by contrast, claims to 'know' the psychic mechanisms, psychosexual aetiology, and symbolic significance of schizophrenic symptoms, but only, I am suggesting, because it recasts disorder as text.

Analyses of Schreber's *Memoirs* are exemplary of the operation of a textual sublime in psychoanalytic discourse more broadly. 'Whatever [its] psychological significance', writes Vincent Crapanzano (1998, p. 739), 'from a literary-discursive point of view it is one of the most challenging texts of the century'.[18] Its seductions, as Louis Sass puts it (1992, p. 244), are many,

> . . . the more closely one reads, the more difficult it becomes to dismiss the hope for achieving some kind of interpretive or empathetic understanding of Schreber's

[17] The issue of narrative is here once again worth noting. Freud's reading of Schreber is, it would seem, more celebrated than Jung's account of Babette's responses to word-association tests because it establishes a coherent, linear narrative of Schreber's delusions.

[18] Or, as Barrett (1998c, p. 471) wryly observes: 'During his illness Schreber suffered the most agonising self-scrutiny, but nothing like the intensity of the posthumous psychiatric scrutiny'.

experiences. The whole structure of his lived world seems to have such specificity and precision; one cannot help but wonder whether it is possible to discover a coherent system lying behind it all.

The interpretative challenge of Schreber's text has been taken up by a staggering number of psychoanalytic and cultural critics, all of whom claim a certain mastery over its contents. Yet the essential enigma of the schizophrenic, bellowing, and long-departed Schreber still remains. In the next section, I will briefly survey the most influential of these analyses of *Memoirs*, not only to demonstrate how wildly divergent each reading is in its interpretation of Schreber's symptomatology, but to argue that this proliferation of scholarly reinterpretations of *Memoirs* testifies to the textual sublimity of schizophrenia within (and beyond) psychoanalysis. According to the logic of the textual sublime, it is not the disorder but the text—literally, the symbolic output—of schizophrenia that is perpetually reframed; the text can be deciphered but the disorder never wholly explained. Of course, the fact that Schreber is dead means that no single account can assert its interpretive superiority through an appeal to therapeutic success. This is widely unacknowledged but diminishes no commentator's interpretive zeal; it only further reinforces the profound schism between the psychotic text and the person to whom it belongs. Aiming to capture the truth of Schreber's delusions, or to 'penetrate' the secrets of his psychosis, the psychoanalytic discourse generated by *Memoirs* continues Freud's approach to schizophrenia as a textual puzzle, and reinforces his view that the schizophrenic patient can only be talked *about* but not talked *to*.

Reading Schreber

Psychoanalysis and (psycho)biography

Freud's 'Psycho-Analytic Notes' established the terms of reference for psychoanalytic readings of Schreber's *Memoirs*, and indeed psychosis in general, until at least the mid-1950s. Perhaps the most frequently cited Freudian analyst of the Schreber case is Maurits Katan. Katan published a number of papers endorsing the tenets of Freud's homosexuality thesis, elaborating on the 'basic masturbatory fantasy' at work throughout Schreber's illness, and suggesting that psychosis occurs when the Oedipal complex fails to contain the 'dangerous passive feminine urge' of the homosexual libido (Katan, 1949, 1950a, b, 1952a, b). However, the translation, by Ida Macalpine and Richard Hunter, of Schreber's *Memoirs*, and their stringent critique of Freud's 'Psycho-Analytic Notes', appear to mark the first major turning point in the psychoanalytic study of both texts. Explicitly challenging the 'taboo of a classic . . . attached to Freud's paper' Macalpine and Hunter take issue with Freud's confused nosology, his (mistaken) treatment of psychosis as an Oedipal psychoneurosis, his selective and self-serving concentration on Schreber's persecutory delusions, and his neglect of the 'other, often much earlier, disturbances of emotion, feeling, association [and] bodily sensations', which occurred during Schreber's pre-psychotic phase and persisted throughout his psychiatric incarceration (Macalpine and Hunter, 1955a, pp. 369–80). Finding in *Memoirs* no evidence to support Freud's thesis that Schreber's psychosis originated from an irruption of homosexual libido, Macalpine and Hunter look beyond the Oedipus complex to explain its aetiology, and in particular his somatic delusions and hypochondria. Like Freud, they suggest that the 'unmanning' fantasy is at the core of Schreber's delusional schema, but instead of viewing it as a castration threat or as evidence of Schreber's homosexuality, they interpret his entire psychosis 'as a reactivation of unconscious, archaic procreation fantasies concerning life, death, immortality, rebirth, creation, [and] self-impregnation . . . accompanied by absolute ambisexuality expressed in doubt and uncertainty about his sex' (Macalpine and Hunter, 1955a, p. 395). For Macalpine and Hunter, it was the intense unhappiness resulting from Schreber's inability to have children (Sabine Schreber suffered six pregnancies resulting in miscarriage or still birth), and not an unconscious homosexual longing for the father, that underscored the archaic procreation fantasy structuring his psychosis.

Macalpine and Hunter's original psychoanalytic rereading of Schreber's *Memoirs* certainly challenged Freudian orthodoxy by pointing towards the pre-Oedipal origins of psychosis. However, their analysis was, for the most part, confined to the text itself. The decisive transformation in Schreber studies was brought about by William G. Niederland's research into an array of other texts pertinent to the Schreber case, in particular, the autocratic pedagogical writings of Daniel Gottlieb Moritz Schreber.[19] Schreber's father, an esteemed and zealous pedagogue, published over the course of his lifetime numerous books on the topic of childrearing in which he advised 'parents and educators [to] use a maximum of pressure and coercion during the earliest years of the child's life' (Niederland, 1984, p. 50).[20] To a twenty-first-century reader, the education system advanced by Moritz Schreber seems at best severe and excessively disciplinarian, and at worst a despotic, sadistic regime guaranteed to scar any child subjected to its principles and practices. Prominent among Moritz Schreber's recommendations to parents is the use of his self-devised

---

[19] Daniel Gottlieb Moritz Schreber—the father of Daniel Paul Schreber, author of *Memoirs*—I shall henceforth refer to as Moritz Schreber.

[20] Note that *The Schreber Case* includes a revised collection of Niederland's publications on Schreber, dating from 1951.

and presumably family-tested prosthetic devices: straps, belts, bars, and hel-
mets worn by children to correct posture, prevent masturbation, and promote
obedience. Niederland argues that the study of these devices and educational
manuals 'enable[s] us—as Freud had suggested—to trace numerous details of
Schreber's delusions to their sources and to correlate a number of hitherto
obscure passages in the description of his delusional system with particular
ideas, principles, and the lifework cherished by the father' (Niederland, 1984,
p. 49). A psychoanalyst by trade, Niederland interprets Schreber's somatic suffering (specifically, the 'compression-of-the-chest-miracle', 'head-being-tied-
together-machine', and various other 'miracles' performed on his eyes and
eyelids)[21] as,

> . . . a highly condensed, symbolized, archaically distorted, yet essentially correct ver-
> sion of many of the paternal physical maneuvers to which the young Schreber was
> subjected, a sort of 'primary-process' catalogue of those remote infantile experiences,
> shaped, altered, and strongly cathected ('deified') by the father–son conflict.

> (Niederland, 1984, pp. 75–80)

Niederland claims that his extensive biographical research uncovers a 'nucle-
us' or 'kernel' of truth in Schreber's delusions (Niederland, 1984, pp. xvi, 101).
What bearing his psychobiographical analysis has on the question of the aetiology of these and other schizophrenic delusions is much less clear, principally
because Niederland struggles to reconcile his historical account of the 'pathological' and abusive father with Freud's insistence upon the intrapsychic, psychosexual origins of paranoia.[22] Niederland does endeavour to confirm Freud's
hypothesis by suggesting that 'the manipulations performed on the child's
body' were both 'punitive' *and* 'seductive', and hence aroused in the young
Schreber deeply contradictory feelings towards his father (Niederland, 1984,
pp. 60, 74). Later, he suggests that the onset of Schreber's psychosis was
a direct result of his professional appointment, the confrontation with his

---

21 Schreber writes that 'From the first beginnings of my contact with God up to the present
day my body has continuously been the object of divine miracles . . . I might say that
hardly a single limb or organ in my body escaped being temporarily damaged by miracles, nor a single muscle being pulled by miracles, either moving or paralyzing it according to the respective purpose. Even now the miracles which I experience hourly are still
of a nature as to frighten every other human being to death . . .'. He goes on to say that
the *'compression-of-the-chest-miracle'*, for example, 'consisted in the whole chest wall
being compressed, so that the state of oppression caused by the lack of breath was transmitted to my whole body' (Schreber, 1955, pp. 131–3).
22 Han Israëls (quoted in Santner, 1996, p. 169) suggests that this is because Niederland's
influence anxiety prevents him from appreciating, or clearly articulating, the sharp distinction between his own findings and those of Freud.

'greatest dread': 'taking the place of the father' and 'assuming an active mascu-line role in real life' (Niederland, 1984, p. 41). However, as Niederland rightly points out, neither these nor Freud's original hypothesis can adequately explain Schreber's 40 years of apparent mental health. Despite illuminating a new symbolic dimension in Schreber's delusional schema, *The Schreber Case* makes no significant methodological departure from psychoanalytic orthodoxy. In a move reminiscent of Freud's abandonment of the seduction theory, Niederland hints at but nowhere posits a *direct, causal* relationship between Schreber's childhood experiences and the onset of his psychosis.

Niederland raised this fundamental question regarding Schreber's psychosis in the early 1950s. Twenty years later, Morton Schatzman answered it resound-ingly in his *Soul Murder: Persecution in the Family* (Schatzman, 1973; see also Schatzman, 1971, pp. 117–207). Whereas Niederland was justifiably wary that a 'conspirational theory' of schizophrenogenic parents is 'simplistic and reduc-tionist' (Niederland, 1984, p. 109), Schatzman insists that Niederland's find-ings 'call for radically *new* hypotheses' and speak to the urgent need for a reappraisal of *Memoirs* as well as a more rigorous investigation of the family life of all people diagnosed with schizophrenia (Schatzman, 1973, pp. 8, xvi, 1, italics in the original). Schatzman's overtly political and passionate discussions of schizophrenia locate him squarely in the antipsychiatry movement. Like R.D. Laing, Schatzman ascribes a considerable agency to the schizophrenic patient: he argues that Schreber's delusional experiences are direct 'images' or 'transforms' of his father's procedures, that they represent an 'ingenious attempt' to negotiate the contradictions inherent in those procedures, and that ultimately Schreber's 'miracles' are not symptoms but memories and re-enactments of his torment (Schatzman, 1973, pp. xii, xiii, 23, 45–7). Schatzman is une-quivocal in assigning Moritz Schreber the role of villain in Schreber's suffering, describing him as 'paranoidogenic' or generative of his son's paranoid states (Schatzman, 1973, pp. 122–4). Schatzman's discussion of the biographical origins of some of Schreber's delusions is certainly dramatic, and suggestive up to a point, although he gives only a cursory account of the psychic mechanisms and processes of schizophrenic symptom formation and his 'conspirational' paranoidogenic-father thesis is, as Niederland might have observed, ill-equipped to explain Schreber's 40 years of apparent normalcy.

If Schatzman approached the Schreber case in the spirit of R.D. Laing, Zvi Lothane is closer to the Thomas Szasz school of antipsychiatry.[23] As I will discuss in the next chapter, Laing and Szasz represent two distinct trends in

---

[23] Lothane (1992, p. ix) refers to Szasz as one of his 'good friends', but does not explicitly identify himself as an antipsychiatrist. Although Lothane cites Niederland as 'the doyen

antipsychiatry: the former dedicated to elucidating the familial, societal, and political causes of 'schizophrenia', the latter more directly concerned with critiquing the institution of psychiatry. Antipsychiatry radically calls into question the existence of schizophrenia (as severe psychic disorder, and especially as disease), and for very different reasons, Schatzman (1973, p. 23) and Lothane (1992, p. 7) categorically reject both psychiatric and psychoanalytic diagnoses of Schreber. Lothane's tome, *In Defense of Schreber*, is an exhaustive biographical study of the Schrebers and the biological psychiatrists who administered the asylums in which Schreber was incarcerated, as well as a multifaceted critique of Schreber studies up to the early 1990s. Most strikingly, Lothane attempts a redemptive re-reading of Moritz Schreber's pedagogic texts, and comes to the conclusion that:

> It is the posture-improving appliances that have procured for Schreber the reputation of a malevolent and sadistic educator. It is due to the horrific imagery *created by the exaggerated descriptions* of these allegedly immobilizing and pain-producing appliances by Niederland, and the even greater distortions by Schatzman, that this legend about Moritz Schreber arose and took root in the popular imagination . . . [and] fictions became historical facts.
>
> (Lothane, 1992, pp. 178–9, my italics)[24]

As the title of his work suggests, Lothane's primary objective is to defend both the Schrebers from the 'character assassinations' made legend by Freud, Niederland, and particularly Schatzman:

> It comes to this: Moritz Schreber and [Daniel] Paul Schreber, father and son, have been the target of gross distortions. The father was made to look like a crank, the son queer and crazy. Both are gross distortions. Both caricatures stem from prejudice and ignorance of the historical facts.
>
> (Lothane, 1992, pp. 438, 7)

Lothane's portrayal of Schreber, by contrast, appears to stem from a strong and almost loving attachment to him: approaching Schreber 'as if [he] had entered into a dialogue with a friend' (Lothane, 1992, p. 5), he views *Memoirs* as a 'glorious' book, 'articulated with intelligence and style,' filled with 'drama and poignancy', and written in the complementary styles of 'ordinary realism

---

of Schreber studies', Eric Santner (1996, p. xiv) later claims that Lothane himself has since become 'the de facto dean of contemporary Schreber studies'.

[24] More than Niederland's 'exaggerated descriptions', Moritz Schreber's own drawings of these devices seem by themselves capable of producing the 'horrific imagery' to which Lothane refers. Nonetheless, Lothane seems rather desperately to insist that in fact '[t]hese appliances were no more menacing than braces for the teeth' (Lothane, 1992, p 180).

and magical realism' (Lothane, 1992, pp. 2, 3). A number of distinct claims emerge in *In Defense of Schreber* to counter further the pejorative label of 'psychotic': Schreber experiences 'daymares' and not delusions; his *Memoirs* are intelligible within the contexts of mysticism and late nineteenth-century philosophy, and are therefore not properly psychotic; Schreber is so remarkable as to be an exception to the norm of psychosis; and Schreber more consistently exhibits symptoms of a depressive syndrome and transvestite fantasies rather than schizophrenia (Lothane, 1992, pp. 384, 393, 431–4).

Lothane's overarching contention is that no one has hitherto considered the '*reality*' of Schreber's long years in mental hospitals and how important this was in itself. For the *Memoirs* are about his adult life, illnesses and hospitalizations' (Lothane, 1992, p. 6, italics in the original). Eschewing psychiatric, psychoanalytic, and Schatzman's paranoidogenetic accounts of Schreber's experience, Lothane nonetheless shares with Schatzman a desire to exonerate Schreber from the 'charge' of mental illness. Accordingly he, too, endeavours to identify the culprits behind his ill-treatment. Although there are just and stringent critiques to be made of the biological psychiatry of the period, Lothane effectively casts Schreber's psychiatrists—Emil Flechsig and Guido Weber (the forensic psychiatrist who ran the Sonnenstein asylum)—as the principal scoundrels in the Schreber tale, including Sabine Schreber in a supportive role to the extent that she conspired with Flechsig and Weber to rob Schreber of his civil liberties. (Here, Lothane echoes Friedrich Kittler's (1990, p. 297) suggestion that 'Schreber's paranoia followed the lead of an insane neurologist'.) Although Schreber refers to Flechsig as his 'soul-murderer', Lothane reserves his most severe criticism for Weber, describing him as an 'adversary', 'actual persecutor', and 'oppressor' who maintained a 'double stranglehold on [Schreber], both medical and juridical' (Lothane, 1992, pp. 295, 300, 277). Weber's professional report to the court (in which he recommended against rescinding tutelage) is apparently indicative of an overt, personal hostility to Schreber; likewise, Sabine's willingness to curtail the legal right of her psychotic husband to manage their finances, and her failure to understand his transformation into a woman, is supposedly evidence of 'the intellectual and spiritual gulf between husband and wife' (Lothane, 1992, p. 452). Fuelled by more than a hint of mean-spiritedness, Lothane's efforts to redeem his 'friend' from accusations of paranoia and schizophrenia are unabashed: 'There was no small amount of truth in Schreber's statement that there was a conspiracy to unman him for he was effectively unmanned insofar as the woman had overpowered him with the assistance of the legal and psychiatric establishments' (Lothane, 1992, p. 456).

Such are the interpretations of Schreber's psychosis motivated by a reappraisal of the psychoanalytic account of unconscious homosexual conflict in paranoia in favour of historical investigation. In the absence of a grounded theory of the schizophrenic psyche, Schatzman and Lothane both imply that *Memoirs* is first and foremost a tale of genuine, biographically verifiable persecution, with the role of tormentor variously assigned to Moritz Schreber and an oppressive family structure, or Flechsig, Weber, and a juridically powerful biological psychiatry. According to these commentators, the 'truth' of Schreber's experience can only be ascertained by decoding the text of *Memoirs* with the master key of documentary evidence. In their recourse to a new set of texts—Moritz Schreber's writings, asylum records, and extra biographical material—these accounts do not challenge but broaden and perpetuate the operation of the textual sublime. There are, however, a significant number of commentators for whom *Memoirs of My Nervous Illness* is valuable not so much as a case study or an exposé of personal suffering, but as a revelation of the political, philosophical, phenomenological, spiritual, and symbolic structures of modernity. 'It can be said', and Lothane (1992, p. 9) says it, 'that the *Memoirs* became a scripture leading to a multifarious exegetical literature that is still growing'. In the writings of, among others, Elias Canetti, Eric Santner, and Louis Sass, Schreber's schizophrenic signification is invested with an unparalleled capacity to symbolize elements of the modern self.[25]

Schreber: power and politics

Many attempts have been made to read Schreber independently of psychiatric, psychoanalytic, and antipsychiatric frameworks by locating him in a genealogy of saints, seers, shamans, and the divinely mad. The Schreber-as-shaman thesis is tentatively advanced by Schatzman (1973, pp. 5, 9) and Lothane (1992, p. 393) but finds its full-blown expression in the work of Brent Dean Robbins (2000). For Robbins, the unmanned Schreber is simultaneously a mystic, poet, proto-feminist, and proto-ecologist. Robbins argues that *Memoirs* is a kind of shamanistic prophecy, a text that teaches those receptive to its message to reject the narrow constrictions of Western masculinist consciousness:

> Out of love for Schreber and with the desire to validate the logos of his pathos, it is possible to read the letter of his memoirs as closely as possible so that, in his difference, he can reveal his being otherwise to us. Having taken up this task, at least upon one reading of Schreber's text, we can discover that he, almost a century ago, had already

---

[25] Deleuze and Guattari's (1982) analysis of Schreber will be examined in detail in Chapter 4.

> given voice to a being otherwise which others, less mad, would also speak and, so doing, change the world. For this task ... we must allow Schreber's being otherwise to disrupt the totality of our self-same existence so that we might hear what he has to teach us.
>
> (Robbins, 2000, p. 138)[26]

Not so, according to philosopher Merold Westphal. Rather than illuminate a transformative pagan spirituality, the Schreber case, in Westphal's view, shows us nothing less than 'the psychology of holy war' (Westphal, 1993, p. 75). Westphal reads Schreber's delusion of being God's wife as an expedient but morally corrupt means of legitimizing his homosexual desires, and just as religion serves to justify 'immoral fantasies in the world of psychotics', so too is it used by war-mongering zealots to legitimize their equally immoral fantasies (Westphal, 1993, pp. 74–5). Continuing the exploration of the religious dynamics in Schreber's delusions, John Farrell (1996, p. 172) argues that Schreber's mind is 'a late battlefield of the Reformation, subject to Catholic proselytizing and Jesuit intrigue, mixed with Jewish conspiracies'. He goes on to suggest that Schreber's delusional structure also draws something from every 'historical resource of paranoia': religious and scientific, class-based, genealogical, macro- and micro-political (Farrell, 1996, p. 174).

From shaman to zealot to paranoid everyman, *Memoirs* has enjoyed a long career of symbolic association with a spiritual and religious discourse. More famous, and more bold, is Elias Canetti's analysis of *Memoirs* as a revelation of the psychology of fascism. In his book *Crowds and Power*, Elias Canetti finds in Schreber's delusional structure no direct connection to shamanism, but on the contrary, 'a precise model of *political* power, power which feeds on the crowd and derives its substance from it' (Canetti, 1962, p. 441, italics in the original). Like many commentators, Canetti contests the psychoanalytic emphasis on

---

[26] Robbins explains the virtues of his methodology in the following passage; however, it must be noted that the 1992 edition of Lothane's *In Defense of Schreber* does *not* contain the quotations attributed to the 1993 edition here: 'With Lothane (1993), a method which truly attempts to comprehend Schreber must be "informed by the ethics of love and love of Schreber ... on his terms, based on the oxymoron that love makes one see more clearly than scientific detachment" (p. 4). One can easily read Schreber's text with clinical distance and simply write him off as deranged and unusual. Yet read with love, Schreber can come alive again as a person who lived, suffered and triumphed, and with a certain level of empathic engagement, we can imagine what it must have been like to be him in his own time, struggling for his freedom. We will never possess Schreber and know him in any totalizing way, but the sheer volume of literature dedicated to the man over the years is a testament to the fact that his story lives on. He still touches us' (Robbins, 2000, p. 136).

Schreber's 'unmanning' and rejects the causal link between homosexuality and paranoia. Instead, he suggests that God's unrelenting attack on Schreber's reason lies at the centre of his persecutions (a point to which we shall return), and insists that the essence of paranoia 'is the *structure* of the delusional world and the way it is *peopled*' (Canetti, 1962, pp. 449–50, italics in the original). It is the religious and political dimensions of Schreber's delusional schema that are fundamentally important, inextricably linked, and most clearly demonstrative of the drive for power that characterizes paranoia. 'Paranoia', Canetti writes, 'is an *illness of power* in the most literal sense', and the delusional structure of the paranoid—as exemplified by Schreber—is identical to the psychic structure of the despot: 'A madman, helpless, outcast and despised, who drags out a twilight existence in some asylum, may, through the insights he procures us, prove more important than Hitler or Napoleon, illuminating for mankind its curse and its masters' (Canetti, 1962, pp. 448, 462, italics in the original).

Canetti introduced to the world a Schreber whose extreme psychic disturbances—his messianic and apocalyptic vision of eternity, bodily experiences of miracles and 'little men',[27] relationship to an equally despotic God, female transformation, and above all, his lust for power—expose the psychological structure of fascism. Without disputing Canetti's thesis, Schatzman (who is compelled, once again, to remind us of the true villain in the Schreber equation) suggests that it is Moritz Schreber whose ideas directly anticipated Hitler's and whose child-rearing practices influenced a generation of Nazis (Schatzman, 1973, pp. 148–54). Lothane, unsurprisingly, vehemently rejects any such suggestion: the 'trend' started by Canetti 'is not just false and preposterous: it is an abuse of a psychiatric diagnosis and an offense to Paul Schreber's memory. It trivializes the complexity of Nazism as a sociohistorical phenomenon by reducing it to a psychiatric formula' (Lothane, 1992, p. 353). Biological psychiatry is, according to Lothane, the only historically accurate link between the Schreber case and Nazism.[28] What links Canetti, Schatzman, and Lothane, despite their

---

[27] Schreber, as I have already noted, discusses at length the various torments visited upon him by 'little men': 'The remarkable thing about it was that souls [of people both living and dead] or their single nerves could in certain conditions and for particular purposes assume the form of tiny human shapes (as mentioned earlier only of a few millimetres in size), and as such made mischief on all parts of my body, both inside and on the surface' (Schreber, 1955, p. 144).

[28] 'Did the dehumanization of psychiatric patients lead logically to the idea of concentration camps and death camps? At the end of the war Sonnenstein was closed down as a psychiatric facility. The last director was under investigation as a war criminal and committed suicide' (Lothane, 1992, p. 301). For a more extensive discussion of the role of Nazi psychiatric institutions in developing the methods of mass murder later used in concentration camps see Torrey and Yolken (2009).

deep divergences, is that they all reinterpret Schreber's psychosis as a problem of power, a problem of far-reaching social, not psychosexual, significance.

Eric Santner joined this increasingly discordant chorus in 1997 with the publication of *My Own Private Germany: Daniel Paul Schreber's Secret History of Modernity*. Santner extends Canetti's analysis beyond the psychological arena: 'I am', he writes, 'convinced that Schreber's breakdown and efforts at self-healing introduced him into the deepest structural layers of the historical impasses and conflicts that would provisionally culminate in the Nazi catastrophe' (Santner, 1996, p. xi). Side-stepping the divisions and politics of victimization in the antipsychiatric camp, Santner argues compellingly that Schreber is subjected to both medico-pedagogic *and* psychiatric regimes of power-knowledge, but argues that *Memoirs* also points to a widespread crisis of symbolic authority in *fin-de-siècle* Germany.

Schreber's appointment as *Senatspräsident* of the court of appeal led, according to Santner, directly to his psychotic break. The 'performative magic' of symbolic investiture failed—it brought Schreber in excessive proximity to the law, and, more importantly, its surplus of power, thus precipitating a psychic crisis:

> Schreber's crisis was a crisis of investiture. He discovered that his own symbolic power and authority as judge—and German man—was founded, at least in part, by the performative magic of the rites of institution, that his symbolic function was sustained by an imperative to produce a regulated series of repeat performances. It was this idiotic repetition compulsion at the heart of his symbolic function that Schreber experienced as profoundly sexualizing, as a demand to cultivate jouissance.

(Santner, 1996, pp. 124–5)

My Own Private Germany is among the most sophisticated analyses of the content of Schreber's delusions largely because the theoretical model it proposes encompasses elements of many previously irreconcilable interpretations of *Memoirs*. Santner links Moritz Schreber's medico-pedagogy with Flechsig's biological psychiatry as two examples of the law operating in excess of its own authority. Schreber's accounts of experiencing soul murder and cultivating voluptuousness are then re-read as attempts to articulate the intensely libidinalizing effects of his overexposure to the disciplinary power of the *'fathers who knew too much'* (Santner, 1996, pp. 86-7, italics in the original).[29] As his delusional obsession with decomposition and degeneration reveals,[30] Schreber discovered rottenness at the core of symbolic identity sanctioned by the law,

---

[29] On the relationship between Moritz Schreber's medico-pedagogy and the Foucauldian concept of disciplinary power, see also Sass (1987b, pp. 101–47).

[30] On this, see also de Certeau (1988, pp. 90–1).

and his delusions are an effort at negotiating this realization (Santner, 1996, pp. xi–xii, 6, 61, 124). Drawing on Sander Gilman's (1996, p. 142) assertion that Schreber's deepest fear was that 'he was turning into an effeminate Jew', Santner continues the passage quoted earlier:

> That [Schreber] experienced this sexualization as feminizing and 'Jewifying' suggests that at the advent of European modernity, 'knowledge' of jouissance was ascribed to women and Jews, meaning that women and Jews were *cursed* with the task of holding the place of that which could not be directly acknowledged: that symbolic identities are, in the final analysis, sustained by *drive*, by performativity-as-repetition-compulsion.
>
> (Santner, 1996, pp. 124–5, italics in the original)

Schreber does not simply reflect a misogynist anti-Semitism culturally prevalent during the period. Rather, his inability to meet the performative demands of authority produced a kind of unconscious identification with '*the symptom that* . . . for German culture more generally . . . materialized the blockage in the smooth functioning of the social body' (Santner, 1996, p. 144, italics in the original).

As Gilman points out, Santner's Schreber is neither a 'prefiguration of the fascist' nor the 'perpetual victim' of power, but a 'canary in the mine shaft whose responses identify the actual victims in the culture in which he lives, women and Jews' (Gilman, 1996, p. 16). In a claim that is at once audacious and problematic, Santner ultimately suggests that *Memoirs* offers real insight into the experiences of the dispossessed:

> To traverse, with Schreber, the fantasy space of *his* own private Germany . . . is to encounter European modernity from the perspective of those figures in whom modern European society 'secreted' its disavowed knowledge of chronic structural crisis and disequilibrium.
>
> Of course, Schreber's fate as a psychotic suggests that one should not, as they say, try this at home; it is, in other words, genuinely maddening to find oneself occupying the place of abjection in the absence of some minimal form of human solidarity.
>
> (Santner, 1996, p. 144, italics in the original)

Santner succeeds in rewriting Schreber's *Memoirs* as a narrative which reveals a crisis besetting the entire social system at the turn of the twentieth century. However, although he persuasively uncovers in *Memoirs* an elite German masculinity-in-crisis (instead of a proto-fascist will to power), the claim that this somehow speaks directly of the experience of women and Jews at the *fin de siècle* seems to me to venture, perhaps unwittingly, into dangerous territory. Through it, Santner seems to present the entire history of modernity—both covert and overt—as a story in which Aryan men are the only protagonists capable of self-representation, and suggests that the dispossessed are, by virtue of their alleged affinity with Schreber, associated with psychosis. This in turn renders his account of psychosis fundamentally problematic, to say the least. Repeatedly citing the crisis of symbolic investiture as the pathogenic factor in Schreber's psychosis, Santner emphasizes the aetiological significance of failed performative, public-sphere identity, but remains unwilling to consider the broader implications of his diagnosis. Certain questions immediately spring to mind: Does psychosis only threaten those whose symbolic investiture brings them too close to the excess or corruption of power? Do subjects who are subordinated within the symbolic order therefore enjoy a relative freedom from psychosis, as if in compensation for a reduced access to power? Or are they already mad, if to be psychotic is in some sense to be the object, not subject, of power? *My Own Private Germany* seems frequently to overstep the parameters implied by its title: by approaching the autobiography of a psychotic male Jurist as nothing less than the palimpsest or unconscious archive of modernity (Santner, 1996, p. 145), Santner ends up implying that Schreber's psychotic break is the prerogative of a white male elite, but that his psychotic experiences resonate with the everyday experiences of women and Jews.

Multifaceted, widely researched, and masterful in its assimilation of previously antagonistic viewpoints, *My Own Private Germany* is nonetheless a high watermark in the post-Freudian quest to decode the symbolic content—and protest—of Schreber's psychosis. I would like to turn now to the work of another equally prominent analyst of *Memoirs of My Nervous Illness*, Louis Sass. Sass explicitly rejects the Freudian approach to psychosis and breaks with the psychoanalytically-inspired tradition of focusing on the symbolic dimensions of Schreber's experience. Instead, he concentrates on the phenomenology of symptomatology and its relationship to modern philosophy, reading Schreber via Wittgenstein as an exemplary 'madman' (Sass, 1994b, p. ix) and in turn an 'exemplary' 'man of modern civilization' (Sass, 1992, p. 246). Although Schreber's delirium revealed to Santner the subtext of *fin-de-siècle* German culture, for Sass every delusional, somatic, and affective experience speaks directly of the structures of modern consciousness. Altogether disregarding the vexed issue of the aetiology of Schreber's schizophrenia, Sass offers us two further incarnations of the world's most quoted psychotic patient—the panoptic and solipsistic Schreber—both 'characterized by an intense and ultimately reifying self-scrutiny, an inner division, and an alienation from self, world, and instinct' (Sass, 1987b, p. 124).[31]

---

[31] In other words, 'Madness, on [Sass's] reading, is neither the psyche's return to its primordial condition, nor the malfunctioning of reason, nor even some inspired alternative to human reason. It is, to be sure, a self-deceiving condition, but one that is generated from within rationality itself rather than by the loss of rationality' (Sass, 1994b, p.12).

Although Sass is highly critical of Foucault's antipsychiatric sentiment in *Madness and Civilization* (Sass, 1987b, p. 106; 1994b, p. 3), he uses Foucault's now famous analysis of Jeremy Bentham's panopticon in *Discipline and Punish* (1977) as the basis for his first reading of *Memoirs*. For Foucault, the panopticon signals a transformation in the operation of power in modernity: instead of the spectacle of public, corporeal punishment, the prisoner in the panopticon is subject to constant surveillance, an effective disciplinary technique because the possibility of always being watched inculcates in the prisoner an ever-vigilant *self*-scrutiny. As Sass notes, Moritz Schreber's educational regime is in essence panoptic, designed to instil obedience in the child through self-monitoring, or the internalization of the gaze of the all-powerful, all-seeing parent (Sass, 1987b, pp. 112–17). Modernity in general and Moritz Schreber's 'depth pedagogy' in particular find their extreme expression in Schreber's schizophrenia, in a split and self-alienated consciousness 'both rent and joined by an inner panopticism' (Sass, 1992, p. 253). Thus, for Sass, Schreber's cosmology—comprising rays, nerves, and a divided God—'demands to be read as a psychological rather than a cosmological vision, as a kind of allegory of the divided state of Schreber's own hyper-aware, acutely reflexive mind' (Sass, 1992, p. 258).[32]

Continuing to address the form, structure, and phenomenology of Schreber's schizophrenic experience—rather than the symbolic content of his delusions and somatic fantasies—Sass moves beyond panopticism in his later work to argue that we can best understand *Memoirs* through the philosophical doctrine of solipsism. Schreber's heightened state of awareness, 'in which he scrutinized the world, and scrutinized his awareness of the world', and the 'affectless, devitalized, or otherwise derealized atmosphere' of his lived world are, according to Sass, in 'perfect accordance with Wittgenstein's analysis of solipsism' (Sass, 1994b, pp. 37, 43, 40). Central to both Schreber's inner panopticism and his schizophrenic solipsism is the idea of an internally and irreparably divided psyche: he simultaneously experiences 'his own consciousness as both a

---

[32] The reifying effects of this schizophrenic inner panopticism are elsewhere noted by Mark Roberts, for whom Schreber's 'psychomechanics' demand to be read as protocyborgian: '"Plugged into" madness, rendered into a machine, strapped into restraints, probed by devices, subjected to the psycho- and electromechanical theories of the time, Schreber was naturally both intensely aware of the fact that he had become a machine and horrified that he was one' (Roberts, 1996, pp. 31–47). John Peters discusses Wolfgang Hagan's more historically grounded view that 'Schreber's fantasies owe much to wireless technology and the now outdated ether-physics, with its dreams of combined thought- and signal-transference' (Peters, 2010, p. 132).

constituted object and the ultimate, constituting subject' (Sass, 1994b, p. 77).[33] The doubling of the 'I' demonstrates for Sass that 'What Schreber lacks is not the observing ego emphasized by ego psychologists but, instead, a fundamental rootedness in the lived-body and the consensual and practical world' (Sass, 1994b, p. 79). Schreber, then, exists at the extremities of Cartesian dualism, and Sass is quick to explore the gendered expression of Schreber's split subjectivity in his concluding analysis of Schreber's 'unmanning'. On this reading, Schreber's delusional schema reproduces the binary opposition of masculine subject and feminine object: transformation into a woman involves, for Schreber, becoming the object and not the subject of awareness. Although as 'soul murder' 'unmanning' is potentially annihilating, it functions as a panacea for Schreber's tormented mind:

> Femininity stands, then, for the sensual as against the intellectual, 'Blessedness' as against the insidious anxieties of 'compulsive thinking', the body as against the self-torturing mind. Tactile voluptuousness is capable of dissolving, at least for a moment, the alienated, scrutinizing consciousness of Schreber's quasi-solipsism . . .

(Sass, 1994b, p. 127)

Reserving his final comments for a wholesale refutation of Freud's reading of *Memoirs*, and schizophrenia more generally, Sass insists that 'A purely libidinal interpretation misses the crucial sense in which schizophrenic fantasies concern not sex but knowledge, expressing a yearning no less intense, and no less pervasive, for being epistemological at its core' (Sass, 1994b, p. 129).

These interpretations of *Memoirs of My Nervous Illness* are, as I have shown, remarkable for their methodological and substantive differences. So, should we view Schreber through a psychoanalytic, psychobiographical, historical, philosophical, or phenomenological lens, or simply with love and compassion? And what does lie at the core of his delusional schema? Is it the homosexual libido, a masturbatory fantasy, or a pre-Oedipal procreation fantasy? Is it the disciplinary power of Moritz Schreber's medico-pedagogy, or Flechsig's biological psychiatry? Is it proto-fascistic despotism, religious paranoia, a failure to take up a powerful position in the symbolic order, or an epistemological crisis? It is relatively easy to be persuaded by these analyses when approaching them individually; viewed collectively, they are impossible to reconcile. Of course, to the literary critic, this is hardly surprising—the text itself cannot contain a final or singular truth because its meaning will always be produced through the process of reading, and so even the most mundane manuscripts

---

[33] There are clear parallels with this reading and Crapanzano's (1998) analysis of Schreber's interlocutionary collapse.

are permanently open to reinterpretation. What *is* surprising is that the canon of Schreber studies should have developed in so literary a fashion.

Although Freud's 'Psycho-Analytic Notes' had—post-Niederland—been forced to relinquish its claim on the truth of Schreber's experience, the psychoanalytic emphasis on deciphering the symbolic significance of *representations* of schizophrenic delusions has made possible a 90-year debate over the meaning of one Jurist's psychosis.[34] It is inconceivable that such a debate could have been ignited and fostered in psychiatric discourse, where the death of the author means that only the retrospective diagnosis of symptoms could be a source of contention. Psychiatry cannot furnish its clinical picture of schizophrenia with decisive evidence of the origins of the disorder which, I have argued, elevates schizophrenia to the status of sublime object. Similarly, commentators within Schreber studies can neither prove the merits of their analysis nor demonstrate the wholesale inadequacy of others, if only because no appeal to the 'truth' of the text itself, let alone Schreber's experience, is possible in this literary mode of interpretation. As it stands in for Schreber's experience, *Memoirs of My Nervous Illness* can therefore be seen as a sublime text within psychoanalytic discourse and for the cultural critics reappraising 'Psycho-Analytic Notes'. Like all literary texts, it supports a proliferation of interpretations, jostling for validity in the absence of an author-patient to authorize or validate any of the narratives offered. What sets it apart from literary texts is its function within the field of psychoanalysis: *Memoirs* is sublime because 'the disciplinary attention' it has garnered works 'to mark the provisional limits and flash points' (Cheetham, 1995, p. 360) of psychoanalysis and related disciplines.

However, *Memoirs* is, as I hope to demonstrate, sublime for another reason, namely that it records Schreber's terrifying experience of the beyond-human, and his constant struggle to assert his rationality against the cosmological forces that would overwhelm him. In the next section of this chapter, through a close reading of *Memoirs*, I will argue that Schreber's autobiographical project and his delusional structure can both be read through the logic of the Kantian sublime, that is, as attempts to reassert rationality in the face of the terror and anxiety aroused by the sublime encounter.[35] Although I am aware that any contribution to Schreber studies cannot escape perpetuating the interpretative trend just described, my purpose is not to provide the definitive interpretation

---

[34] In one of the latest contributions to this debate, McGlashan (2009, p. 480) makes the point that because 'pharmacotherapy that has truncated extended periods of active positive psychotic symptoms', Schreber's ongoing importance to understanding acute psychosis is assured.

[35] I should make absolutely clear at this point that I am *not* making any claims about schizophrenic experience more generally.

of *Memoirs* but to demonstrate that Schreber, like the theorists so far discussed, has recourse to the sublime to describe his schizophrenic experience. Not only do psychiatrists, psychoanalysts, and antipsychiatrists frame schizophrenia as sublime, the world's most famous and most quoted psychiatric patient shares their tendency. Concentrating on the structure of Schreber's delusional system and the way that system is described and contextualized, my analysis does not address the question of schizophrenia's aetiology and onset, nor does it consider extra-textual biographical material, the theme of sexual identity, or Schreber's capacity to symbolize this or that aspect of modern consciousness. The significance of this contribution to Schreber studies lies not only in the attention paid to an aspect of *Memoirs* all too frequently overlooked—the crisis of rationality that I suggest occupies centre stage in the text—but also in the connections drawn between the obsession with reason, the dynamics of the sublime and the discourse of Schreber studies. Like those of many critics before me, my reading of Schreber takes as its starting point Freud's 'Psycho-Analytic Notes', specifically, Freud's failure to account for Schreber's crisis of rationality.

A sublime Schreber

Freud, as I have shown, accords psychosexual disturbance a primary role in the symptomatology and aetiology of Schreber's psychosis. He refers only twice and in passing to Schreber's constant struggle to prove his sanity to God. First cited as evidence of Schreber's ambivalent and rebellious attitude towards God-as-the-father, it is later produced as confirmation of Schreber's infantile sexual urge:

> Finally, we come to enforced thinking to which the patient submitted himself because he supposed that God would believe he had become an idiot and would withdraw from him if he ceased thinking for a moment. This is a reaction . . . to the threat of fear of losing one's reason as a result of indulging in sexual practices and especially in masturbation. Considering the enormous number of delusional ideas of a hypochondriacal nature which the patient developed, no great importance should perhaps be attached to the fact that some of them coincide word for word with the hypochondriacal fears of masturbators.

(Freud, 1981, pp. 56–7)

Schreber's compulsive thinking—which continued without respite—is in one swift move explained and dismissed as mere masturbatory fantasy.[36] 'No other part of his delusions is treated by the patient so exhaustively, one might

---

[36] Maurits Katan would later publish a series of papers (see especially 1949, 1950a) arguing that a homosexual masturbatory fantasy was not only present during all phases of Schreber's illness, but actually precipitated it.

almost say so insistently, as his alleged transformation into a woman' (Freud, 1981, p. 32)—Freud's exclusive focus on what Schreber calls 'unmanning' is possible only because he overlooks the frequency and significance of Schreber's apparently onanistic delusions that God is continually searching for confirmation Schreber has succumbed to dementia. This is a point already noted by Canetti, Sass, and Crapanzano.[37] However, as I will argue, this delusion is in fact central to Schreber's behaviour and symptomatology, his feelings towards God, indeed his entire project in *Memoirs*; it can, moreover, be more usefully interpreted not as masturbatory hypochondria but as integral to Schreber's representation of his experience as sublime.

Schreber does not hesitate to describe his psychosis as a revelation of the sublime. Alongside distinctly 'gruesome' visions of the end of the world, Schreber writes of having been filled with 'the most sublime ideas about God and the Order of the World', ideas that in his own estimation surpass any historical conceptions of the holy (Schreber, 1955, pp. 79, 86, 54). As his introductory remarks indicate, his is an experience that exceeds the limits of comprehension:

> I cannot of course count upon being *fully* understood because things are dealt with which cannot be expressed in human language; they exceed human understanding. Nor can I maintain that *everything* is irrefutably certain even for me: much remains only presumption and probability. After all I too am only a human being and therefore limited by the confines of human understanding; but one thing I am certain of, namely that I have come infinitely closer to the truth than human beings who have not received divine revelation.

(Schreber, 1955, p. 41, see also 117, italics in the original)

Although his delusions defy even Schreber's complete understanding, he nevertheless offers a number of reasons as to why he is compelled to record them. According to Lothane, the English title *Memoirs of My Nervous Illness* is an inaccurate translation that fails to do justice to the underlying rationale of Schreber's project. His translation of the full title—*Great Thoughts of a Nervous Patient with Postscripts and an Addendum Concerning the Question: 'Under what Premises Can a Person Considered Insane be Detained in an Asylum Against His Own Declared Will?'* (Lothane, 1992, p. 7, italics in the original)—highlights more dramatically both Schreber's grandiosity and his direct engagement with

---

[37] Canetti, for example, suggests that the real aim of Schreber's imagined conspirators 'was the destruction of Schreber's reason, and this they persisted in for years. They wanted to turn him into an imbecile, to push the illness of his nerves to the point where he would appear permanently incurable. Could there be any prospect more terrible for a human being as highly gifted as he thought himself?' (Canetti, 1962, p. 439, see also Sass, 1992, p. 248; Crapanzano, 1998).

the legal and moral questions surrounding his tutelage. A further practical function of *Memoirs* is that it facilitates his return to the 'civilized' world by informing family and friends of his religious beliefs and their impact on his behaviour (Schreber, 1955, p. 41). However, these considerations appear secondary to his desire to have the truth of his experience recognized, analysed, and legitimized by the scientific establishment. In his 'Open letter to Professor Flechsig', Schreber states that his aim is 'solely to further knowledge of truth in a vital field, that of religion', but later he indicates that with Flechsig's confirmation, the religious dimensions of his experience would 'gain universal credence and would immediately be regarded as a *serious scientific problem to be investigated in every possible way*' (Schreber, 1955, pp. 33, 35, italics in the original). Schreber's contradictory imperative is to elicit scientific confirmation of his supernatural experience. Cognizant of how potentially difficult this might be, he concludes *Memoirs* in the hope that empirical study will uncover physical evidence of his sublime transformation:

> I can do no more than *offer my person as object of scientific observation for the judgment of experts. My main motive in publishing this book* is to invite this. Short of this I can only hope that at some future time such peculiarities of my nervous system will be discovered by *dissection of my body*, which will provide stringent proof.

> (Schreber, 1955, p. 251, italics in the original)

Schreber repeatedly calls attention to how his experience exceeds language, but does not abandon the search for a discourse that might provide a vocabulary and an epistemological framework through which to establish the truth of his delusions. Biological psychiatry is among the first disciplines to be found wanting. Noting that some of Kraepelin's technical observations regarding symptom formation are valuable for his own ideas, Schreber nonetheless rails against the attendant discussion of patients' deteriorating rational faculties (Schreber, 1955, pp. 89–90).[38] The question of approaching 'delusional' experience with the 'right kind of reason' is brought to the fore:

> He who in Kraepelin's sense (p. 146) understands 'sound experience' simply as the denial of everything supernatural, would in my opinion lay himself open to the reproach of allowing himself to be led only by the shallow 'rationalistic ideas' of the

[38] Schreber, quoting Kraepelin, then writes almost testily that 'the total content of the present work will hardly show anything *in my case* which justifies speaking of "the inability of the patient to use earlier experiences to correct thoroughly and accurately his new ideas" (p. 146), or of "faulty judgement", which Kraepelin (p. 145) says "invariably accompanies delusions". I trust I have proved that I am not only not "controlled by fixed and previously formed ideas", but that I also possess in full measure the "capacity to evaluate critically the content of consciousness with the help of judgement and deduction"' (p. 146).

period of enlightenment of the 18th century, which after all are mostly considered to have been superseded, particularly by theologians and philosophers, and also in science.

(Schreber, 1955, p. 90, italics in the original)

Just as an outmoded biological psychiatry fails to account for the supernatural, theology is likewise ill-equipped to explain in broadly accepted terms what Schreber insists is scientific evidence of his 'unmanning'. Again, to assert the reality of his transformation into the world's redeemer, he appeals to the condition of his body, 'which on examination shows recognizable feminine characteristics convincing to everybody' and is open to observation by 'any serious specialist whose motive is scientific interest and not mere curiosity' (Schreber, 1955, pp. 203, 207). On matters more holy, like the creation of the world, Schreber is understandably less confident of scientific vindication and falls back on a defensive optimism.[39] He may lack the means to prove his beliefs scientifically (Schreber, 1955, p. 184) and to assert them as religious truth, but, as befits a once-distinguished jurist, Schreber has no difficulty conducting his struggle to be believed at the level of rhetoric. Weber's report from 1899 makes clear that in spite of his rigid delusional system, Schreber's mental faculties were intact and his intelligence uncompromised (Weber, 1955, p. 271). Indeed, as Octave Mannoni observes, 'Schreber devotes all his mad efforts to proving that he himself is alive and in full possession of his intellectual faculties. The project of writing a book is precisely one of these efforts, and the book itself will constitute proof against God and Flechsig' (Mannoni, 1988, p. 57).

Memoirs includes direct appeals to Flechsig, physicians, and others whose professional expertise would lend support to Schreber's ideas and his release, as well as innumerable appeals to the implied reasonableness of his general readers. This is an example of one such petition, again related to the truth value of the physical:

This [that I 'once had a different heart'] as indeed the whole report about the miracles enacted on my body, will naturally sound extremely strange to all other human beings, and one may be inclined to see in it only the product of a pathologically vivid imagination.

[39] 'I cannot be expected to furnish scientific proof of this fundamental idea; I do not intend writing a scientific treatise on the history of the evolution of the universe. I only wish to relate what I have experienced and learned, and draw a few legitimate conclusions in the light of this knowledge. I expect confirmation of my fundamental idea mainly from my own personal fate and fortune as they will develop in the future; the time will come when other human beings will also have to recognize as a fact that my person has become the centre of divine miracles. I would then have to leave to other people to elaborate scientifically the conclusions I have hinted at and perhaps to correct some details' (Schreber, 1955, p. 94).

> In reply I can only give the assurance that hardly any memory from my life is more certain than the miracles recounted in this chapter. What can be more definite for a human being than what he has lived through and felt on his own body?

(Schreber, 1955, p. 132)

That clarity of judgement also persisted *within* Schreber's delusional system is evidenced by his decision to accept his unmanning both as divine duty *and* strategic choice:

> Since [that realization] I have wholeheartedly inscribed the cultivation of femininity on my banner, and I will continue to do so so far as consideration of my environment allows, whatever other people who are ignorant of the supernatural reasons may think of me. I would like to meet the man who, faced with the choice of either becoming a demented human being in male habitus or a spirited woman, would not prefer the latter. Such and *only such* is the issue for me. The pursuit of my previous profession, which I loved wholeheartedly, every other aim of manly ambition, and every other use of my intellectual powers in the service of mankind, are now all closed to me through the way circumstances have developed.

(Schreber, 1955, p. 149, italics in the original)

Even if, following Freud, Schreber's entire cosmological system is an elaborate unconscious strategy through which the ego can accept his homosexual libido, it is still significant that Schreber describes it as a choice between transsexuality and dementia, a choice that entails the abandonment of previously cherished intellectual pursuits. It is not simply that Schreber is articulate or intelligent *in* his madness; it is that he makes every effort to present a reasonable and rational account *of* his utterly fantastic experiences.

Having established the centrality of reason to Schreber's autobiographical project—the reasons offered for producing the text, as well as appeals made throughout it to the reasonableness of its author and readers—we can now turn to the crisis of rationality that occupies prime position *within* his delusional schema. The central cosmological conundrum is this: human beings with nerves as highly excited as Schreber's exert an irresistible power of attraction for God, but in succumbing to this attraction, God endangers his own existence. God can extricate himself from this 'nerve-contact' only, it appears, by receiving confirmation that Schreber is demented. God is persistent in his efforts to prove Schreber a dement and this constant testing is experienced as persecution. Schreber therefore insists that 'All the attacks made over the years, on my life, my bodily integrity, my manliness and my reason, were and still are based on the same idea: to withdraw again as far as possible from the power of attraction of my over-excited nerves, which far surpasses anything that has ever existed before' (Schreber, 1955, p. 119). Again and again (Schreber, 1955, pp. 78, 79, 114, 119, 131), this litany of attempted persecution is repeated, each time crowned by the attack on reason. Schreber divides his stay at Sonnenstein into two periods distinguished by the severity of these attacks. At first, believing the world had ended and was populated only by 'fleeting-improvised-men', he reports horrific bodily and mental tortures. The list of behaviours or symptoms Schreber describes as direct attempts to demonstrate his rational faculties to God is impressive. It includes compulsive thinking, the 'writing down-system' (compulsive writing), constant speaking aloud and noise-making, banging on the piano or reading during meals, insomnia, bellowing, reciting historical and geographical facts in French, and even the retention of faeces (Schreber, 1955, pp. 68, 69, 123, 160, 162). Schreber does not, as Freud would seem to imply, spend most of his time cultivating soul-voluptuousness; he is engaged in constant intra-psychic battle. After this first and overwhelming year, Schreber gradually came to suspect that the world had not in fact been destroyed and that God would not succeed in his persecutory project. His delusional system then stabilized and although 'miracles' like the ones mentioned earlier continued unabated, they became less severe.

Schreber's representation of a panoply of persecutory divine beings further reinforces the connection between the crisis of rationality and the sublime. In his delusional system, Schreber constructs a vast, potentially infinite cosmic reality, in which God figures as a distant being capable of penetrating Schreber's mind. Regardless of whether God is a sublimated symbol of the father or, following Sass, a symbol of panoptic consciousness, the way in which Schreber explains their relationship in spatial terms contributes to his already stated conviction that God is sublime. After creating the world, God 'retired to an enormous distance', a position from which, in accordance with 'the Order of the World', he dealt only with corpses (Schreber, 1955, pp. 191, 75). Schreber's highly excited nerves attract and threaten to entangle God but whereas proximity to an exceptional human carries the risk of divine annihilation, proximity to a dement poses no such danger. As he cannot discontinue 'nerve-contact' with God, Schreber must constantly suffer the above-mentioned tests of his reason, which he perceives as an invasion of his mental autonomy: 'I also ought to have the right of being master in my own head against the intrusion of strangers' (Schreber, 1955, p. 175). What mediates the relationship between God and Schreber—preserving their close contact but ensuring that God's plan cannot be successful—is the Order of the World, which 'reveals its very grandeur and magnificence by denying even God Himself in so irregular a case as mine the means of achieving a purpose contrary to the Order of the World' (Schreber, 1955, p. 78). (In a footnote, Schreber explains that the Order of the

World is the inherently constructive relationship of God to human beings; God's attempted *destruction* of a man's reason is therefore an internal contradiction and bound to fail (Schreber, 1955, p. 79).[40])

The following passage—significant for its uncharacteristically confused prose—details Schreber's frustration with God's failure to recognize his own limitations, and gives an indication of just how incessantly intrusive God's nerves ('rays') are:

> It seems to be impossible for God to draw a lesson for the future from such an experience, perhaps because of some qualities innate in His nature. For these phenomena are repeated in exactly the same way year in year out, day after day, particularly in the attempt to withdraw at first sight (in the twinkle of an eye) which every pause in my thinking activity (when the not-thinking-of-anything-thought starts), and the assumption that I have then succumbed to dementia; this is usually expressed in the fatuous phrase 'Now he should (*scilicet* think or say) I will resign myself to the fact that I am stupid', followed in senseless monotony like a barrel-organ by all the other tasteless forms of speech 'Why do you not say it (aloud)?' or 'But then for how much longer' (*scilicet* will your defence against the power of the rays still be successful) etc., etc., : this goes on until I proceed to take up some new occupation which proves my undiminished mental powers. It is an extremely difficult question even for me to explain the inability on the part of God to learn by experience.

> (Schreber, 1955, p. 154)

Paradoxically, this perpetual internal dialogue is a form of mental stimulation that encourages Schreber's methodological, reasoned discourse: the upshot of answering such irritating questions all the time is that 'I am unavoidably forced to give myself an account of the reason and purpose of every single job' (Schreber, 1955, p. 179). God in his stubbornness may never cease to be suspicious that he is dealing with a person bereft of intelligence (Schreber, 1955, p. 247), but, speculating on his future towards the end of *Memoirs*, Schreber writes:

> All I can say with absolute certainty is something *negative, namely* that God will never succeed in his purpose of destroying my reason. I have been absolutely clear on this point for years . . . with it the main danger which seemed to threaten me during the early years of my illness is removed. Can there be any prospect more terrible for a human being so highly gifted in such various ways, as I may say of myself without conceit, than the prospect of losing one's reason and perishing an imbecile? Hence anything which might befall me seemed more or less trivial, once I had gained the absolute conviction through years of experience that all attempts in this direction were

---

40 Crapanzano offers a detailed discursive analysis of the Order of the World as 'the Third', or 'laws and their embodiments that govern communicative and other interpersonal encounters' between the self and other, or Schreber and his God (Crapanzano, 1998, p. 749).

predestined to fail, as within the Order of the World not even God has the power to destroy a person's reason.

(Schreber, 1955, pp. 211–12, italics in the original)

Secure in the knowledge that his relationship with an aggressive God is safeguarded and mediated by the Order of the World, Schreber can then go on to express his hopes that his complete transformation into a woman will eventuate, and his role as the world's redeemer will be fully realized.

Schreber's perpetual (re)assertion of his rationality is a core feature of his delusional system as well as of the text in which it finds expression, and in both positions it serves to construe his psychosis as an experience at the threshold of the sublime. For the subject of the Kantian sublime, feelings of emotional powerlessness in the presence of the boundless facilitate a delightful affirmation of the rational faculty; this is a linear process culminating in conceptual mastery, an undoing and reassertion of the rational self. Schreber, by contrast, seems condemned to exist in a kind of time loop at its threshold, forever striving to assert his rational faculty—to God, his physicians and readers—but disbarred from the pleasures of mental security. *Memoirs* is a struggle to establish and defend sufficient distance from Schreber's inner cosmology; his obsession with defending, reasserting, and proving reason constitutes, I would argue, the most significant recurring theme within the text. Secure in the knowledge that the Order of the World deems one man's reason too important to be destroyed by God, *Memoirs of My Nervous Illness* concludes with Schreber's megalomaniac expectation that,

... a very special palm of victory will eventually be mine. As possibilities I would mention that my unmanning will be accomplished with the result that by divine fertilization offspring will issue from my lap, or alternatively that great fame will be attached to my name surpassing that of thousands of other people much better mentally endowed.

(Schreber, 1955, p. 214)

Schreber died childless, physically ill, and acutely psychotic, but it may have pleased him to know that he would become the world's most famous sufferer of paranoid schizophrenia, heralded as brilliant by virtually every one of his numerous commentators.

Lacan: the sublime structure of psychosis

More than any clinical case study or asylum-based research, *Memoirs of My Nervous Illness* is pivotal to the psychoanalytic construction of schizophrenia as a sublime text. As we have seen, the sublime is doubly present within Schreber's text: it is an experience to which Schreber is perpetually condemned and it also provides the structure through which his delusional system is articulated. Deploying psychotic signification as an unproblematic metonym for the complexities of schizophrenic experience, analysts of *Memoirs* in turn construe schizophrenia itself as a sublime text, ripe for interpretation but fundamentally inaccessible to analytic or transferential influence. Jacques Lacan is no exception. That Schreber should feature so prominently in his third seminar, *The Psychoses*, appears unsurprising, especially when he observes that 'Of all the literary productions of the type that plead a cause, of all the communications of those who, having gone beyond the limits, have spoken of the psychotic's alien experience, Schreber's work is certainly one of the most remarkable' (Lacan, 1993, p. 10). However, unlike Freud, Lacan had by the mid-1950s a long professional history of working with paranoid–schizophrenic patients and his engagement and fascination with psychosis was far from limited to the study of autobiography (Roudinesco, 1997, p. 80). Indeed, Lacan's first and only case study, *Le Cas Aimée*, was published in his 1932 doctoral thesis, *On Paranoiac Psychosis in Its Relation to Personality*. It appears significant, then, that although Lacan had ready access to a wealth of case material, including his own, he should construct his theory on the texts of Schreber, Freud, and Ida Macalpine, as Marcelle Marini (1992, p. 159) observes. Once again, *Memoirs* displaces clinical experience as the source and test of psychoanalytic accounts of schizophrenia: it is 'a document whose guarantees of credibility are unrivalled' and, as Lacan endeavours to demonstrate in 'On a question preliminary to any possible treatment of psychosis', its structure 'will prove to be similar to the process of psychosis itself' (Lacan, 1966, p. 201). Before discussing Lacan's reading of *Memoirs* in more depth and its elaboration of a new relationship between schizophrenia and sublimity, I want to look first at the context in which Lacan situates his contribution to the psychoanalytic study of psychosis, that is, his critique of Freud.

Despite casting himself as Freud's true disciple, Lacan is unequivocal in his rejection of Freud's account of paraphrenia. Questioning both the selective interpretation of Schreber's delusional system and the broader theoretical model Freud derived from his analysis of the case, he writes:

> Does the entire delusion consist of the dialogue of this unique Schreber, who, with his enigmatic partner, the Schreberian God, is the new starting point for the regeneration of humanity through the birth of a new Schreberian generation? No, it doesn't. Not only is this not the whole delusion, but it's quite impossible to understand it entirely at this level.
>
> [In 'Psycho-Analytic Notes'] the entire dynamics of the Schreber case are explained to us on the basis of the ego's efforts to escape from a so-called homosexual drive

threatening its completeness . . . The narrowing of perspective, the clinical inadequa-
cies of this construction, are self-evident.

(Lacan, 1993, pp. 106, 105, see also 307–12)

Lacan distinguishes his approach to the question of psychosis from Freud's
in a number of important ways. First, in the introductory seminar Lacan makes
clear that the thorny issue of nosology is beyond his concern. Rather than pre
varicate over the differences between schizophrenia, paraphrenia, and paranoia, he states simply that the psychoses 'correspond to what has always been
called and legitimately continues to be called *madness*' (Lacan, 1993, p. 4)
(although here, as in so many other psychoanalytic accounts of psychosis, the
paranoid–schizophrenic narrative functions as the privileged object of investigation). Lacan's apparent indifference to psychiatric taxonomy contrasts
sharply, however, with his insistence on a fundamental difference between
neurosis and psychosis, and on the need for a radically revised approach to the
latter. Thus Lacan praises Freud for his interpretive skill—'it's the genius of
the linguist who sees the same sign appear several times in a text, begins from
the idea that this must mean something, and manages to stand all the signs of
this language right side up again'—but cautions that this kind of 'symbolic-
order' reading 'leaves the fields of the psychoses and the neuroses both on the
same level' (Lacan, 1993, pp. 10–11). Fundamental to establishing the different
'levels' of neurosis and psychosis is the status of the unconscious. Freud, like
Jung before him, insisted that psychotic patients openly display the unconscious 'secrets' otherwise hidden by those with neurosis, and thereby sought to
justify basing his analysis of paraphrenia exclusively upon written testimony.[41]
Although Lacan concurs that psychotic signification is of paramount importance to the diagnosis, if not analysis, of psychosis, he explicitly challenges the
idea that it should be interpreted as a forthright symbolic revelation of the
unconscious:

> It's classically said that in psychosis the unconscious is at the surface, conscious. That
> is even why articulating it doesn't seem to have much effect . . . Translating Freud, we
> say—the unconscious is a language. Its being articulated doesn't imply its recognition,
> though. The proof of this is that everything proceeds as if Freud were translating a
> foreign language, even carving it up and reassembling it. The subject is, with respect to
> his own language, quite simply in the same position as Freud. If it's ever possible for

---

[41] Recall that for Freud (1981, p. 9), psychosis 'is precisely a disorder in which a written
report or a printed case history can take the place of personal acquaintance with the
patient'.

someone to speak in a language that he is totally ignorant of, we can say that the psychotic subject is ignorant of the language he speaks.

(Lacan, 1993, pp. 11–12, see also 191–2)[42]

Psychosis cannot, according to Lacan, be approached as one would a neurosis: although there is 'great satisfaction in rediscovering certain neurotic symbolic themes in psychosis . . . one really must recognize that it only covers a tiny bit of the picture' (Lacan, 1993, p. 106). Again, unlike Freud, and the majority of commentators since Freud, Lacan is uninterested in finding a new way to decrypt or unscramble Schreber's schizophrenic code. Instead, he turns his attention to the status of the code or utterance itself, and proposes a radically new way of approaching psychosis *through* language, and through the question of the father underpinning Freud's research.

If psychosis cannot be properly understood in terms of homosexual libido, narcissistic regression, psychoneurosis, or the hieroglyphic presentation of the unconscious, how then is it to be defined? To answer this question, Lacan turns to a primordial stage of psychic development, to the process by which the child's 'imaginary register—that of visual images, auditory, olfactory, and other sense perceptions of all kinds, and fantasy—is restructured, rewritten, or "overwritten" by the symbolic' (Fink, 1997, p. 88). The origins of psychosis lie in the subject's failure to enter the realm of signification:

Prior to all symbolization—this priority is not temporal but logical—there is, as the psychoses demonstrate, a stage at which it is possible for a portion of symbolization not to take place. This initial stage precedes the entire neurotic dialectic, which is due to the fact that neurosis is articulated speech, insofar as the repressed and the return of the repressed are one and the same thing. It can thus happen that something primordial regarding the subject's being does not enter into symbolization and is not repressed, but rejected.

(Lacan, 1993, p. 81)

'Not repressed, but rejected'—Lacan here refers to a psychic mechanism peculiar to psychosis.[43] Foreclosure, a translation of Freud's *Verwerfung*, is the

---

[42] Lacan (1993, p. 132) later expands on this point: 'This discourse, which has emerged in the ego, shows itself . . . to be irreducible, unmanageable, incurable. In short, it could be said that the psychotic is a martyr of the unconscious, giving this term *martyr* its meaning, which is to be a witness. It's an open testimony. The neurotic is also a witness to the existence of the unconscious, he gives a closed testimony that has to be deciphered. The psychotic, in the sense in which he is in a first approximation an open witness, seems arrested, immobilized, in a position that leaves him incapable of authentically restoring the sense of what he witnesses and sharing it in the discourse of others'.

[43] Russell Grigg (1999, p. 70) notes that Lacan, in an analysis of Joyce published 20 years after *The Psychoses*, revised his theory of foreclosure to be 'the universal condition of the

process by which a grounding signifier is expelled or refused, thus creating a 'gap or fissure' in the subject's entire signifying system (Richardson, 1988, p. 24). Psychosis arises then from a rupture or hole in a symbolic order structured by phallic signification:

> It is an accident in this register and in what takes place in it, namely, the foreclosure of the Name-of-the-Father in the place of the Other, and in the failure of the paternal metaphor, that I designate the defect that gives psychosis its essential condition, and the structure that separates it from neurosis.

> (Lacan, 1966, p. 215)

The Name-of-the-Father is a complex concept: a substitute for the Desire-of-the-Mother, it is a symbolic intervention in the imaginary mother–child dyad, an intervention that may or may not be enacted by a biological father or father figure. The Name-of-the-Father is experienced as the loss or castration upon which the child's entry into language and Oedipal development depends. As Lacan explains:

> The Oedipus complex means that the imaginary, in itself an incestuous and conflictual relation, is doomed to conflict and ruin. In order for the human being to be able to establish the most natural of relations, that between male and female, a third part has to intervene, one that is the image of something successful, the model of some harmony. This does not go far enough—there has to be a law, a chain, a symbolic order, the intervention of the order of speech, that is, of the father. Not the natural father, but what is called the father. The order that prevents the collision and explosion of the situation as a whole is founded on the existence of this name of the father.

> (Lacan, 1993, p. 96, see also 210)

In psychosis, the foreclosure of the Name-of-the-Father fundamentally alters the subject's relationship to language: 'If the neurotic inhabits language, the psychotic is inhabited, possessed, by language', so it is in the register of speech that the phenomenology of psychosis appears (Lacan, 1993, pp. 250, 36). Lacan is at pains to emphasize, however, that schizophrenic neologisms cannot be treated as unconscious hieroglyphs, *pace* Freud; rather, such signifiers have 'the property of referring essentially to meaning *as such*', that is, they remain 'irreducible' (Lacan, 1993, p. 33, italics in the original). Lacan offers the following explanation of how psychotic hallucinations and delusions differ structurally from the neurotic symptoms arising from repression:

> Let's start with the idea that a hole, a fault, a point of rupture, in the structure of the external world finds itself patched over by psychotic fantasy. How is this to be explained? We have at our disposal the mechanism of projection.

---

symptom'. This revision, however, has no direct bearing on the arguments presented here.

> Projection in psychosis is . . . the mechanism that makes what has got caught up in the *Verwerfung*—that is, what has been placed outside the general symbolization structuring the subject—return from without.

> (Lacan, 1993, pp. 45, 47)

One of Lacan's most famous statements on psychosis—'whatever is refused in the symbolic order, in the sense of *Verwerfung,* reappears in the real' (Lacan, 1993, p. 13, see also 136)—encapsulates his account of the psychotic symptom: it comes to the subject from a place beyond the imaginary or symbolic registers, from the Real of unrepresentable experience.

Psychotic symptoms erupt when something happens to make apparent the hole in the symbolic, for example, when someone appears in the place of the Name-of-the-Father, a place which is impossible or non-existent for the psychotic patient. If the psyche is a structure consequent upon our subjection to and habitation of language, it follows that the foreclosure of the Name-of-the-Father is the decisive factor in the establishment of a psychic structure, which may or may not be revealed through psychotic symptomatology. Once determined, this psychic structure cannot be altered: 'the paternal function is considered to be all or nothing: either a father (as noun, name or "No!") *has* been able to take on all the symbolic function or he has not. There are no in-betweens' (Fink, 1997, p. 82, italics in the original). (Or, to put it crudely: 'psychosis is like pregnancy: you have it or you don't' (Hill, 1997, p. 110)). So if no psychic structure can be changed, what exactly can Lacanian psychoanalysis offer the psychotic patient? Given that the fissure in the symbolic register cannot be remedied, the reconstitution of the subject can only be attempted in the realm of the imaginary. In the words of Bruce Fink (1997, p. 101): 'The goal, superficially stated, is to return the imaginary to the stable state that characterized it prior to the psychotic break'. However, as Lacan offers no insight in *The Psychoses* or elsewhere into how this might be achieved, it seems that he has little interest in or enthusiasm for radically revising the pessimism with which psychoanalysts have approached the treatment of psychosis.[44]

---

[44] Marcelle Marini wryly observes that Lacan 'was more interested in understanding the apparently incomprehensible than in creating a liberating psychotherapy' (Marini, 1992, p. 31). Rodney Kleiman, Director of the Freudian School of Melbourne, has suggested that the analyst offers someone with psychosis recognition that they 'reveal the truth about man's [sic] subjection to language': 'When they ask, "Am I mad?" . . . is there a way of replying which says to them this—"That what you are saying is of value in a discursive sense because at the very least it's a commentary on meaning of man's relationship to language". What would they do with that? [. . .] What it does is say there's a point to what you have to say' (Kleiman, 2003). Eugenie Georgaca's (2001) case study of a literature

It should be clear even from this brief account of Lacan's theory of psychosis why Schreber's *Memoirs* should occupy pride of place in its explication. Over the course of *The Psychoses,* Lacan consistently refers to Schreber's delusions to illustrate the mechanisms of psychosis and the structural importance of the paternal metaphor.[45] I have already dealt at length with competing interpretations of specific aspects of Schreber's delusional system; my concern here is to pinpoint the major claims Lacan makes regarding its origins. According to Freud, Schreber's second encounter with Flechsig caused an upsurge of homosexual libido, releasing a previously repressed desire for his father and brother. Similarly, Lacan is forced to posit a double origin in order to address the issue of how Schreber, despite his underlying psychotic psychic structure, lived an apparently normal, even successful, life until the onset of his second 'nervous illness'. As the foreclosure of the Name-of-the-Father occurs during infancy, the subject will subsequently,

> . . . have to bear the weight of this real, primitive dispossession of the signifier and adopt compensation for it, at length, over the course of his life, through a series of purely conformist identifications with characters who will give him the feeling for what one has to do to be a man.

> The situation may be sustained for a long time this way, psychotics can live compensated lives with apparently ordinary behavior considered to be normally virile, and then all of a sudden, mysteriously, God only knows why, become decompensated. What is it that suddenly renders insufficient the imaginary crutches which have enabled the subject to compensate for the absence of the signifier? How does the signifier as such again lay down its requirements? How does what is missing intervene and question?

> (Lacan, 1993, p. 205)

In other words, what event *reveals* the psychotic structure or precipitates the psychotic break? Lacan identifies two experiences that occurred immediately prior to the onset of Schreber's psychosis—his repeatedly thwarted expectations of paternity and his prestigious appointment to a court presided over by men 20 years his senior—suggesting that '[u]ltimately the question is whether or not the subject will become a father' (Lacan, 1993, pp. 320–1). If the question was thus raised, it was unable to be answered; indeed, it exposed a gaping hole where the Name-of-the-Father should otherwise have been. Acknowledging that 'every author has in fact attempted to explain the onset of Schreber's delusion with reference to the father' (Lacan, 1993, p. 212), Lacan's distinction is to

----

teacher diagnosed as psychotic gives an excellent account of how Lacan's theory of psychosis can be more practically applied in the clinical context.

[45] Like Freud, however, Lacan appears singularly uninterested in Schreber's struggle to prove his rationality to God.

place the emphasis on the symbolic function of the Father, rather than on Schreber's libidinal attachment to Moritz Schreber, or his childhood persecution. For Elisabeth Roudinesco, this distinction reconciles any lingering debate over how to interpret *Memoirs* in the wake of Niederland's research:

> With this sophisticated abstract formula, Lacan brilliantly solved the problem that all other commentators on the *Memoirs of My Nervous Illness*, including Freud, had puzzled over before him. All of them had noticed the link between the father's educational creed and the son's delusions, but Lacan was the first to build a theory on it and to define its functioning in the autobiographical ravings of a crazy narrator. The younger Schreber's pen described a universe full of instruments of torture strangely resembling the apparatuses recommended in the books bearing the name of D. G. M. Schreber—the 'name-of-the-father' excluded from or censored out of both the *Memoirs* and the memory of the son.

(Roudinesco, 1997, p. 290)

The case presented here is, in my view, exaggerated and inaccurate. Although Lacan certainly laid the theoretical foundations for work such as Santner's *My Own Private Germany,* nowhere in *The Psychoses* does he discuss in any depth the medico-pedagogic regime of Moritz Schreber or its impact on the young Schreber. Moreover, to insist on the importance of early childhood experience would contradict the claim that the foreclosure of the Name-of-the-Father occurs at the time the infant enters the register of speech. The importance of Lacan's third seminar, I would suggest, extends well beyond his reading of *Memoirs of My Nervous Illness*, even as it reinforces that latter's status as a sublime text in psychoanalytic discourse. The significance of *The Psychoses* for the broader question of psychoanalytic accounts of schizophrenia lies in its stark portrayal of schizophrenic signification—and indeed psychosis itself—as sublime.

The operation of the textual sublime—the textualization of schizophrenia—is more apparent in Lacan's work than in any other psychoanalytic oeuvre. Marini has already argued that his reliance on textual rather than clinical material in *The Psychoses* is problematic: 'Lacan would study texts about texts concerning the case of Schreber; the few allusions to his own patients, whom he had met only once, were not enough to redeem this seminar from being a reading of texts of texts' (Marini, 1992, p. 33). For Freud, the paraphrenic display of unconscious material rendered the substitution of autobiography for interpersonal encounter acceptable, if not desirable. Having already rejected this reading of psychosis, Lacan offers a far more elaborate theoretical justification for why it is that Schreber's manuscript appears to be more valuable than an in-person appearance. Lacanian psychoanalysis is, even by comparison with competing psychoanalytic traditions, singularly focused on language and the

appearance of the symptom in the symbolic register.[46] The question of schizophrenia's non-verbal manifestations is raised by him only to be dismissed:
even though 'the by no means metaphysical question arises of what is really
going on in the lived experience of the psychotic', he states clearly: 'We are not
yet in a position to give an answer and perhaps at no time will the question ever
have any meaning for us' (Lacan, 1993, p. 67). Easily dispensed with at first,
this apparently unmeaningful question later resurfaces in a discussion of
Memoirs of My Nervous Illness. I have already noted the propensity of commentators on this text to overlook the conditions of its production, specifically, its status *as* memoir. Lacan, too, observes that Schreber presents his
delusional system to the reader many years after its onset and concedes:

> In this respect I have some reservations, legitimate ones, since something that we may
> suppose is more primitive, prior, originary, escapes us—the lived experience, the
> famous ineffable and incommunicable lived experience of psychosis in its primary or
> fertile period.

> (Lacan, 1993, p. 118)

However, he then urges us to 'abandon the idea, implicit in many systems,
that what the subject puts into words is an improper and always distorted
enunciation of a lived experience that would be some irreducible reality'
(Lacan, 1993, p. 118). It is, after all, in the symbolic order that psychosis is
made apparent. What is significant, according to Lacan, is not whether or not
a particular aspect of lived experience or psychotic speech can or cannot
be *understood*: 'What, on the contrary, is altogether striking is that it's inaccessible, inert, and stagnant with respect to any dialectic' (Lacan, 1993, p. 22). If
'understanding', in the sense of interpersonal empathy, is inconsequential if
not impossible, then all that remains to be done is scrutinize psychotic discourse. Here, Lacan effectively makes Schreber the bellowing madman super-
fluous to the analysis of *Memoirs*, and by implication, the flesh-and-blood
patient to the analysis of psychosis.

Lacan takes the psychoanalytic textualization of schizophrenia to the
extreme, but his portrayal also reproduces elements of psychiatry's framing of

---

[46] As Dylan Evans notes, this almost exclusive emphasis on the analysand's speech is justified on three main grounds: 'Firstly, all human communication is inscribed in a linguistic
structure; even "body language" is, as the term implies, fundamentally a form of *language*, with the same structural features. Secondly, the whole aim of psychoanalytic treatment is to articulate the truth of one's desire in speech rather than in any other medium;
the fundamental rule of psychoanalysis is based on the principle that speech is the only
way to this truth. And thirdly, speech is the only tool which the analyst has; therefore, any
analyst who does not understand the way speech and language work does not understand
psychoanalysis itself' (Evans, 1996, pp. 97–8).

schizophrenia as sublime. Although he squarely opposes Jaspers's account of the importance of interpersonal 'understanding' in psychiatric and psychological practice, Lacan paradoxically appears to be more closely aligned with Jaspers than with many other psychoanalysts. In addition to criticizing Freud's attempt to translate the 'meaning of madness', both Jaspers and Lacan insist that the sublime (unknowable, inaccessible, ineffable, or unrepresentable) is central to the structure of schizophrenia. 'Not only can man's being not be understood without madness, it would not be man's being if it did not bear madness within itself as the limit of his freedom' (Lacan, 1966, p. 215). Psychosis in these accounts reveals—and threatens to rupture—ontological boundaries. Not only do schizophrenic delusions and hallucinations appear from beyond the threshold of the symbolic, Lacan's theory of psychosis also condemns the sufferer herself to exist in an unrepresentable and unspeakable psychic space. It is the idea of radical exteriority, a 'psychotic abyss outside the symbolic domain' (Lacan quoted in Žižek, 1999, p. 273), which clearly pays homage to a vision of the schizophrenic sublime as exceeding the limits of 'normal' subjectivity. Although the psychic structure of psychosis and the mechanisms of its operation can be theorized, Lacan, like Jaspers, repeatedly highlights the futility of attempting to interpret the ineffable psychotic utterance, or decipher the central, incomprehensible mystery of schizophrenia:

> At the heart of the psychoses there is a dead end, perplexity concerning the signifier. Everything takes place as if the subject were reacting to this by an attempt at restitution, at compensation. Fundamentally the crisis is undoubtedly unleashed by some question or other. Which is . . . ? I've got no idea. I suppose that the subject reacts to the signifier's absence by all the more emphatically affirming another one that as such is essentially enigmatic.

> (Lacan, 1993, p. 184)

Delusions may be 'legible' but 'there is no way out', presumably for both the psychotic analysand and the analyst (Lacan, 1993, p. 104). Classical psychoanalysts negotiated this impasse by reading or rewriting the psychotic literary outpour as an essentially immutable neurotic narrative; Lacan, on the other hand, consistently emphasizes the problem of legibility in such a way as to exacerbate its structural singularity and distinction from neurosis.

Lacan's theory of psychosis thus maps a twofold relationship between schizophrenia and sublimity. First, it repeats and heightens the already established logic of the textual sublime. If psychoanalysis has, since Jung, shown that psychotic delusions can be interpreted, it has been unable to demonstrate that such interpretation has any psychotherapeutic value, intent, or consequence. Lacan raises the stakes here: once it is manifested discursively, the psychic structure of psychosis can be identified and explained but *never* altered.

The defining characteristic of the psychotic psychic structure, the foreclosure of the Name-of-the-Father, is precisely that which makes the psychoanalytic 'treatment' of schizophrenia impossible. Secondly, although Lacan's psycho-analytic theory of the origins of psychosis deploys a model of the psyche radically different from any advanced in psychiatry, it nevertheless reaffirms the psychiatric view of schizophrenic phenomena as bizarre, beyond comprehension, resistant to psychotherapeutic treatment, and fundamentally distinct from other forms of psychic disturbance. In short, although there is no theoretical convergence between Lacanian psychoanalysis and psychiatry in the subject of schizophrenia, at the level of metatheory both frame psychosis as sublime.

A brief comparison between *The Psychoses* and the model of schizophrenia advanced by Lacan's contemporary, Melanie Klein, highlights the way in which his approach to psychosis departs from psychoanalytic tradition to reinforce the dominant (i.e. psychiatric) perception of schizophrenia as sublime. Klein is the strongest advocate both of the psychoanalytic 'regressive hypothesis' of schizophrenia and of an *un*sublime psychosis; she argues that schizophrenia is a latent possibility for every individual as it is a regression to the 'paranoid–schizoid position' of earliest infancy (Klein, 1952, p. 294). A necessary stage in psychic development, the paranoid–schizoid position is so called because 'anxieties characteristic of psychosis arise which drive the ego to develop specific defence-mechanisms' also seen in schizophrenia: the ego responds to the 'anxiety of being annihilated by a destructive force within' and subsequent fear of persecution by subdividing itself and splitting internal and external objects (Klein, 1952, pp. 292, 297, 317). Failure to work through the paranoid–schizoid position and progress to the depressive position has dire immediate and long-term consequences:

> If states of splitting and therefore of disintegration, which the ego is unable to overcome, occur too frequently and go on for too long, then in my view they must be regarded as a sign of schizophrenic illness in the infant, and some indications of such illness may already be seen in the first few months of life. In adult patients, states of depersonalization and of schizophrenic dissociation seem to be a regression to these infantile states of disintegration.

> (Klein, 1952, p. 302)

Defining psychosis as the return to a chaotic pre-Oedipal, pre-linguistic stage of psychic development, Klein downplays the importance of interpreting or decoding schizophrenic speech in symbolic terms. Instead, she concentrates on the other challenges schizophrenia raises for the analyst: 'It is generally agreed that schizoid patients are more difficult to analyse than manic–depressive types. Their withdrawn, unemotional attitude, the narcissistic elements in their object-relations [and] a kind of detached hostility which pervades the whole relation to the analyst create a very different type of resistance' (Klein, 1952, p. 313). Klein's emphasis on the interpersonal and affective dimension of schizophrenia is reinforced by frequent references to her clinical experience, and although she does offer a brief account of Schreber's psychic splitting, she is not party to the general psychoanalytic love affair with *Memoirs of My Nervous Illness*. By theorizing schizophrenia as psychic regression to an earlier phase in ego development, undertaking analysis with infants as well as adults, and concentrating on the non-verbal signs of the disorder, Klein offers an account of psychosis that could hardly be more opposed to Lacan's. On this model, we are all at least potentially a little bit schizophrenic, and the suggestion of a continuum between psychosis and a myriad of other disorders[47]—unimaginable in Lacanian psychoanalysis—frames schizophrenia in terms not of the sublime but of the quotidian.

Schizophrenia and the problem of the father

Klein's 'Notes on Some Schizoid Mechanisms' is an exception to the rule of psychoanalytic accounts of psychosis. As I have endeavoured to demonstrate in this chapter, the psychoanalytic incursion into psychiatric territory has yielded a variety of competing models of schizophrenia metatheoretically linked through the logic of the textual sublime. From *The Psychology of Dementia Praecox* to *The Psychoses*, analysts have claimed to master the meaning of madness and hence dispel schizophrenia's aura of sublimity, while simultaneously locating the schizophrenic patient in an unknowable realm beyond psychoanalytic reach. The many attempts to discover in Schreber's *Memoirs* literary proof of a particular paradigm of psychosis are further evidence that schizophrenia must be construed as a text or interpretive puzzle in order to be (psycho)analysed. Thanks to the significant number of rival readings of the Schreber case already in circulation, *Memoirs* has become something of a sublime text within its own interdisciplinary arena, and it is therefore strangely fitting that Schreber's experience, and his representation of that experience, can also be understood through the sublime. However, it is in Lacan's third seminar, I have argued, that schizophrenia, framed as a disorder of signification, is most clearly connected to the sublime, and it is to this text that I want to return in the final part of this chapter in order to consider the

---

[47] Klein points to an 'inherent relation' between hysteria and schizophrenia, and suggests that 'the group of schizoid or schizophrenic disorders is much wider than has been acknowledged', and should even be extended to include 'certain forms of mental deficiency' (Klein, 1952, pp. 295, 303).

questions Lacan's work raises regarding the relationship between schizophrenia, sublimity, and gender.

A key point of contention between Lacan and Klein is the role assigned to parents in aggravating or forestalling the drama of foreclosure or fixation at the paranoid–schizoid position. For Klein, the only protagonists in the inchoate pre-Oedipal stage of the paranoid–schizoid position are the infant and the mother, or more accurately, the infant's fragmented experience of the mother's body as the good and bad breast. If 'the mother's love and understanding of the infant can be seen as the infant's greatest stand-by in overcoming states of disintegration and anxieties of a psychotic nature' (Klein, 1952, p. 302), it stands to reason that a *lack* of maternal care would exacerbate such anxieties, possibly resulting in fixation at this stage (Mann, 1994, pp. 70–1). American ego psychologists and British object-relations theorists subsequently developed Klein's implied link between schizophrenia and poor mothering into a robust, if now discredited, theory of the schizophrenogenic mother (Willick, 2001, p. 33). Lacan, too, construes the mother–infant relationship as problematic, but only insofar as *paternal* intervention fails to rupture the dyad. Of course, Lacan conceives of paternal intervention in symbolic terms—it is the foreclosure of the Name-of-the-Father that determines the psychotic psychic structure—but this event is not entirely unrelated to the presence or absence of a father figure in the infant's life. To what extent, then, do individual parents, or societies at large, bear responsibility for the failure of the paternal function?

In order to address this question, it is necessary to re-examine the status of the Name-of-the-Father in Lacan's theory of psychosis; specifically, to consider whether it is *the* master signifier that 'grounds or anchors the symbolic order as a whole' (Fink, 1997, p. 79) or one among many possible 'quilting points' at which 'the signified and the signifier are knotted together' (Lacan, 1993, p. 268). The quilting point, or *point de capiton*, is an upholstery term: it refers to the point at which the cover and the stuffing are joined to each other independently of the frame of the furniture. Like the unbound fabric and filling of a chair, 'the relationship between the signified and the signifier always appears fluid, always ready to come undone'; it is the quilting points that create the impression that signifier and signified are bound together and meaning is fixed. Psychosis can be conceived of as a division of signifier and signified produced by the absence of such button ties:

> I don't know how many there are, but it isn't impossible that one should manage to determine the minimal number of fundamental points of insertion between the signifier and the signified necessary for a human being to be called normal, when they are not established, or when they give way, make a psychotic.

(Lacan, 1993, pp. 261, 268–9)

However, in the case of Schreber, Lacan identifies only one such dysfunctional 'point of insertion':

> To all appearances President Schreber lacks this fundamental signifier called *being a father*. This is why he had to make a mistake, become confused, to the point of thinking of acting like a woman. He had to imagine himself a woman and bring about in pregnancy the second part of the path that, when the two were added together, was necessary for the function of *being a father* to be realized.

> (Lacan, 1993, p. 293)

So, although Lacan shows the foreclosure of the Name-of-the-Father to be the decisive factor in Schreber's psychosis, is it necessarily the case that the paternal signifier is the *only* point relevant to the formation of a psychotic psychic structure? Marcelle Marini argues persuasively that Lacan's failure to explain the role of other quilting points is a significant shortcoming of his theory of psychosis; the foreclosure of the Name-of-the-Father is, she suggests, so intimately connected to the case of Schreber that it is 'impossible to know if this concept would truly work in the case of Aimée or in the crime of the Papin sisters, which Lacan had previously studied' (Marini, 1992, pp. 159–60, 41–2).[48] What is clear is that whereas hysteria—via Lacan's analysis of the Dora case—involves the question '*What is it to be a woman?*' (Lacan, 1993, p. 175), psychosis— via Schreber's '*being a father*'—becomes a problem fundamentally related to the symbolic function of the father.

Bruce Fink makes this point explicit: 'to reject the father's role, to undermine the father's current symbolic function, will lead to no good; its consequences are likely to be worse than those of the father function itself, increasing the incidence of psychosis' (Fink, 1997, p. 111). Contemporary society, in his view, is marked by just such a decline, if not crisis, in patriarchal authority:

> Combined with the de facto increase in the divorce rate and the consequent increase in the number of children being raised solely by their mothers, and with the growing antiauthoritarian attitude toward children among men (no doubt at least in part encouraged by certain modern-day feminist discourse), the paternal function seems to be in danger of extinction in certain social milieus.

> (Fink, 1997, p. 110)

Fink here suggests that the paternal function is not merely symbolic, but directly related to the roles assigned to and fulfilled by heterosexual men in raising children, and in turn that a 'crisis' of masculinity can be causally linked

---

[48] Grigg disagrees on this point, arguing that for Lacan 'it is *only* when what is foreclosed is specifically concerned with the question of the father, as in Schreber's case, that psychosis is produced' (Grigg, 1999, p. 54, my italics).

to an increase in psychosis. Although it is not uncommon to suggest that Moritz Schreber was a 'paranoidogenic' father, as does Schatzman, Fink takes the argument to a new level. Here, 'the father' has been emasculated by a new social order, which must bear ultimate responsibility for the increased number of psychotic individuals it produces.[49] Is this the paranoia of a persecuted patriarch speaking? Unsupported by any sociological or psychological research, Fink's claims are anti-feminist and overstated. More disturbingly, they are not as controversial an interpretation of Lacan as they might appear. In a 1938 article on the family, Lacan pointed to 'the contemporary social decline in the paternal imago (clearly visible in the images of absent fathers and humiliated fathers) as the cause of current psychopathological peculiarities' (Evans, 1996, p. 61),[50] which goes some way to explaining his conviction in 1955 that the question of psychosis had attained a greater 'degree of acuteness or urgency' (Lacan, 1993, p. 81) than in Freud's day. And by 1966, 'paternal inadequacy', as well as the mother's relation to the person and speech of the father, was clearly implicated in the development of a psychotic psychic structure (Lacan, 1966, p. 218). The question remains, 40 odd years later, (how) has this situation changed?

If Freud first identified the father as the love object at the centre of the paraphrenic drama, Lacan's thesis assigns the father and the paternal function unparalleled agency in the determination of psychosis. As is well documented, psychoanalysis has since its earliest days associated hysteria with 'the feminine'. I would argue that in the work of Freud and Lacan the connection between psychosis and 'the masculine' is equally as strong, in no small part because both analysts defer to Schreber's delusional system as the exemplary psychotic text. More than in any psychiatric account, schizophrenia here is *aetiologically* linked to a symbolic and to some extent individual *failure* in normative heterosexual masculinity. This issue warrants further investigation on a scale that is, unfortunately, beyond the scope of the current project. What *is* important to note at this juncture is that in attributing to schizophrenia this

[49] In his enthusiasm for explaining schizophrenia as a consequence of changing gender relations in the twentieth century, Fink does not mention the fact that schizophrenia has been shown to be more or less stably distributed across global populations, regardless of cross-cultural variations in the symbolic status of the father (Miller and Mason, 2002, p. 35).

[50] In the article in question—'The Family: The complex, a concrete factor in familial psychology. Familial complexes in pathology'—Lacan offers 'unconditional praise of the "paternalist" family', 'vibrant regrets over "the social decline of the paternal image"... and over the increased role of the mother or of woman' according to Marini (1992, p. 144).

kind of symbolic agency, psychoanalysis at a structural level anticipated the production in cultural theory of a notion of schizophrenia imbued with social significance. We are now in a position to examine in more detail the way in which clinical theory—psychiatric but especially psychoanalytic—has been interrogated and re-imagined by cultural theory. And there is no better place to begin than with the most impassioned, polemical of these discourses: antipsychiatry.

Part 2

Cultural theory

Chapter 3

Antipsychiatry: schizophrenic experience and the sublime

The antipsychiatry movement of the 1960s and 1970s marked a decisive turning point in the history of representing schizophrenia: it reconceptualized in subjective terms psychiatry's sublime object. With varying degrees of subtlety and sophistication, antipsychiatric thinkers challenged the clinical pictures of psychosis offered by psychiatrists and psychoanalysts, suggesting that schizophrenic symptomatology is not baffling, bizarre, or otherwise unfathomable, but on the contrary rich in meaning. Instead of approaching schizophrenia as the expression of a disease process, genetic aberration, neurological abnormality, libidinal upsurge, or psychic structure, antipsychiatric thinkers focussed on the person as an embodied subject bound by history, geography, and social class; a person whose 'madness' was fundamentally social in character, and therefore had to be understood in the context of the family, the welfare state, the total institution or patriarchal Western culture at large. 'Rescuing', as it were, the schizophrenic patient from the relatively closed world of the clinic or the asylum, antipsychiatric discourse re-framed 'the schizophrenic' as a figure now capable of sustaining multiple and sometimes contradictory *symbolic* roles. And in opening up schizophrenia to associations and functions far beyond those circumscribed by psychiatry, antipsychiatry also called in to question schizophrenia's status as sublime.

This chapter analyses the way schizophrenia is represented, mobilized, and politicized in an antipsychiatry movement characterized by diversity and disavowal. For the purposes of this analysis, and although none of its many theoretically divergent practitioners embrace the label, I use the term 'antipsychiatry movement' to refer to the work of Erving Goffman (1973), Michel Foucault (1993), Thomas Szasz (1972; 1976), and R.D. Laing (1990), as well as to the various countercultural movements across Europe and America which protested against the institutions of psychiatry and psychoanalysis.[1] I will

---

[1] This critique was also vigorously mounted by Anglo-American feminists, especially in the wake of Phyllis Chesler's widely celebrated *Women and Madness* (1972). Highlighting the patriarchal nature of psychiatry's pathologization of woman and its oppressive

argue that while framing schizophrenia in social and subjective terms appears antithetical to psychiatry's construction of schizophrenia as sublime, the divergent discourses loosely assembled under the rubric of antipsychiatry enact a more complex critique of the psychiatric model of schizophrenia than one of simple opposition.

Antipsychiatrists have proposed three distinct responses to psychiatry's elevation of schizophrenia to the status of sublime object. The first and perhaps the most immediately obvious is the wholesale repudiation of any association between schizophrenia and sublimity found in the work of Thomas Szasz, Erving Goffman, and Thomas Scheff. Concentrating on Szasz's 1976 monograph on schizophrenia, I will argue that by rejecting the medical model of mental illness and establishing a continuum between so-called schizophrenic and normal behaviour, this position effectively denies that any person or experience can be 'intrinsically' psychotic. Psychiatric diagnosis is all that distinguishes people diagnosed as schizophrenic from the distressed, deviant, or disenfranchised. The second antipsychiatric reinterpretation of schizophrenia, like many of its psychoanalytic counterparts, oscillates between rejecting and reinforcing schizophrenia's sublimity. R.D. Laing's *The Divided Self* is the exemplary text here: although its existential-phenomenological account of schizophrenia seeks primarily to render schizophrenia intelligible, something of the 'essential mystery' of psychotic experience is preserved as its defining characteristic. Finally, there is the contention, advanced variously by Laing, Cooper, and Foucault, that schizophrenia is more than a sublime object; that it is, in fact, an experience of the sublime, the transcendent, and the liberating. This third response, then, paradoxically confirms the psychiatric attitude towards schizophrenia at the precise moment when the disorder is completely redefined in spiritual, non-clinical terms.

In order to grasp the subtleties and significance of these diverse antipsychiatric accounts of schizophrenia, however, it is important first to locate antipsychiatry within its broad historical context and to understand how the movement as a whole utilized schizophrenia in its multifaceted assault on psychiatric theory and practice. This in turn demands that we revisit the thorny issue of language with respect to schizophrenia. The antipsychiatry movement of the 1960s and

---

institutional response to women's suffering, feminist theorists and activists called for radically new ways of understanding madness and healing distress. Although their claims clearly overlap with the extremely male-dominated antipsychiatry movement, feminists by and large tended to engage the category of madness rather than schizophrenia (see Busfield, 1996; Russell, 1995; Ussher, 1991). Given the focus and expressed intentions of the present study, Anglo-American feminist critiques of madness and psychiatry, powerful as they continue to be, are for this reason not examined in depth.

1970s played a vital if not decisive role in creating the discursive and political space for subsequent survivor and service-user movements, critical psychology, and post-psychiatry to flourish. The activists, clinicians, patients, and mental health professionals working in and through the legacy of antipsychiatry have now, for the most part, rejected the noun 'schizophrenic' as a pejorative, stigmatizing, and dehumanizing label, which reduces the person to their illness (COPE Initiative, 2010). However, when it comes to writing and thinking about the antipsychiatry movement itself, as well as the cultural theory that is the focus of the rest of this book, the concept of 'the schizophrenic' is not one that can be jettisoned, ignored, or otherwise willed away. Antipsychiatrists gave Anglo-American culture the figure of 'the schizophrenic'—a figure invested with multiple and sometimes contradictory political meanings, a figure charged with a potent symbolic function, a figure whose cultural status *far exceeds* the experiences of any individual. When I use the term 'the schizophrenic', then, I am referring to an almost mythical and certainly at times over-determined *figure*. I am not making claims about the experience of people who have received this diagnosis, nor am I in any way seeking to intervene in clinical and philosophical debates about what schizophrenia really is or is not. My quotation marks signal both that I am using the language of others and that there is nothing natural or self-evident about a category that is both constructed and highly contested.

A brief overview of antipsychiatry

Antipsychiatrists may be the most well known and widely published opponents of mainstream psychiatry, but they were by no means the first or the only critics of what went on in asylums, clinics, and universities in the name of psychological science. Ever since its earliest days as a fledgling medical discipline, psychiatry has encountered some form of vibrant opposition to its practices.[2] It will not be surprising to learn that Daniel Paul Schreber is again one of the most famous first-hand critics of biological psychiatry. In addition to reporting attempted 'soul murder' and physical abuse during his incarceration, Schreber in a lengthy appendix to his 1903 *Memoirs of My Nervous Illness* addressed himself to the pertinent question: 'In what circumstances can a person considered insane be detained in an asylum against his declared will?' Although Schreber's physicians, Emil Flechsig and Guido Weber, did not feel compelled to answer to the arguments of a declared lunatic, they *were* forced

---

[2] Nick Crossley is one of the foremost analysts of opposition to psychiatry in the UK (Crossley, 1998, 1999, 2002, 2004, 2005, 2006; Crossley and Crossley, 2001). For a more global perspective see McLean, 1995; Nelson et al., 2006; Nelson et al., 2007.

to defend publicly the scientific legitimacy of psychiatry in the face of escalating attacks on its moral credibility. Indeed, revising insanity laws, improving asylum conditions, reinstating patient rights, and supervising psychiatrists and lawyers were such contested issues in turn-of-the-century Germany that they became the focus of parliamentary inquiry (Lothane, 1992, p. 222, see also pp. 273, 288–90). Far from fading into obscurity, these issues are still relevant to contemporary debates in and around Western psychiatry. Contemporary mental health charities, activists, and advocacy groups,[3] for example, in addition to providing direct support to patients or 'consumers' and their families, undertake comprehensive media monitoring, promote 'stigma-busting' and other anti-discrimination practices, and advocate for improvements to all aspects of mental health services. Whereas some campaign specifically for increased education on mental health issues to ensure that mental disorders are understood to be medically legitimate diseases of the brain, others are vocal in highlighting the limitations of the biomedical model and advance a range of alternative ways of understanding distressing experience. Today, as in Schreber's day, such groups issue powerful calls for reform, addressing their demands as much to a society deemed ignorant and intolerant of the reality of mental illness as to the psychiatric system in question. These examples can only hint at how consistently controversy has plagued psychiatry, its subjects and objects of analysis. Yet it is not overstating the point to suggest that psychiatry's scientific credentials, history, and ethical standing have been more fiercely and more frequently contested than those of any other branch of medicine (Healy, 2002, p. 173; Porter and Micale, 1994, p. 4).

In contrast to patient-driven critiques of biological psychiatry, however, the antipsychiatry movement was primarily a theory-driven critique of a psychiatry on the brink of a psychopharmacological revolution. Among the most influential events in post-War psychiatry were the discovery of the first antipsychotic drug, chlorpromazine, in 1952, and its rapid distribution; the unprecedented increase in asylum admissions, peaking in the mid-1950s; the subsequent trend towards deinstitutionalization within the same decade; the considerable influence of psychoanalytic theory in the treatment and definition of severe psychic disorders; and the significant diagnostic divergences between national psychiatries (Healy, 2002, pp. 96–112; Shorter, 1997). The most

---

[3] Such groups are diverse in their aims, interests, and agendas, and many operate at the local level. Among the most prominent groups are: internationally, the World Network of Users and Survivors of Psychiatry and the Hearing Voices Network; in America, the National Alliance on Mental Illness and the National Coalition of Mental Health Consumer/Survivor Organizations; and in the UK, Mind, SANE, the National Schizophrenia Fellowship, Rethink and the Mental Health Foundation.

powerful critiques of psychiatry emerged in response to these paradigm shifts in both the conceptualization and management of psychological disorders. Though they each strenuously disavowed the label 'antipsychiatrist',[4] Goffman, Foucault, Szasz, and Laing were swiftly established as the antipsychiatry movement's foundational theorists (Kotowicz, 1997; Porter and Micale, 1994; Sedgwick, 1982). Reappraising the status of madness and the mad, they staked out the intellectual and political territory of antipsychiatry by redrawing the boundaries of sociology, philosophy, psychiatry, and psychoanalysis.

Schizophrenia was, of course, one of the principal grounds upon which antipsychiatrists fought, and the movement challenged the dominant psychiatric account of schizophrenia in two distinct arenas. The first of these was the clinic itself: antipsychiatrists rejected the medical model of mental illness; focused public attention on psychiatry's inability to produce a definitive account of the aetiology of schizophrenia (let alone treat it successfully); and proposed radical new ideas about the nature and origins of mental disorder. As we have seen, since its clinical debut in 1896, psychiatrists and psychoanalysts had argued that schizophrenia was variously caused by viral infection, an upsurge of homosexual libido, defective heredity, neurochemical imbalances, psychic regression to an infantile paranoid–schizoid position, obstetric complications, and the foreclosure of the Name-of-the-Father. Over the first half of the twentieth century, clinicians sought to manage schizophrenic symptoms using insulin-coma therapy, straitjackets, neuroleptic or antipsychotic drugs, sterilization and castration, regular beating, electroconvulsive or 'electric shock' treatment, 12-step programmes, psychotherapy, fasting, frontal lobe lobotomy, and 'mega-vitamin therapy'.[5] Antipsychiatrists were as quick to point out inconsistencies in this impressive list of competing hypotheses and therapies as they were to add to them. As we shall see, they variously, and passionately, argued that schizophrenia was really a label applied to non-normative behaviour, a rational response to psychiatric incarceration, and a direct product of maternal and family relationships if not capitalist society in general.

---

[4] Of these, Thomas Szasz is by far the most sweeping: 'I reject the term *antipsychiatry* because it is imprecise, misleading, and cheaply self-aggrandizing' (Szasz, 1976, p. 48). It would appear, however, that despite repeated insistence that he is 'anti-coercion, not antipsychiatry' (Szasz, 2010), Szasz is destined to remain forever associated with the movement he so detests.

[5] Many of these treatments for schizophrenia are of course well known. On the use of castration and sterilization by biological psychiatrists in early twentieth-century Germany, see Lothane, 1992, p. 210. On the sterilization of patients in mental hospitals in 1950s America, see Whitaker, 2002, p. 142. On psychiatric advocacy of vitamin cures, fasting, physical violence, and 12-step programmes as treatments for schizophrenia see Szasz, 1976, pp. 112–9.

In short, the disorder's origins were to be found everywhere but in biology. David Cooper's 1967 definition of schizophrenia is exemplary of the shift in interest from the schizophrenic individual to a schizophrenogenic world:

> *Schizophrenia is a micro-social crisis situation in which the acts and experiences of a certain person are invalidated by others for certain intelligible cultural and micro-cultural (usually familial) reasons, to the point where he is elected and identified as being 'mentally ill' in a certain way, and then is confirmed (by a specifiable but highly arbitrary labelling process) in the identity 'schizophrenic patient' by medical or quasi-medical agents.* This statement, it will be noted, refers to extreme disturbance (crisis) in a group and says nothing about disorder in a 'schizophrenic' person.

(Cooper, 1970, p. 16, italics in the original)

The antipsychiatry movement not only exposed the definitional chaos surrounding schizophrenia but also introduced to it new, politically charged ways of interpreting the most severe of mental disorders.

Antipsychiatry further challenged psychiatric and popular perceptions of schizophrenia by repositioning the schizophrenic patient as a key protagonist in the political arena. According to one historian, 'the schizophrenic, along with women, homosexuals, low-paid workers, prisoners, and army conscripts, became part of "the oppressed"' (Postel and Allen, 1994, p. 387) and took on a potent role as society's 'ultimate underdog' (Healy, 2002, p. 148; Sedgwick, 1982, p. 102). The significance of the symbolic function of 'the schizophrenic' was guaranteed by the high profile of antipsychiatry within the broader countercultural movements of the period. Never celebrated for its uniformity, antipsychiatry appeared in a diverse range of political guises across a number of national contexts. In 1967, for example, leading British antipsychiatrists convened a two-week congress in order to tackle what they perceived as an 'emerging global crisis' (Burston, 1996, p. 105). The 'Dialectics of Liberation' was an all-male 'star-studded Left-Wing line-up' (Laing, 1994, p. 135) of 'academics, economists, psychiatrists, political activists, literary critics, anthropologists, sociologists, theatrical directors and Buddhist monks'; Stokely Carmichael, Herbert Marcuse, Allen Ginsberg, and R.D. Laing most famously among them (Mullan, 1999, p. 105). Across the channel in May 1968, students attacked the department of psychiatry at the University of Paris and forced the resignation of Jean Delay, the man who first demonstrated chlorpromazine's antipsychotic properties (Healy, 2002, pp. 176–7). Condemning 'chemical straitjackets' as insidious and oppressive, they waved placards proclaiming 'Schizophrenics are the Proletariat' (Postel and Allen, 1994, p. 387). More revolutionary even than their French counterparts were the patients of the university clinic in Heidelberg. In 1970 they were accused by authorities of using terrorist tactics to demand the restructuring of their mental hospital, and when the SPK, or Socialist Patients' Collective, later disbanded, many of its members joined the Red Army Fraction (Kotowicz, 1997, pp. 79–81; Patientenkollektiv(H); Huffman). The *Semiotext(e)* Schizo-Culture convention in New York 1975—attended by hundreds, including Jean-François Lyotard, Michel Foucault, Gilles Deleuze, and Félix Guattari—was perhaps the last major antipsychiatric event.[6] In denouncing the role that psychiatry played in furthering the advanced capitalist agenda, antipsychiatrists across Europe and America mobilized 'the schizophrenic' either as the apotheosis of the oppressed, an exemplary militant in the fight against oppression, or as a figurehead for psychic and political emancipation.[7]

The broader arguments, politics, and personalities of the antipsychiatry movement have been well documented elsewhere; having thus briefly situated antipsychiatry within its psychiatric and social contexts, my central task in this chapter is to examine the way in which schizophrenia has been framed in key antipsychiatric texts. With the exception of Foucault, whose *Madness and Civilization* I discussed in detail in Chapter 1, antipsychiatrists did not deal exclusively in general, trans-historical concepts like madness or psychosis but focused specifically on schizophrenia as 'the major problem area' of post-War psychiatry (Cooper, 1970, pp. 9, 11). Although antipsychiatrists uniformly rejected the medical models of schizophrenia (Bolton, 2008, pp. 103–5), placing an emphasis on the social (the interpersonal psychiatric exchange, the family, capitalist society) as either schizophrenogenic, or as responsible for constructing a false mythology of schizophrenia, they did not uniformly contest schizophrenia's status as the sublime object of psychiatry. The rest of this chapter endeavours to understand the antipsychiatric models of schizophrenia most prominent in the popular and critical imaginations as following one of three responses to the construction of schizophrenia as sublime within psychiatric discourse. We begin with Thomas Szasz's polemical attack on psychiatry's sublime object.

---

[6] For more on the Schizo-Culture convention itself see Schwarz and Balsamo (1996) and Lotringer and Cohen (2001). The convention also gave rise to a special issue of *Semiotext(e)* called *Schizo-Culture* (1978). A radical, exuberant, multidimensional publication, the journal features stories, interviews, artworks, poetry, parodied advertisements, photo essays, hand-written notes, and articles by many stars of antipsychiatry and the avant-garde, among them, Michel Foucault, Kathy Acker, William Boroughs, David Cooper, Ulrike Meinhof, Gilles Deleuze, and Jean-François Lyotard. It also includes 'The Boston Declaration on Psychiatric Oppression' of 1976.

[7] See Donnelly (1992), in particular Giovanni Jervis 'Psychiatrists and Politics', a revised version of the paper presented at the 1967 Dialectics of Liberation Conference. See also Boyers and Orrill (1972).

Thomas Szasz and anti-sublime schizophrenia

A psychoanalyst and emeritus professor of psychiatry, Thomas Szasz is an American civil libertarian and outspoken opponent of orthodox, or what he calls 'involuntary', psychiatry. Szasz's critique of the entire psychiatric enterprise began in 1961 with the aptly titled *The Myth of Mental Illness* (1972) and has continued unabated for nearly 50 years. His central contention—neatly summarized in a 2001 publication—is that there is no such thing as a mental illness, and that psychiatry perpetuates to its own advantage a fundamental category mistake:

> When we negate the distinction between physical objects and social beings, between bodies and persons, the concept of disease ceases to be limited to the dysfunction of cells, tissues, and organs and expands to include personal conduct. This enables persons deputized by the state as its agents (psychiatrists) and informants (family, teachers, students, employers) to transform any behavior they deem troublesome into a mental illness requiring psychiatric intervention. The result is an erosion of privacy, dignity, liberty and responsibility.[8]

(Szasz, 2001, p. 97)

Szasz's major contribution to the antipsychiatric literature on psychosis is his book *Schizophrenia: The Sacred Symbol of Psychiatry*, and he lists its objectives as follows:

> In this book I shall try to show how schizophrenia has become the Christ on the cross that psychiatrists worship, and in whose name they march into battle to reconquer reason from unreason, sanity from insanity; how reverence toward it has become the mark of psychiatric orthodoxy, and irreverence toward it the mark of psychiatric heresy; and how our understanding of both psychiatry and schizophrenia may be advantaged by approaching this 'diagnosis' as if it pointed to a religious symbol rather than to a medical disease.

(Szasz, 1976, p. xiii)[9]

----

[8] Szasz's career, his principal claims and ongoing concerns as well as his contribution to psychiatry, is compellingly documented in a series of radio interviews and discussions featured on the Australian ABC radio programme *All in the Mind* (Mitchell and Szasz, 2009a, b; Mitchell et al., 2009). The relevance of Szasz's work to the project of critical psychiatry has also been debated in a recent issue of *Philosophy, Psychiatry & Psychology* (Bracken and Thomas, 2010a, b; Ratcliffe, 2010; Szasz, 2010). For a sympathetic appraisal of Szasz's capacity to out-argue his critics, see Cresswell (2008).

[9] After his keynote presentation at the 13th annual International Network for Philosophy and Psychiatry conference (Manchester, July 2010), I asked Szasz whether he thought schizophrenia was still 'the sacred symbol of psychiatry'. 'More than ever', he replied, beaming.

'"Schizophrenic" is a concept wonderfully vague in its content and terrifyingly awesome in its implications', he writes, and 'its meaning is the more powerful because it is inscrutable' (Szasz, 1976, pp. xiii, 87). Although there are clear parallels between my reading of schizophrenia as the sublime object of psychiatry and Szasz's 'sacred symbol' analogy, his thesis depends upon a mind–body dualism that is crude and absolute: he rejects both the validity of schizophrenia and the discipline of psychiatry on the grounds that illness can *only* be defined in corporeal terms. In the absence of any demonstrable physical aberration, the diagnosis of schizophrenia is for Szasz similar to the charge of un-Americanism; consequent not upon 'empirical or scientific' observation but 'ethical and political decision making' (Szasz, 1976, pp. 115, 3). Kraepelin and Bleuler—the fathers of modern psychiatry and the first to identify schizophrenia as a disease entity—therefore come to be seen alongside Freud as 'conquistadors and colonizers of the mind of man', 'religious-political leaders and conquerors', and 'wardens' who practised 'psychiatric slavery' at the behest of an entire society eager to sequester and punish its misfits (Szasz, 1976, pp. 21–3, 35, 38).

Szasz's wholesale rejection of psychiatry's disease model begs the question of what exactly he thinks schizophrenia is. Although at no point does he explicitly offer a positive definition of schizophrenia, references scattered throughout the text add up to a fairly suggestive portrait of the 'so-called schizophrenic': 'incompetent', 'self-absorbed', and 'socially inadequate or impaired', s/he disturbs others, speaks in socially unacceptable metaphors, and leads a 'disordered', 'aimless', and 'useless' life (Szasz, 1976, pp. 136, 182, 36, 14, 74). To put it differently,

> . . . what we call 'sanity'—what we mean by 'not being schizophrenic'—has a great deal to do with competence, earned by struggling for excellence; with compassion, hard won by confronting conflict; and with modesty and patience, acquired through silence and suffering.
>
> (Szasz, 1976, pp. 82–3)

Schizophrenia, on this model, is a moral choice conceptualized in narrowly individualist terms. At pains to emphasize 'patient' agency, Szasz clearly views the schizophrenic patient as one whose freely chosen failure in life reflects only their refusal to face its vicissitudes and negotiate its rhetorical codes (Vatz and Weinberg, 1994, p. 313). The refusal—to be stoic, to suffer in silence in the name of self-improvement—that is constitutive of schizophrenia is enacted in a social space unaffected by systemic inequalities. As Peter Sedgwick argues, the social-Darwinist or twentieth-century Herbert Spencer in Szasz 'is content to redefine out of existence the structured social problems of the exploited communities of America' and offers no 'generalised sympathy for people in trouble' (Sedgwick, 1982, pp. 163–4).[10] Szasz the civil libertarian is nonetheless a committed campaigner for the peoples' right to be protected from 'psychiatric rape' (Szasz, 1976, p. 49) or involuntary commitment, and to be emancipated from enslavement in the psychiatric system. Psychiatry has—much like an abusive husband in an arranged marriage, to paraphrase from another of Szasz's analogies—deprived the person it diagnoses as schizophrenic of her rights and freedoms. But setting empathy aside once again, we must also,

> ... acknowledge that mental patients have exploited their positions as slaves, and that the only way to overcome their subjection is by both economic and personal independence from psychiatrists. This means that 'psychotics' should not expect to be supported by psychiatrists (society) as patients, but must support themselves by work saleable in the marketplace. To the extent that women and 'psychotics' cannot, or do not, so liberate themselves, they will remain enslaved to men who 'love' them and psychiatrists who 'treat' them.

> (Szasz, 1976, p. 176)

Only when financially solvent and hence morally upright can people diagnosed as schizophrenic win legitimacy as clients of Szasz's preferred model of private, fee-paying 'contractual' psychiatry.

If the person diagnosed with schizophrenia is in fact a free, rational, and autonomous agent who chooses to lead a disordered life, what can schizophrenia have to do with the sublime? The answer is very little. Szasz's audacious critique of the medical model of schizophrenia is certainly cogent in places, and in my view he is right to point out that psychiatry elevates schizophrenia to something approaching a sacred status. David Rosenhan's famous 1973 study 'On Being Sane in Insane Places' supports the argument that American psychiatry during the mid-1970s was anything but scientifically rigorous when over-diagnosing schizophrenia (Rosenhan, 1975).[11] However, so total is Szasz's repudiation of psychiatry that he ends up throwing the baby out with the bath water, so to speak. In rejecting schizophrenia and its sublime associations, he redefines its symptoms as signs merely of quotidian distress or disturbance,

---

[10] Szasz has remained adamant on this point. Where there is almost universal consensus that it is difficult to dispute the suffering of those diagnosed with mental illness, Szasz maintains on the contrary that it is 'easy' to do so on the grounds that 'most people who psychiatrists characterise as "seriously mentally ill" do not suffer: they make others suffer' (Szasz, 2004, p. 51).

[11] In the study, eight 'normal' people admitted themselves to mental hospitals complaining of hearing voices. Seven received a diagnosis of schizophrenia. Once admitted, the 'pseudopatients' ceased feigning any symptoms, but remained in hospital for an average of 19 days before being discharged as 'schizophrenics in remission'.

unremarkable variations of everyday behaviour. This effectively denies that there is any such thing as a psychotic experience, much less an ontology of schizophrenia. Sedgwick is again critical of this move: severe mental illness is 'to be sure, a social status: but, before that, it is a private hell. Szasz attains his role as proxy spokesperson for the rights of the mental patient by ignoring, simply, what it is to be a mental patient' (Sedgwick, 1982, p. 158). The reason that Szasz's 'so-called schizophrenic' has all the characteristics of a work-dodging, truculent teenager is principally because delusions, hallucinations, anhedonia, alogia, and other hallmark symptoms of schizophrenia are not among them. Szasz's model—the negation of psychiatry's sacred symbol—certainly deserves to be thought of as 'anti-sublime'; the more pressing question is whether it says anything more about the experience of schizophrenia than it does about the experience of adolescence or long-term unemployment.

Szasz is probably the most famous and undoubtedly the most politically contentious advocate of an anti-sublime social–constructivist model of schizophrenia, but he was not alone. In *Asylums: Essays on the Social Situation of Mental Patients and other Inmates*, Erving Goffman produced compelling sociological evidence that the asylum itself was deeply implicated in the development of its inmates' symptomatologies. The ritualized, dehumanizing practices of the 'total institution' induce self-defensive responses, which are then interpreted as symptoms of an underlying psychopathology, whereas they are better understood within the complex social context of the closed asylum community. Like Szasz, Goffman casts doubt over psychiatry's scientific and moral legitimacy, and confines himself to a strictly sociological model of mental illness in which 'the psychiatric view of a person becomes significant only in so far as this view itself alters his social fate' (Goffman, 1973, p. 119). The category of schizophrenia becomes a 'magical' way of redefining the patient's behaviour as a single entity eligible for 'psychiatric servicing' (Goffman, 1973, p. 326). A sociologist, and not a critical social theorist (Sedgwick, 1982, p. 63), Goffman concentrates primarily on the immediate microcosm of face-to-face interpersonal exchange and seldom locates the process of psychiatric diagnosis and treatment within its broader social and political contexts. *Asylums* was nonetheless a determining influence on the development of a more radical antipsychiatric position under the rubric 'labelling theory'. In his 'Schizophrenia as Ideology', Thomas Scheff advances the work of Szasz and Goffman in an unmistakably polemical direction:

> The concepts of mental illness in general—and schizophrenia in particular—are not neutral, value-free scientifically precise terms but are, for the most part, the leading edge of an ideology embedded in the historical and cultural present of the white

> middle class of Western societies. The concept of illness and its associated vocabulary—symptoms, therapies, patients, and physicians—reify and legitimate the prevailing public order at the expense of other possible worlds.
>
> (Scheff, 1975b, p.6)

Psychiatry, in constructing schizophrenia as its sublime object, implies always that *there is something more* to the disorder, an elusive or enigmatic essence that has yet to be understood. The foundational metatheoretical gesture of Szasz, Goffman, and Scheff, by contrast, is the insistence that schizophrenia is perfectly comprehensible, that it is *nothing more than* a label deployed with great effect in specific social contexts.[12] These theorists may not agree on how the diagnosis/label of schizophrenia reflects or intersects with broader issues of power, subject formation, and the maintenance of social order, but the insistence upon an anti-sublime schizophrenia is pivotal to each of their antipsychiatric projects.

Between two sublimes: schizophrenia and *The Divided Self*

'If what makes "schizophrenic" utterances "symptoms" is that they are incomprehensible, do they still remain "symptoms" after they are no longer incomprehensible?' (Szasz, 1976, p. 15). This question, posed in passing by Thomas Szasz, goes straight to the heart of R.D. Laing's career-long interest in schizophrenia. Renowned as the founder of Kingsley Hall, an experimental therapeutic community established in 1965, Laing, a Glaswegian psychiatrist-cum-countercultural-hero, has at one time or another held or been attributed the full gamut of antipsychiatric positions on schizophrenia.[13] Of particular interest to this discussion of antipsychiatry, schizophrenia, and the sublime are the analyses of psychosis outlined in his two most celebrated publications: *The Divided Self: An Existential Study in Sanity and Madness* and *The Politics of Experience*. In the latter book—published during the Vietnam War at the height of his fame and popular appeal—Laing presents schizophrenia as an experience of the sublime, a portrayal I will address in more depth in the next section. The earlier *The Divided Self*, by contrast, has a very different 'basic purpose': 'to make madness, and the process of going mad, comprehensible' (Laing, 1990, p. 9).

---

[12] The issue here could also be construed as a distinction between schizophrenia as unknowable ontology versus schizophrenia as oppressive ideology. Unlike Foucault, Szasz, Goffman, and Scheff seem optimistic about the individual's capacity to oppose psychiatric ideology.

[13] For an overview of these see *Janus Head* 'Special Issue: The Legacy of R. D. Laing' (2001), in particular Burston (2001a, b) and Bortle (2001).

Heralded, not without cause, as 'a classic of psychiatric literature' (Kotowicz, 1997, p. 25), *The Divided Self* also holds a place of distinction in *antipsychiatric* literature as it locates schizophrenia between multiple sublimes—the anti-sublime just discussed, the textual sublime of psychoanalysis, and the disciplinary sublime of psychiatry as figured in the work of Karl Jaspers.

The Divided Self sets out an existential–phenomenological model of psychosis. Schizophrenia is the intensification of a schizoid state characterized by psychic splitting, or rents between the self and the world, between the mind and the body, and between the true inner self and the outer 'false-self system'.[14] The schizoid state is one of extreme ontological insecurity wherein anxiety—specifically concerning the engulfment, implosion, and petrification of the self—reigns. Its 'symptoms' are therefore best seen as strategies for guarding against the destruction of personality or the annihilation of the self:

> If the individual cannot take the realness, aliveness, autonomy, and identity of himself and others for granted, then he has to become absorbed in contriving ways of trying to be real, of keeping himself or others alive, of preserving his identity, in efforts, as he will often put it to prevent himself losing his self.

(Laing, 1990, pp. 42–3)

Laing's analysis of the divided self unfolds through a series of case studies, vignettes, and vivid accounts of schizoid despair and isolation. His strategy is to orient the reader within the life world of the patient (Laing, 1990, p. 26). Where catatonic, hebephrenic, and paranoid symptoms are only meaningful to psychiatrists as signs of an underlying disease process or evidence of psychic *mal*function, to Laing they are rational, coded communiqués that can only be understood by returning the person diagnosed as schizophrenic to her existential status as a being among others. Through detailed examples, otherwise fragmented or nonsensical schizophrenic speech is translated into an eloquent commentary on damaged, and damaging, interpersonal relations. Laing therefore elucidates an anti-sublime model of schizophrenia on two distinct levels. The major theoretical claim of *The Divided Self* is that schizophrenia is intelligible: as the exacerbation of schizoid psychic states with which we all have some familiarity, it is therefore something with which we can empathize.[15] But Laing further portrays schizophrenia as anti-sublime in the sense that it is an emotionally and psychically devastating experience, which threatens to destroy

---

[14] See Laing, 1990, pp. 17, 69, 94–105. Here, Laing is indebted to Klein (1952).

[15] This emphasis on a continuum between normalcy and psychosis is shared by Szasz, Scheff, and Goffman, although they do not concede a schizophrenic ontology; it is also evident in Melanie Klein's theory of schizophrenia as psychic regression to the paranoid–schizoid position.

rather than reinvigorate the self. (This is of course the direct inverse of his thesis in *The Politics of Experience* that schizophrenia is the sublime transcendence of egoic existence.) If we recall that Kant and Burke both distinguished the sublime from the 'simply terrifying', it becomes clear that in all 'his separateness and loneliness and despair' (Laing, 1990, p. 38), Laing's 1960 'schizophrenic' far from resembles the self-affirmed subject of the sublime or the spiritual voyager 'he' would later become.

Laing's existential model posits an anti-sublime schizophrenia twice over, even if the question of *understanding* schizophrenia is not as easily resolved in *The Divided Self* as appearances and reputation might suggest. Laing's attempted synthesis of psychoanalysis and Jasperian phenomenological psychiatry creates considerable tension with regard to the vexed issue of comprehensibility. As I discussed in Chapter 1, Jaspers maintained that schizophrenia's defining characteristic is the impression created in the observer:

> It is easier to describe the common factor [among schizophrenic patients] in subjective terms, that is, in terms of the effect on the observer, rather than try to do so objectively. All these personalities have something baffling about them, which baffles our understanding in a peculiar way; there is something queer, cold, inaccessible, rigid, and petrified there, even when the patients are quite sensible and can be addressed and even when they are eager to talk about themselves. We may think we can understand dispositions furthest from our own but when faced with such people we feel a gulf which defies description.
>
> (Jaspers, 1972, p. 447)

Like Jaspers, Laing held that '*sanity or psychosis is tested by the degree of conjunction or disjunction between two persons where the one is sane by common consent.* The critical test of whether or not a patient is psychotic is a lack of congruity, an incongruity, a clash, between him and me' (Laing, 1990, p. 36, italics in the original). Where Laing departs from the framework of phenomenological psychiatry is in his conviction that this seemingly alien experience can in fact be understood. This interpretive impulse—the effort to decipher the content of the psychotic utterance rather than simply register its formal features—is, as Laing acknowledges, shared by classical psychoanalysis. Once an object of interpretation, schizophrenia is now construed as a textual puzzle: 'The difficulties facing us here are somewhat analogous to the difficulties facing the expositor of hieroglyphics, an analogy Freud was fond of drawing; they are, if anything, greater' (Laing, 1990, p. 31).[16] We have seen that schizophrenia is framed as a sublime text in psychoanalytic discourse through a double

---

[16] Lacan (1993, p. 10) makes the same observation: '[Freud] deciphers [*Memoirs of My Nervous Illness*] in the way hieroglyphics are deciphered'.

gesture—it is declared amenable to endless reinterpretation but fundamentally beyond therapeutic reach. Laing's distinction in *The Divided Self* is to suggest that the therapist should endeavour to comprehend not just the content of the schizophrenic utterance but its status within the overall context of the patient's experience:

> Like the expositor [of ancient texts], the therapist must have the plasticity to transpose himself into another strange and even alien view of the world. In this act, he draws on his own psychotic possibilities, without forgoing his sanity. Only thus can we arrive at an understanding of the patient's *existential position*.

> (Laing, 1990, p. 34, italics in the original)

A sufficiently empathetic therapist can understand schizophrenic experience, and, moreover, Laing suggests understanding itself has a distinct therapeutic value. Or so it would appear. This contention is immediately followed, however, by Laing's appeal to the underlying—or intrinsic—sublimity of schizophrenia:

> What is required of us? Understand him? The kernel of the schizophrenic's experience of himself must remain incomprehensible to us. As long as we are sane and he is insane, it will remain so. But comprehension as an effort to reach and grasp him, while remaining within our own world and judging him by our own categories whereby he inevitably falls short, is not what the schizophrenic either wants or requires. We have to recognize all the time his distinctiveness and differentness, his separateness and loneliness and despair.

> (Laing, 1990, p. 38)

Schizophrenia therefore traverses a conceptually confused territory in *The Divided Self*. It is anti-sublime in so far as psychotic experience can be rendered intelligible, and anti-sublime insofar as one can empathize with that experience. Yet schizophrenia here, as in Jaspers's *General Psychopathology* and many psychoanalytic accounts, retains its status as a disorder that is *in essence* ultimately beyond understanding.

Schizophrenia as sublime experience

Despite, or perhaps even because of, its internally conflicted thesis on the incomprehensibility of schizophrenia, *The Divided Self* is a compelling account of 'schizophrenic' experiences of the world, the demands of others, embodiment, psychic splitting, and simple survival in the face of ontological insecurity. In his next book, the 1964 *Sanity, Madness and the Family*, Laing switched the focus from intrapsychic despair to interpersonal conflict; schizophrenia was now an intelligible response to a maddening family. By 1967, Laing's paradigms of schizophrenia had again developed and multiplied. One of the most striking and consistent themes in *The Politics of Experience* is the rejection of the assumption that normality is desirable:

> ... social adaptation to a dysfunctional society may be very dangerous. The perfectly adjusted bomber pilot may be a greater threat to species survival than the hospitalized schizophrenic deluded that the Bomb is inside him. Our society may itself have become biologically dysfunctional, and some forms of schizophrenic alienation from the alienation of society may have a sociobiological function that we have not recognized.
>
> (Laing, 1967, p. 120)[17]

It is within this dichotomy of 'normal, impoverished, and inauthentic' versus 'schizophrenic' experience that Laing elaborates and endorses a number of contradictory definitions of psychosis. Following Goffman and anticipating Scheff, he argues that schizophrenia is a label applied within institutional and interpersonal contexts, emphasizing, but without offering further explanation, that 'the label is a social fact and the social fact a *political* event' (Laing, 1967, p. 120, italics in the original). In praise of Gregory Bateson's theory of the schizophrenic double bind, Laing also suggests that schizophrenia is as much a property of the modern nuclear family as it is of the individual.[18] Although he later disavowed this position (Laing, 1985, pp. 8–9), Laing in 1967 was unrelenting in his indictment of the schizophrenogenic family[19] and saw schizophrenic symptoms as '*a special strategy that a person invents in order to live in an unlivable situation*' (Laing, 1967, p. 114, italics in the original). An ever-expanding field of

---

[17] The change in Laing's thinking is also apparent in his Preface to the 1964 edition of *The Divided Self*: 'Thus I would wish to emphasize that our "normal" "adjusted" state is too often the abdication of ecstasy, the betrayal of our true potentialities, that many of us are only too successful in acquiring a false self to adapt to false realities' (Laing, 1990, p.12). This view was also taken up by Scheff (1975a, p.18): 'Perhaps the time has come to consider the possibility that the reality that the so-called schizophrenics are out of touch with is so appalling that their view of the world may be more supportive to life than conventional reality.'

[18] '... *no* schizophrenic has been studied whose disturbed pattern of communication has not been shown to be a reflection of, and reaction to, the disturbed and disturbing pattern characterizing his or her family of origin' (Laing, 1967, p. 114, see also 65). This view was shared by Laing's friend and colleague David Cooper, who went so far as to argue that 'schizophrenia, it if means anything, is a more or less characteristic mode of disturbed group behaviour. There are no schizophrenics' (Cooper, 1970, p. 43).

[19] 'The family's function is to repress Eros; to induce a false consciousness of security; to deny death by avoiding life; to cut off transcendence; to believe in God, not to experience the Void; to create, in short, one-dimensional man; to promote respect, conformity, obedience; to con children out of play; to induce a fear of failure; to promote a respect for work; to promote a respect for "respectability"' (Laing, 1967, p. 65).

inquiry—and culpability—sees a progression from the individual to the family and finally to society at large:

> Questions and answers have so far been focused on the family as a social subsystem. Socially, this work must now move to further understanding, not only of the internal disturbed and disturbing patterns of communication within families, of the double-binding procedures, the pseudo-mutuality, of what I have called the mystifications and the untenable positions, but also to the meaning of all this within the larger context of the civic order of society—that is, of the *political* order, of the ways persons exercise control and power over one another.

> (Laing, 1967, p. 114, italics in the original)

The Politics of Experience here gestures towards the political territory suggested by its title; however, despite claiming that 'the social system, not single individuals extrapolated from it, must be the object of study' (Laing, 1967, p. 114, italics in the original), Laing does not proceed far in his implied critique of a schizophrenogenic modern society. Instead, and in what appears to be a complete about-face, he argues that the 'desperately and urgently required project for our time' is the exploration of 'the inner space and time of consciousness', and schizophrenic consciousness in particular (Laing, 1967, p. 127).

It is towards the end of *The Politics of Experience* that Laing elucidates his famous account of schizophrenia as an ecstatic voyage into 'inner space' (Laing, 1967, p. 127). 'Madness need not be all breakdown. It may also be breakthrough. It is potentially liberation and renewal as well as enslavement and existential death' (Laing, 1967, p. 133). Future generations, Laing assures us, 'will see that what we call "schizophrenia" was one of the forms in which, often through quite ordinary people, the light began to break through the cracks in our all-too-closed minds' (Laing, 1967, p. 129).[20] Once defined by Laing as an ontology of existential despair and isolation, then as a disturbance in the realm of the interpersonal, psychosis is now, in a shift back from the social to psychic interior, analogous to religious and mystical revelation. Indeed, schizophrenia even eclipses sanity as the preferred mode of being: 'Can we not see that *this voyage is not what we need to be cured of, but that it is itself a natural way of healing our own appalling state of alienation called normality*?' (Laing, 1967, p. 136, italics in the original). *The Politics of Experience* culminates in this vision of schizophrenia as a Romantic experience of the sublime—a transcendent loss of self followed by the recovery of authenticity, an essential or original form of

---

[20] This is foreshadowed in *The Divided Self*: 'I am aware that the man who is said to be deluded may be in his delusion telling me the truth, and this in no equivocal or metaphorical sense, but quite literally, and that the cracked mind of the schizophrenic may *let in* light which does not enter the intact minds of many sane people whose minds are closed' (Laing, 1990, p. 27).

being unmarred by modernity and techno-scientific rationality. In keeping with the late 1960s zeitgeist, Laing's schizophrenia-as-enlightenment thesis captured the public imagination on a politico-spiritual level in part because of its clear rejection of 'negative' medical models of madness. However, because it not only preserves, but also heightens and celebrates, the 'essential mystery' of schizophrenia, Laing's reading of schizophrenia as sublime experience can actually be seen to reinforce its status in psychiatric discourse. This is antipsychiatry's translation of sublime object into sublime ontology: bypassing any discussion of individual case histories or symptomatological profiles, *The Politics of Experience* posits schizophrenia not as comprehensible in personal, psychological terms (as for the early Laing, and many psychoanalysts) but as an essentially unmappable form of spiritually superior being. In psychiatry, schizophrenia's sublimity both incites and unsettles scientific investigation, thus facilitating the expansion of the discipline. In Laingian antipsychiatry, one should not so much interrogate schizophrenia as revere its role in facilitating the expansion of the psyche.

Outside its countercultural context, Laing's celebration of insanity as a spiritual journey of ego loss seems at best romantic and naive. Yet at Peter Sedgwick notes, within only a few years of *The Politics of Experience* 'virtually the entire left and an enormous proportion of the liberal-arts and social-studies reading public was convinced that R.D. Laing and his band of colleagues had produced novel and essentially accurate renderings of what psychotic experience truly signified' (Sedgwick, 1982, p. 6). Zbigniew Kotowicz also notes that Laing was 'elevated to stardom' by its publication and 'came to be perceived as a maverick guru of schizophrenics, a leader of society's vanguard who, through experiences of transcendental reality, would break out of the vicious circle in which the modern capitalist society imprisons its citizens' (Kotowicz, 1997, p. 2). As I have already suggested, analysts of antipsychiatry, Sedgwick and Kotowicz included, seldom probe or problematize its oppositional stance against mainstream psychiatry. Ironically, it is Thomas Szasz who, in his vitriolic critique of Laing and the socialist aspirations of Kingsley Hall, points out that Laingian antipsychiatry 'is, in some ways, the mirror image of the cult of modern institutional psychiatry. As in psychiatry the core concept, the sacred symbol, is "schizophrenia," so in antipsychiatry it is "authenticity"' (Szasz, 1976, p. 57),[21] an authenticity that is obtainable, so Laing maintains, through the schizophrenic voyage. Szasz continues:

> The antipsychiatrists' lack of imagination in inverting not only the logic and the vocabulary, but even the trappings, of psychiatry, and appropriating them all as their

---

[21] Would that Szasz thought through the implications of this critique with reference to his own work.

own 'original' theoretical principles and therapeutic methods provokes, in me at least, only contempt and pity.

(Szasz, 1976, p. 76)

Although I obviously do not share Szasz's sentiment, I agree that Laing's account of schizophrenia as an experience of the sublime does invert the logic, the vocabulary, and the trappings of psychiatry, but would argue that this says more about the inherent flexibility of psychiatry's clinical picture of schizophrenia than it does about any failure of imagination on Laing's part.

Underlying this chapter's analysis of the antipsychiatry movement, schizophrenia, and the sublime has been the supposition that to stake a claim on schizophrenia—as distinct from madness in general, or even from psychosis—is also to comment on its status in psychiatric and psychoanalytic discourse. In the case of antipsychiatry, a focus on psychological metatheory reveals three distinct trends. Szasz's position explicitly divests schizophrenia of any associations with the sublime, but in so doing it also denies that there is any such thing as a schizophrenic *experience* that can be meaningfully distinguished from everyday malingering. The intermediary view—Laing's analysis of schizophrenia in *The Divided Self*—hinges on the issue of understandability, paradoxically framing schizophrenic experience as anti-sublime (wholly intelligible) and sublime (because essentially beyond comprehension). Laing's subsequent valourization of schizophrenia *as* sublime experience resolves this tension by assigning schizophrenia an ontological status that is at once transcendent, mystical, and superior to an alienated existence. In so doing, it exposes and affirms psychiatry's construction of schizophrenia as sublime. Although there is no denying that antipsychiatric accounts of the origins of schizophrenia were theoretically at odds with the received wisdom of the day, the elasticity of psychiatry's definition of schizophrenia—a disease with no empirically certain cause or cure—was such that most of these could simply be absorbed into the grab bag of already competing theories. It would appear that antipsychiatrists either struggled to escape framing schizophrenia as a sublime or unknowable disorder, or succeeded in demystifying the psychiatric account of schizophrenia only to render the term virtually meaningless.

The sublime, then, offers a flexible framework through which to understand how the antipsychiatric critique of psychiatry and psychoanalysis remains complicit with these discourses at a 'meta' level. The significance of the antipsychiatry movement is not limited to the short-lived appearance of polemics, political conviction, and passion in the clinical setting. As Nick Crossley observes, while no one was forced to agree with antipsychiatry, and many in the medical establishment did not, 'nobody could carry on as before after antipsychiatry. The field of psychiatric contention was opened up for new, more critical trains of thought. The ground has moved and the paradigm shifted' (Crossley, 2006, p. 123). In addition to opening up new patient and survivor movements, one of the lasting achievements of antipsychiatry was to transform the ways in which schizophrenia could be conceptualized in non-clinical contexts. If schizophrenic symptoms registered particular effects of capitalism, psychiatric disciplinary power, families, and social life at large on the subject, or else were a means of rejecting or transcending the entire messy business of modernity, 'the schizophrenic' was suddenly available to take on multiple, potent, and hitherto unexploited symbolic roles. Of these, arguably the most notorious was as a revolutionary subject. Turning next to Deleuze and Guattari's analysis of capitalism and schizophrenia, we can see how the antipsychiatric critique of psychiatry extends to an anti-Oedipal critique of the whole psychological enterprise.

A final observation to close what is a pivotal chapter within the overall argument of this book. The narrative trajectory of *The Sublime Object of Psychiatry*—which flows from clinical psychiatry, to psychoanalysis, to antipsychiatry and cultural theory, concluding in the imaginative worlds of literary fiction—is, as I have emphasized repeatedly, by no means the only story that can or should be told about the concept of schizophrenia. Jonanathan Metzl's powerful book *The Protest Psychosis: How Schizophrenia Became a Black Disease* is an interdisciplinary study of the complex 'confluence of social and medical forces', which effected 'schizophrenia's rhetorical transformation from an illness of white feminine docility to one of black male hostility' in America during the civil rights era (2009, p. xv). Stokely Carmichael, who participated in the 1967 'Dialectics of Liberation' conference in London, is a key figure in Metzl's study (see especially pp. 121, 133–4) and represents the central point of overlap between our two very different accounts of how schizophrenia has been conceptualized across clinical and cultural domains throughout the twentieth century. Institutionalized racism, racialized diagnostic categories, protest, resistance, violence, hostility, marginalization, criminality, gender, race, and bodies are central concepts in *The Protest Psychosis*. It is telling that they hardly figure at all in the work of the cultural theorists under consideration in the next few chapters. Indeed, as we shall see, one of the hallmarks of what I have been calling cultural theory's 'figure of the schizophrenic' is that there is little sense at all of being a figure, of being embodied. One of the questions Metzl's work raises, and to which we shall return, is to what extent the highly abstracted 'figure of the schizophrenic' in cultural theory is therefore inextricably (if still invisibly) tied to whiteness.

Chapter 4

Anti-Oedipus and the politics of the schizophrenic sublime

To begin, a quotation:

> The schizo carries along the decoded flows, makes them traverse the desert of the body without organs, where he installs his desiring-machines and produces a perpetual outflow of acting forces. He has crossed over the limit, the schiz, which maintained the production of desire always at the margins of social production, tangential and always repelled . . . These men of desire—or do they not yet exist?—are like Zarathustra. They know incredible sufferings, vertigos, and sicknesses. They have their specters. They must reinvent each gesture. But such a man produces himself as a free man, irresponsible, solitary, and joyous, finally able to say and do something simple in his own name, without asking permission; a desire lacking nothing, a flux that overcomes barriers and codes, a name that no longer designates any ego whatever. He has simply ceased being afraid of becoming mad. He experiences and lives himself as the sublime sickness that will no longer affect him. Here, what is, what would a psychiatrist be worth?

> (Deleuze and Guattari, 1982, p. 131)

Anti-Oedipus: Capitalism and Schizophrenia (1982) is one of the most notorious philosophical works of the late twentieth century.[1] A collaboration between French philosopher Gilles Deleuze and Italian psychoanalyst and activist Félix Guattari, it was, as Ian Buchanan so beautifully puts it, an 'intellectual cluster bomb' lobbed into the fray of post-1968 French theory (Buchanan, 2008, p. 21). Deleuze and Guattari claim to have written their book for 15- to 20-year olds (Deleuze, 1990, pp. 7–8), and offer it as a tool for political struggle rather than a philosophical tract to be digested in its entirety. Whether *Anti-Oedipus* reached, engaged or mobilized into action its intended teenage audience I do not know, but it did succeed in sending shock waves through the academic establishment. Quite apart from its sensationalism—the scandalous treatment of Freud and Marx, striking but difficult style, intellectual hybridity, and almost manic exuberance—it played a decisive role in

---

[1] And has been cited over 2700 times in peer-reviewed publications in English (Google scholar search, 17 November 2010).

promoting schizophrenia as a paradigm through which to understand subjectivity in the late capitalist era.

Anti-Oedipus capitalized on the momentum of the antipsychiatry movement, extended its critique of psychiatric and psychoanalytic practice, and intensified its valorization of 'the schizophrenic' (or 'schizo') as a revolutionary and revelatory figure. Deleuze and Guattari's work marks a new moment in the history of revolutionary struggle, a moment in which *all* forms of social order (including class-based oppositional politics, identity politics, and even identity itself) are rejected as covertly totalitarian (Plant, 2001, p. 1097). In order to be true to its naturally rebellious state, desire had to be freed from the systems which sought to contain and redeploy it in the service of capitalism. Rather than reinvigorate or even redefine the revolutionary subject of Marxism, Deleuze and Guattari therefore advocated abandoning the notion of integrated subjectivity altogether, mobilizing instead the micro-political, machinic productivity of the unconscious in the struggle against capitalism.

Enter schizophrenia. Schizophrenia, in *Anti-Oedipus*, is a process of psychic deterritorialization which liberates desire from the straitjacket of Oedipus, a process that is simultaneously the realization of capitalism and its potential undoing. Schizophrenia provides the primary conceptual vehicle for Deleuze and Guattari's articulation of a radically decentred, desiring, and revolutionary form of (non)subjectivity, as well as the basis for a 'materialist psychiatry' that views desire in terms of production and production in terms of desire (Deleuze, quoted in Deleuze and Guattari, 1990, p. 17; see also Deleuze and Guattari, 1982, p. 5). Breaking with the psychoanalytic fixation on Oedipus, neurosis, and psychic interiority, Deleuze and Guattari's schizoanalysis aims 'to de-oedipalize the unconscious', 'to demonstrate the existence of an unconscious libidinal investment of sociohistorical production' (Deleuze and Guattari, 1982, pp. 81, 98) and 'to get revolutionary, artistic, and analytic machines working as parts, cogs, of one another' (Deleuze and Guattari, quoted in Deleuze 1990, p. 23).

Rather than locate *Anti-Oedipus* within its usual contexts—post-Marxism, post-modernism, the events of May 1968, and the oeuvre of Deleuze—this chapter approaches the text from the perspective of the interdisciplinary debates about schizophrenia that have so far been the focus of this book. With the publication of *A Thousand Plateaus* (volume two of *Capitalism and Schizophrenia* (1987), but a tome in which references to schizophrenia are practically non-existent), and the end of the antipsychiatric era, academics have evinced little interest in *Anti-Oedipus*'s many and complex representations of schizophrenia, and to my knowledge no one has engaged in any depth with the question of why Deleuze and Guattari assign this specific psychopathology such a central role in their analysis. My reading of schizophrenia in *Anti-Oedipus* considers how Deleuze and Guattari use schizophrenia strategically, but not unproblematically, to reconceptualize a revolutionary (non)subject, and to challenge psychoanalytic, antipsychiatric, and, by extension, psychiatric models of psychic health.

It is now not uncommon for Deleuze and Guattari's use of schizophrenia to be dismissed out of hand as deeply misguided or even something of an embarrassment.[2] Examining the portrayal of schizophrenia in *Anti-Oedipus* in the detail it deserves, however, enables us to identify two major tensions in their account of its subversive potential. The first concerns the relationship between the revolutionary form of schizophrenia distinct from its clinical counterpart. Deleuze and Guattari's thesis depends upon drawing a hard and fast distinction between a revolutionary form of schizophrenia ('the schizo') and its pathological correlates ('the paranoid' and 'the schizophrenic'). Focusing on the internal contradictions present in Deleuze and Guattari's reading of Schreber's *Memoirs* (1955), I will argue that because the differentiation of these three forms of anoedipal subjectivity is in fact highly unstable, it is almost impossible to safeguard dynamic modes of schizophrenic (non)subjectivity from descending into paralysis or pathology. The second area of tension is found at the level of metatheory, in the way Deleuze and Guattari make their model of agency contingent upon schizophrenia's association with the sublime. Schizophrenia's political efficacy—its capacity not simply to represent capitalism but to destroy it—is for Deleuze and Guattari a function of its sublimity, of being outside and beyond representation, capitalism, Oedipus, identity, and psychoanalytic reach. The key question here is how effective a politics founded on the sublime could be. In what follows, then, my aim is to demonstrate that in its proximity to clinical accounts of psychosis, Deleuze and Guattari's model of a revolutionary form of schizophrenia is doubly problematic: first because it cannot be defended against becoming 'mere' pathology, and secondly because its political efficacy is dependent on, and I suggest limited by, its association with the sublime.

---

2 Although the launch of a new journal, *Deleuze Studies,* and two publications of Deleuze and Guattari's work from this period may well reverse this trend. As the name suggests, *The Anti-Oedipus Papers* (Guattari, 2006) is primarily a collection of the letters and notes sent by Guattari to Deleuze during the course of writing the book. Deleuze annotated and returned the letters, which read at times as a veritable collage of ideas. One of the highlights of *Two Regimes of Madness* (Deleuze, 2006) is the brief piece 'Schizophrenia and Society', written in 1975 for the *Encyclopaedia Universalis.* It is undoubtedly the most succinct and accessible account of their view of schizophrenia, and, in my view, puts an end to many of the misconceptions surrounding their attitude towards the term.

Introducing schizophrenia and capitalism

Although their critique of psychoanalysis owes much to Michel Foucault's *Madness and Civilization* (1993), Deleuze and Guattari eschew trans-historical terms like madness, unreason, and even psychosis, instead staking their claim on that quintessentially twentieth-century psychopathology: schizophrenia. The authors' attachment to psychiatric taxonomy belies their irreverence towards the psychiatric establishment—unpacking the term 'schizophrenia' in *Anti-Oedipus* requires not that we understand neural circuitry or theories of heredity, but the double or paradoxical operation of capitalism. According to Deleuze and Guattari, the capitalist machine is constantly breaking down codes and dismantling historically meaningful social structures to permit the free flow of capital and labour. At the same time, in order to function, it must reterritorialize the social sphere, re-establish 'artificial' codes and re-channel desire. Deleuze and Guattari identify two poles of libidinal investment possible under capitalism—one paranoid molar (the drive to restore or re-impose meaning, codes, and structures), the other a 'molecular schizophrenic line of escape' (Deleuze and Guattari, 1982, p. 315). Schizophrenia, then, is the process of psychic and social deterritorialization unleashed by capitalism; it is capitalism's 'deepest tendency' but its absolute limit, 'its difference, its divergence, and its death' (Deleuze and Guattari, 1982, p. 245).[3] Because it knows no 'I' and no ego, schizophrenia is synonymous with a true or original desire, which precedes the Oedipal configuration of mother–father–child. Schizophrenia is disjunction as opposed to synthesis, reality as opposed to representation, an 'either ... or ... or' of seemingly unlimited possibilities (Deleuze and Guattari, 1982, pp. 12, 76, ellipses in the original).

Deleuze and Guattari outline three figures produced by or in relation to schizophrenia-as-process: 'the schizo', 'the paranoid', and 'the schizophrenic'. 'The schizo' is the realization or embodiment of the process of schizophrenia.

---

[3] 'What we are really trying to say', write Deleuze and Guattari (1982, p. 34), 'is that capitalism, through its process of production, produces an awesome schizophrenic accumulation of energy or charge, against which it brings all its vast powers of repression to bear, but which nonetheless continues to act as capitalism's limit. For capitalism constantly counteracts, constantly inhibits this inherent tendency while at the same time allowing it free rein; it continually seeks to avoid reaching its limit while simultaneously tending towards that limit. Capitalism institutes or restores all sorts of residual and artificial, imaginary, or symbolic territorialities ...', which is why the boundary-less schizophrenia functions as its absolute limit. As Jean-François Lyotard (1977, p.25) notes, 'Schizophrenia is called the *absolute limit*, because if it ever happened, it would be force undistributed in a libidinal network, pure liquid inflexion'.

He (for in *Anti-Oedipus*, 'the schizo' is always assigned the masculine pronoun) is the 'universal producer'; an atheist, nomad, and orphan; a figure who explodes the 'Oedipal genealogy' and traverses deterritorialized space with an idiosyncratic set of co-ordinates (Seem, introduction to Deleuze and Guattari, 1982, p. xxi). Because the 'code of delirium or of desire proves to have an extraordinary fluidity', 'the schizo', like a digital virus, is subversive and continually on the move; 'he deliberately *scrambles all the codes*', parodying, parroting, and breaking apart the social systems he inhabits (Deleuze and Guattari, 1982, p. 15, italics in the original). Revolution is 'the schizo's' prerogative: he 'deliberately seeks out the very limit of capitalism: he is its inherent tendency brought to fulfilment, its surplus product, its proletariat, and its exterminating angel' (Deleuze and Guattari, 1982, p. 35). Deleuze and Guattari contrast this dynamic, romantic figure with two further anoedipal subjects: 'the paranoid' and 'the schizophrenic'. 'The paranoid' directly opposes the process of schizophrenia by overcoding desire, viewing the entire world through the prism of an individual ego, and reinstating a master or 'despotic' signifier as the source of all meaning. Although from the perspective of psychiatry schizophrenia has always encompassed paranoia as a subtype, *Anti-Oedipus* shares the psychoanalytic tendency to differentiate paranoia from schizophrenia, but goes further in positioning the two in diametric opposition. What, then, of 'the schizophrenic', the 'artificial', or the 'sick' schizo? For Deleuze and Guattari, 'the schizophrenic' is the *interruption* of schizophrenia-as-process; the outcome of trying and failing to break through social and psychic repression. 'The hospital schiz, the great autistic one, the clinical entity that "lacks" Oedipus', is like an 'immense transfixed hippopotamus who will not come back up to the surface' (Deleuze and Guattari, 1982, p. 136). Catatonic, a body without organs,[4] impassive, and withdrawn, 'the schizophrenic' is 'the schizo' who has been re-absorbed or trapped in the capitalist system (Deleuze and Guattari, 1982, p. 245).[5]

---

[4] For Deleuze and Guattari, 'The full body without organs is the unproductive, the sterile, the unengendered, the unconsumable' (Deleuze and Guattari, 1982, p. 8). It is not a body as such, or the image of a body, but designates a 'zero-degree of intensity, a moment of antiproduction fed back into the process of production' (Bogue, 1989, p. 93). Deleuze and Guattari borrow the term from Antonin Artaud's 1946 poem 'To Have Done with the Judgement of God' (Artaud, 1976).

[5] It is seldom acknowledged that Deleuze and Guattari were not the first to emphasize a structural continuity between schizophrenia and capitalism. Joseph Gabel's *False Consciousness*, first published in French in 1962, synthesized clinical psychiatry and Marxism to draw a 'sociopathological parallelism' between schizophrenia and false consciousness. Drawing on the work of his mentor Eugene Minkowski (an existential-phenomenological psychiatrist who was an important influence also for R.D. Laing and

Sidelining and sanitizing schizophrenia

Broadly speaking, the academic establishment has responded to the concept of schizophrenia and its clinical connotations in *Anti-Oedipus* fleetingly or with marked discomfort (see Braidotti, 2005; Colebrook, 2002, 2006; Patton, 2001). Deleuze and Guattari's critics have dismissed their use of psychiatric terminology as 'uncritical, illegitimate, and simply imprecise' (Rajchman, 1977, p. 46); 'irresponsible and insensitive to the human costs of this illness' (Glass, 1993, p. 15) and plausible only as myth or fantasy (Elliott, 2002, pp. 157–63; Frank, 2001, p. 1272).[6] Those more sympathetic to Deleuze and Guattari's project have eschewed literalism in favour of a tropic reading of their work, insisting that the schizophrenia Deleuze and Guattari write about has nothing to do with the schizophrenia that affects on average one in one hundred people. Sylvère Lotringer, who devoted an entire issue of *Semiotext(e)* to *Anti-Oedipus*, therefore defines schizophrenia 'loosely, and not clinically, as the uncontrollable, polymorphous movement of desire' (Lotringer, 1977, p. 8), whereas Brian Massumi sees it as 'the enlargements of life's limits through the pragmatic proliferation of concepts' (Massumi, 1992, pp. 1, 92). Eugene Holland's otherwise authoritative work on *Anti-Oedipus* goes furthest in this figurative tradition (see Holland, 1985–1986; 1988; 1998; 1999). Despite Deleuze and Guattari's many references to psychiatric, psychoanalytic, antipsychiatric,

---

Louis Sass), Gabel argued that: 'Schizophrenia ... in fact clearly represents a form of reified consciousness, characterized on the existential level by a deterioration of dialectical praxis, and on the intellectual level by a de-dialecticization of cognitive functions, a phenomenon described long ago by E. Minkowski as *morbid rationalism* [1927]. The appropriate rationality of false consciousness, characterized by a loss of the dialectical quality of thought is therefore clearly a social form of morbid rationalism; inversely, I consider the onset of schizophrenia as an individual form of false consciousness. The mental state therefore constitutes a real bridge between the areas of social and clinical alienation; it is a form of alienation both in the Marxist sense and in the psychiatric meaning of the term' (Gabel, 1976, p.xx–xxi). Deleuze and Guattari reference one of Gabel's independently published case studies but curiously do not refer to *False Consciousness*, even though Gabel's use of schizophrenia to show the congruence between psychiatric and social forms of alienation resonates with their account of 'the schizophrenic' as described above. For a comprehensive introduction to Gabel's work, see Sica (1995).

6   If anything, Gabel's work, though much less widely read, was even more vehemently rejected: 'Gabel's identification of schizophrenia, reification, ideology, and false consciousness is ultimately ludicrous [. . .] and it is a travesty of Marxist thought to conflate the highly complex notion of ideology with such an extreme form of mental illness as schizophrenia' (Swingewood, 1977, p. 224).

fictional, and autobiographical accounts of schizophrenia,[7] Holland argues that a better analogy for this deterritorializing process is improvisational jazz. 'When references are made . . . in *Anti-Oedipus* . . . to schizophrenia as the principle of freedom', Holland writes, 'readers should think of jazz, which represents a fulfilment of the process of schizophrenia' and 'an ideal instance of human relations and interpersonal dynamics' (Holland, 1999, p. xi). Although Holland's metaphor is not wholly incompatible with the spirit of schizophrenia-as-process (even if it is, as he acknowledges, insufficiently political), it completely misses the specificity, and hence the complexity, of Deleuze and Guattari's account of schizophrenia's different manifestations.

If there is one compelling reason immediately to be wary of efforts to sanitize schizophrenia in *Anti-Oedipus*, and of critics seeking to divest the term of its potentially unpleasant clinical connotations, it is Félix Guattari (see Guattari, 1996c). Beyond his collaboration with Deleuze, Guattari is perhaps best known as a militant antipsychiatrist and a forceful critic of the residual humanism and perceived political weaknesses of the antipsychiatry movement. Although sympathetic to Laing, Guattari saw in his retreat to mysticism a failure to realize the potential of his earlier theoretical insights, and dismissed the Kingsley Hall experiment as misguided in its reinstatement of Oedipal structures and its emphasis on decoding the secrets of psychosis (Guattari, 1996a, d). He writes:

> Let's hope that Laing, who has sought to dissociate himself in an exemplary fashion from the traditional role of the psychiatrist, returns to the concrete struggle against the repression of the mentally ill and that he will be able to define more rigorously the conditions of a revolutionary psychiatric practice, that is, of a non-utopian psychiatry that is susceptible to being taken up en masse by the avant garde of mental health workers and by the mentally ill themselves.

> (Guattari, 1996d, p. 51)

Guattari admired aspects of the institutional reforms achieved by Italian antipsychiatrist Franco Basaglia, but thought it important never to lose sight of the madness of madness and the dangers of reducing mental alienation to social alienation (Guattari, 1996b, p. 44). According to Gary Genosko, Guattari considered Germany's radical SPK (*Sozialistisches Patienten Kollektiv*) exemplary of the ideals of antipsychiatry because they 'established an inextricable

---

[7] These include references to the psychiatric textbooks of Kraepelin and Bleuler; the work of Freud, Lacan, Tausk, Jung, Klein, and others in the psychoanalytic tradition; the antipsychiatric case studies and political treatises of Laing and Cooper; the 'schizophrenic' style and sensibility of the Beat poets, DH Lawrence, Henry Miller, and Samuel Beckett; and finally, to the autobiographical accounts of schizophrenia published by Antonin Artaud, Vaslav Nijkinsky, and Daniel Paul Schreber. It is perhaps little wonder that 'the schizo', in *Anti-Oedipus*, should bear the masculine pronoun.

link between political struggle and mental illness, making madness the concern of everyone' (Genosko, introduction to Guattari, 1996c, pp. 4, 7). In addition to his involvement in the antipsychiatry movement, Guattari's concern for madness also encompassed a strong therapeutic dimension, for as a practising Lacanian analyst, he spent almost 40 years working with psychotic patients at the Clinique de la Borde. In an interview in the year *Anti-Oedipus* was published, Guattari went so far as to identify one of his four major intellectual influences as "'a sort of schizoid background or discourse'". "'I'd always liked schizophrenics, been drawn to them'", he said, "'You have to live with them to understand this. Schizophrenics do at least, unlike neurotics, have real problems'" (Guattari quoted in Deleuze and Guattari, 1990, pp. 14–15). With one half of cultural theory's most dynamic duo so intimately involved with the 'problem' of schizophrenia, it becomes difficult to sustain the claim that they use the term arbitrarily or remain wholly insensitive to its lived reality, regardless of how shocking their use of the term 'schizophrenia' may now appear to some.

Guattari's extensive clinical experience with and academic attraction to schizophrenia should also prompt us to suspect that 'the schizo'—and its anoedipal 'others', 'the paranoid' and 'the schizophrenic'—do not float as free from clinical discourse as many a Deleuzoguattarian might suggest (see Bogue, 1989, p. 8). Indeed, it is arguable that the three forms of anoedipal subjectivity identified by Deleuze and Guattari are in fact loosely adapted from schizophrenia's three original diagnostic categories—hebephrenia, paranoia, and catatonia. The similarities between Deleuze and Guattari's process of schizophrenia and hebephrenic (now called 'disorganised' or 'undifferentiated') schizophrenia are particularly suggestive. Kraepelin identified hebephrenia as the most common form of schizophrenia, particularly prominent in younger people who 'exhibit a marked restlessness', 'leave their work, stroll about or travel from place to place', and 'indulge in illicit and promiscuous intercourse' (Kraepelin, 1981, p. 231). Although Kraepelin's tone here is disapproving rather than celebratory, it is not difficult to see how this description of hebephrenia resonates with the antics of 'the schizo':

> In *conduct* and *behavior*, the most characteristic symptom is that of childish silliness and senseless laughter . . . At one moment patients are increasingly headstrong, at the next as supremely tractable. They neglect their personal appearance, perform all sorts of outlandish and foolish deeds, such as prowling about all night, setting fire to buildings, throwing stones to break windows, and travelling about without evident purpose. [. . .] The patients are very often seen to converse with themselves, sometimes aloud, while associated with this there is almost always silly laughter.
>
> (Kraepelin, 1981, p. 234)

If the symptomatology is a match with 'the schizo', so too is the hebephrenia patient's failure to be productive in a capitalist economy, for even if they recover, 'the patients fail to employ themselves profitably. They spend much time in reading, evolving impractical schemes, and pondering over abstract and useless questions' (Kraepelin, 1981, p. 240).

With these clinical antecedents in mind, and in order to develop a more accurate and nuanced understanding of the multiple forms of schizophrenia in *Anti-Oedipus*, our focus now turns to Deleuze and Guattari's direct engagement with competing clinical accounts of psychosis. It should come as no surprise that the key figure here is again Daniel Paul Schreber. Deleuze and Guattari introduce us to Schreber in the first paragraph of *Anti-Oedipus* and return to him repeatedly: he is at the forefront of their efforts to explain schizophrenia and at the heart of their quarrel with psychoanalysis. Tracking Schreber through the labyrinth of *Anti-Oedipus*, we can see that the point at which the distinctions between 'the schizo', 'the paranoid', and 'the schizophrenic' should be most obvious is in fact the point at which they begin to collapse.

Deleuze, Guattari, Schreber

Deleuze and Guattari's engagement with *Memoirs of My Nervous Illness* is as much a strategic repudiation of psychoanalytic accounts of psychosis as it is a close reading of Schreber's autobiography. In Chapter 2, I discussed at length the detail of Freud's and Lacan's interpretation of the case of Schreber; here, a brief summary of their positions will suffice. In his reading of *Memoirs*, Freud singled out Schreber's feelings of persecution, and his belief that God was transforming him into a woman, as the two most salient facets of a vastly complex delusional system. In Schreber's case, writes Freud, 'The exciting cause of his illness . . . was an outburst of homosexual libido; the object of this libido was probably from the very first his doctor . . . and [Schreber's] struggles against the libidinal impulse produced the conflict which gave rise to the symptoms' (Freud, 1981, p. 43). Freud goes on to argue that Schreber's assumption of a feminine attitude towards God 'had its roots in a longing, intensified to an erotic pitch, for his father and brother' (Freud, 1981, p. 50)—it is, in short, the father complex, which gives rise to psychosis. For Lacan, by contrast, the origin of psychosis lies not with homosexual longing, but with the subject's failure to enter the realm of phallic signification. The child's entry into language and Oedipal development depends on the symbolic intervention of the Name-of-the-Father in the imaginary mother–child dyad. For psychotic patients, this intervention has failed: 'It is an accident in [the symbolic] register', 'the foreclosure of the

Name-of-the-Father' and 'the failure of the paternal metaphor that . . . gives psychosis its essential condition, and the structure that separates it from neurosis' (Lacan, 1966, p. 215).

Lacan suggests that Schreber's early promotion and his failure to have children raised the question of whether or not he would become a father (Lacan, 1993, pp. 320–1). Once asked, this question was unable to be answered; it exposed a hole where the Name-of-the-Father would otherwise have been, a hole which flagrant psychotic symptoms try unsuccessfully to fill. Lacan astutely observed that 'every author has . . . attempted to explain the onset of Schreber's delusion with reference to the father' (Lacan, 1993, p. 212). The relevance of paternity and paternal authority to the Schreber case was in the 1950s given a new twist by William Niederland, who revealed that Schreber's father advocated an authoritarian, disciplinarian, and deeply patriarchal pedagogical programme, regulating his children's posture, slumber, and play through straps, braces, and other restrictive devices (see Niederland, 1984; Schatzman, 1973). Were Schreber's delusions of persecution not so delusional after all? By the time *Anti-Oedipus*'s was published, the paternal-paranoid reading of Schreber had reached its zenith in Elias Canetti's *Crowds and Power* (1962). Canetti persuasively argued that Schreber's extreme psychic disturbances—corporeal miracles, enslavement by a despotic God, but most significantly, his drive for power—were a naked revelation of the psychology of fascism.

Freud, Lacan, Niederland, and Canetti all offered compelling readings of Schreber's paranoid symptomatology, but as we have seen, the issue of how best to account for the greater complexity of Schreber's delusional system is still far from resolved. In Chapter 2, I argued that the psychoanalytic emphasis on the symbolic significance of psychotic symptoms—a practice nowhere more clearly displayed than in studies of *Memoirs*—produces schizophrenia itself as a sublime text subject to endless re-interpretation. Deleuze and Guattari's intervention in the Schreber debate is central to *Anti-Oedipus* and short-circuits the textual sublime in two ways. First, in refusing to cast the father in the principal pathogenic role, Deleuze and Guattari claim to rescue Schreber from being 'posthumously oedipalized' (Deleuze and Guattari, 1982, p. 57) at the hands of Freud, Lacan, and other psychoanalysts. 'How does one dare reduce to the paternal theme a delirium so rich, so differentiated, so "divine" as the Judge's . . .?' they ask (Deleuze and Guattari, 1982, p. 56). Dogmatic in its adherence to orthodoxy, psychoanalysis,

> . . . continues to ask its questions and develop its interpretations from the depths of the Oedipal triangle as its basic perspective, even though today it is acutely aware that this frame of reference is not adequate to explain so-called psychotic phenomena.

> The psychoanalyst says that we must *necessarily* discover Schreber's daddy beneath his
> superior God, and doubtless also his elder brother beneath his inferior God.
>
> (Deleuze and Guattari, 1982, p. 14, italics in the original)

Deleuze and Guattari not only critique as narrow and repressive the Oedipal framework at operation here, but more radically, at a metatheoretical level, they reject the psychoanalytic approach to psychic phenomena as encoded texts. To interpret delusions as literature, they argue, misses the point.[8] Rather than scrutinize delusion for proof of an underlying trauma sustained in infancy, or aim to uncover the psychosexual symbolism of a particular hallucination, the schizoanalyst acknowledges what 'Judge Schreber would not deny', namely, that 'every delirium is first of all the investment of a field that is social, economic, political, cultural, racial and racist, pedagogical, and religious' (Deleuze and Guattari, 1982, p. 274). Schreber cannot be understood via Oedipus, the father complex, or the Name-of-the-Father because he is, for the authors of *Anti-Oedipus*, 'the schizo' par excellence.

Schreber's status in *Anti-Oedipus* as the exemplary 'schizo' is clear from the playful and irreverent opening paragraph:

> Judge Schreber has sunbeams in his ass. *A solar anus.* And rest assured that it works: Judge
> Schreber feels something, produces something, and is capable of explaining the process
> theoretically. Something is produced: the effects of a machine, not mere metaphor.
>
> (Deleuze and Guattari, 1982, p. 2, italics in the original)

This is 'schizo' as universal producer—out for a stroll (never mind that it is within the grounds of the Sonnenstein asylum), plugged into the world, dissolving the boundaries between self and other, interior and exterior. This is 'the schizo' whose somatic hallucinations we must view literally, not as literature, for: 'The breasts on the judge's naked torso are neither delirious nor hallucinatory phenomena: they designate, first of all, a band of intensity, a zone of intensity on his body without organs' (Deleuze and Guattari, 1982, p. 19). Deleuze and Guattari continue:

> Nothing here [i.e. in the case of Schreber] is representative; rather, it is all life and lived
> experience: the actual, lived emotion of having breasts does not resemble breasts, it
> does not represent them . . . Nothing but bands of intensity, potentials, thresholds,
> and gradients. A harrowing, emotionally overwhelming experience, which brings the
> schizo as close as possible to matter, to a burning, living centre of matter. . .
>
> (Deleuze and Guattari, 1982, p. 19)

---

8 Although Deleuze and Guattari's references to Schreber make it appear as though he is personally known to them, they fail to acknowledge here that, like Freud, they can *only* know Schreber through/as the text of *Memoirs*.

The fragmented body lashed by sensory intensities does not stand *for* anything, just as Schreber's 'nerve-contact' with (among others) 'the Pope', '240 Benedictine Monks', 'a Viennese nerve specialist', 'a baptized Jew and Slavophile' (Schreber, 1955, p. 70) has nothing to do with the closed circuit of the domestic Oedipal drama and everything to do with history. Before 'being crushed in the psychiatric and psychoanalytic treadmill', 'all delirium possesses a world-historical, political, and racial content, mixing and sweeping along races, cultures, continents, and kingdoms' (Deleuze and Guattari, 1982, pp. 274, 88, see also 352, 362, 365). The psychological interpretation of psychotic symptoms is therefore misguided, as Guattari elsewhere suggests,

> . . . it is illusory to hope to recover raw desire, pure and simple, by embarking on a search for the knots hidden in the unconscious and the secret keys of interpretation. Nothing can unravel, by the sole magic of the transference, the real micropolitical conflicts in which the subject is imprisoned; no mystery, no hidden universe. There is nothing to discover in the unconscious. The unconscious is something to be built.

> (Guattari, 1996d, pp. 51–2)[9]

Schreber, like Samuel Beckett's characters and the narrators of Beat fiction, lives out this de-personalized, de-psychologized desire in an untrammelled form. Forget the confines of the nursery or the Greek amphitheatre; 'the schizo' is connected to the world. It is no longer a question of *fin de siècle* Germany or even of modernity per se: 'No one has ever been as deeply involved in history as the schizo, or dealt with it in this way. He consumes all of universal history in one fell swoop' (Deleuze and Guattari, 1982, p. 21).

Deleuze and Guattari pitch 'schizo' Schreber against the oedipalized paranoid Schreber of Freud and Lacan, but do they successfully reconcile Schreber's fantastically rich delusional structure with his account of years of incarceration, with his periods of catatonic stupor, and with his own experience of mutism and autistic withdrawal? Rhetorical questions regarding the relationship between 'the schizo' and 'schizophrenic' are posed no less than eight times in *Anti-Oedipus* (Deleuze and Guattari, 1982, pp. 24, 67–8, 88, 91, 123, 130, 136, 319, 362), hinting at an element of authorial anxiety on this score. 'Schizo' and 'schizophrenic' are certainly portrayed as polar opposites: the former is a 'free man, irresponsible, solitary, and joyous . . . a desire lacking nothing, a flux that overcomes barriers and codes, a name that no longer designates any ego whatever' (Deleuze and Guattari, 1982, p. 130); the latter, the sick 'schizophrenic', is an immense transfixed hippopotamus, a static dead-end, a pitiable creature confined to an asylum. 'The schizophrenic' is the interruption or blockage of the process of schizophrenia; someone whose attempted psychic breakthrough

---

[9] But *not* built through the acts of representation or interpretation.

culminated in psychic breakdown. Is it possible, then, even by Deleuze and Guattari's own criteria, to say with certainty that Schreber is all 'schizo' and not at all 'schizophrenic'?

Such a claim, as I discussed at length in Chapter 2, captures only a fraction of Schreber's experience. In *Memoirs*, Schreber himself spares no detail in recounting his mental agony and anguish, manifested at times in long periods when he made 'absolute passivity' his duty (Schreber, 1955, p. 145). Furthermore, despite the obvious limitations of the psychoanalytic emphasis on paternity, Schreber's delusional system is neither as diverse nor as arbitrary as *Anti-Oedipus* implies. Central to Schreber's paranoid world-view is an unrelenting attempt to re-channel desire in a heavenly duty towards God, and to prove to a sceptical scientific and psychiatric establishment the validity of his divinity and the truth of his master code. Addressing then-contemporary legal and psychiatric issues, Schreber's delirium is also not as universally valid as Deleuze and Guattari would suggest, but is framed within a modern positivist logic. In addition, at different stages of his 'nervous illness', Schreber displays many if not all of the symptoms of hebephrenia, paranoia, and catatonia, Kraepelinian psychiatry's three subtypes of dementia praecox. Deleuze and Guattari posit a resolute distinction between 'the schizo'—their hebephrenic hero—the proto-fascistic 'paranoid' and the catatonic 'autistic rag'. However, if Schreber can simultaneously be thought of as schizo-revolutionary, paranoid-fascist, *and* as a catatonic hippopotamus, it becomes virtually impossible to sustain the idea of a radical discontinuity between 'schizo', 'schizophrenic', and 'paranoid'. These anoedipal figures not only seem far less removed from the clinic than their critics claim, but also far more closely connected than Deleuze and Guattari allow. And, as we shall see, if the boundaries between revolution and catatonia are potentially so porous, the political efficacy Deleuze and Guattari attribute the process of schizophrenia is in turn called into question.

A politics of the sublime

If the first and hitherto unacknowledged problem with Deleuze and Guattari's account of revolutionary schizophrenia is its interconnectedness with (distinctly non-revolutionary) paranoia and catatonia, the second major tension can be found at the level of metatheory. Although there are of course significant methodological and theoretical divergences between and within the fields of psychiatry, psychoanalysis, and many forms of antipsychiatry, all approach schizophrenia as an aberration, an exception to the norm that is the result of a neurological, psychobiographical, or sociological problem.[10] By arguing that it

---

[10] The exception here is Laingian antipsychiatry, which I discuss in more detail later.

is the direct or unfettered expression of a naturally rebellious desire, Deleuze and Guattari depathologize the process of schizophrenia and imply that the search for its origins *as pathology* is no longer necessary. In the most general sense, the claim that schizophrenia is a deterritorializing process analogous as well as antagonistic to the operation of capitalism swiftly dismisses the interdisciplinary debate concerning its aetiology.

Assuming rather than demonstrating the obvious inadequacy of psychiatry's accounts of schizophrenia, Deleuze and Guattari, as the title of their book suggests, identify psychoanalysis and not psychiatry as the discourse worthy of attack. Guattari 'had always liked' 'schizophrenics', Freud had always 'hated' them (Deleuze and Guattari, 1982, p. 23),[11] and it is possible that this perceived hostility to schizophrenia immediately qualified it as an object of theoretical interest. Deleuze and Guattari use Schreber—who was for Freud and Lacan the paradigmatic case of psychosis—to expose the structural limitations of psychoanalysis on multiple fronts. Theoretically, they reject Oedipus (the idea that the father complex or Name-of-the-Father plays a determining part in psychosis); metatheoretically, they challenge the very assumption that schizophrenic symptoms are amenable to the kind of literary analysis so important to psychoanalysts. Psychoanalysis, by its own admission, can only offer to psychotic patients an Oedipal interpretation of paranoid symptomatology; schizoanalysis, as the case of Schreber makes clear, has no truck with interpretation (psychobiographical or otherwise) or with the production of schizophrenia-as-text.[12] But there is yet another layer here: the fact that the process of schizophrenia is beyond the therapeutic, and to some extent analytic, reach of psychoanalysis is, I would argue, precisely what makes it politically attractive to Deleuze and Guattari.[13] Exceeding the theoretical and therapeutic

---

[11] Freud, in a letter to Istvan Hollos in 1928 (quoted in Dupont, 1988, p.251) wrote "'I did not like those patients . . . They made me angry and I find myself irritated to experience them so distant from myself and from all that is human. This is an astonishing intolerance which brands me a poor psychiatrist'". Guattari in an interview observed that "'Many inner struggles in the psychoanalytic movement would be understood if Freud's fundamental hostility toward psychosis were finally acknowledged'" (Guattari and Munster, 1977, p. 79).

[12] Even if this move, as I suggested earlier, belies the fact that Schreber is known to Deleuze and Guattari only as and through texts.

[13] Derrida makes a similar observation with regard to Foucault's choice of focus in *Madness and Civilization*: 'If Foucault . . . mentions, under the name of madness, only schizophrenia and psychosis, it is because psychoanalysis most often approaches these only in order to acknowledge its own limit: a forbidden or impossible access. This limit defines psychoanalysis. Its intimacy with madness par excellence is an intimacy with the least intimate, a nonintimacy that relates it to what is most heterogeneous, to that which in no

parameters of psychoanalysis is evidence that schizophrenia-as-process is not (perhaps can not be) co-opted by the social order; proof of its disruptive and hence revolutionary potential. The schizoanalytic *valorisation* of the anoedipal, disconnected, ego-less nature of the schizophrenic process depends in part, I am suggesting, on its status as sublime within the psychoanalytic discourse Deleuze and Guattari seek to contest.

Deleuze and Guattari's 'schizo' is exemplary as a revolutionary figure only in so far as 'he' exists outside the structures of psychic and social repression. In the broadest sense, their schizo-as-outsider radicalizes R.D. Laing's model of schizophrenia as an experience of the sublime, a transcendent experience, a voyage into inner psychic space. 'I am aware', wrote Laing in *The Divided Self*, 'that the man who is said to be deluded may be in his delusion telling me the truth, and this in no equivocal or metaphorical sense, but quite literally, and that the cracked mind of the schizophrenic may *let in* light which does not enter the intact minds of many sane people whose minds are closed' (Laing, 1990, p. 27). Pursuing the theme of schizophrenia as enlightenment, Laing famously asserted in *The Politics of Experience* that 'what we call "schizophrenia" was one of the forms in which, often through quite ordinary people, the light began to break through the cracks in our all-too-closed minds' (Laing, 1967, p. 129). The potency, agency, and oppositionality assigned to the 'schizo' by Deleuze and Guattari testifies to the influence of Laing's account of schizophrenia as a form of emancipation, a mode of being closer to the truth of human existence (or desire) than so-called normality, and a subjective state which contains within it the potential to dismantle the codes of capitalism.

So, Deleuze and Guattari extend the antipsychiatric celebration of schizophrenia as a sublime experience, while simultaneously utilizing and challenging the account of schizophrenia as a sublime text subject to psychoanalytic interpretation but not therapeutic intervention. The 'schizo' *works* as a paradigm for revolutionary desire—to the extent that it does—*because* of schizophrenia's association with the sublime in clinical discourses. However, as I have argued, the porous or unstable boundaries between the 'schizo', 'paranoid', and catatonic 'schizophrenic' make a politics based on schizophrenia highly problematic. If every 'schizo' is in danger of becoming an 'immense transfixed hippopotamus', then escaping Oedipus and embracing the flux of desire is not without significant risks. The agency of 'the schizo' cannot be guaranteed. It is not clear, ultimately, *what* exactly interrupts the process of schizophrenia—transforming 'schizo' into 'schizophrenic'—and consequently

---

way lets itself be interiorized, nor even subjectified: neither alienated, I would say, nor inalienable' (Derrida, 1978, p. 107).

it remains unclear whether anything can be done to forestall or avoid this.[14] Like sides of a mobius strip, 'schizo' and 'schizophrenic' are too closely connected, too intimately interlinked to be meaningfully separated.

Even if this tension were able to be resolved, schizophrenia's association with the sublime presents further significant problems for the radical politics Deleuze and Guattari espouse. Schizophrenia may be capitalism's 'deepest tendency' but more importantly it is also, according to Deleuze and Guattari, 'its difference, its divergence, and its death' (Deleuze and Guattari, 1982, p. 245). To gain and maintain this revolutionary agency, schizophrenia must in some sense remain resolutely exterior to capitalism; it must exceed the boundaries of social and psychic organization, refuse interpretation and interpretive closure, resist therapeutic intervention and theoretical representation. This is certainly an anti-fascist mode of being, as Foucault famously declared in the preface to *Anti-Oedipus*, but it is anti almost everything else as well. This model takes the concept of micro-politics to new extremes, radically undermining all forms of collective and individual political action. As Anthony Elliott notes, at the most basic level 'blueprints for social and political transformation will be unsuccessful because such activity and planning will necessarily involve a paranoiac encoding of desire' (Elliott, 2002, p. 160). Similarly, Reidar Due worries that the idealized 'schizo' is 'so radically immanent within its own circuits of desire that it can hardly be given the political task of challenging existing forms of power' (Due, 2007, p. 115). Hence the conundrum: to be revolutionary, the process of schizophrenia must be sublime, but to be politically effective and not simply anarchic, it must—even if partially and provisionally—reconstitute social, psychic, and organizational boundaries.

Schizophrenia, in *Anti-Oedipus*, does not function as a single notion, a thing to be appraised in isolation. It is, rather, a concept that connects a new vision of subjectivity to capitalism, to the revolution, to the antipsychiatric politics of the day, and to a psychoanalysis found wanting on multiple fronts. Deleuze and Guattari's work is distinctive in what we might broadly term 'postmodern'

---

[14] This is a point worth emphasizing. 'What makes the schizophrenic ill, since the cause of the illness is not schizophrenia as a process? What transforms the breakthrough into a breakdown?' (Deleuze and Guattari, 1982, p. 362) The answer, for Deleuze and Guattari, is that 'capitalist production is constantly arresting the schizophrenic process and transforming the subject of the process into a confined clinical entity' (Deleuze and Guattari, 1982, p. 245). Or, as Buchanan puts it, 'it is not the schizophrenic process that makes the schizo ill . . . but the environment in which he or she finds himself in' (Buchanan, 2008, pp. 35–6). In my mind, the failure to specify what, precisely, in the capitalist environment causes 'the schizo's' breakthrough—sometimes but not always—to end in schizophrenic breakdown, is the most pressing unanswered question to be addressed to *Anti-Oedipus*.

theory: they alone assign the 'schizo' a heroic role as the one who escapes psychic repression, remains true to desire, and has the potential to push capitalism to and past its limits. However, their model remains free from contradiction only on the condition that any and all previous notions of how radical political action might function effectively are completely reimagined. Sublimity, they imply, is the precondition of political action and not, in fact, an indication of its impossibility. It is precisely this contradiction that subsequent postmodern theorists challenge through their claim that 'the schizophrenic' is not the hero but the casualty of the postmodern. *Anti-Oedipus* played a crucial role in the development of schizophrenia as a topos in postmodern cultural theory by linking schizophrenia to capitalism and focussing attention on the fragmentation of the modern self. And, as we will see in Chapter 6, as Deleuze and Guattari's 'schizo' becomes the victim of late capitalist postmodernity, schizophrenia drifts further from its clinical origins and its antipsychiatric oppositionality, rendering paradoxical its ongoing association with the sublime.

Chapter 5

Schizophrenia, modernity, postmodernity

Only the real conflict of the conditions of existence
may serve as a structural model for the paradoxes of
the schizophrenic world.

(Foucault, 1976, p. 84)

Part Two of this book has so far identified three far-reaching effects of the
antipsychiatric project, broadly conceived. First, it issued a multifaceted critique of the psychiatric and psychoanalytic approaches to schizophrenia: Laing,
Szasz, Deleuze, Guattari, and others contested not only the methodology and
therapeutic practices of these disciplines but also their theoretical foundations.
The second and perhaps less obvious effect of the antipsychiatry movement
was to leave *un*challenged elements of psychological metatheory. As I have
argued, with the exception of Thomas Szasz's work, antipsychiatric accounts
of schizophrenia as sublime experience remain complicit with, and consequently fail to confront, the psychiatric and psychoanalytic production of
schizophrenia as a sublime object and text. Finally, and perhaps most significantly, through the figure of 'the schizophrenic' or 'schizo', antipsychiatric
theorists radically politicized schizophrenia, highlighting its aetiological, structural, and symbolic associations with capitalist society and culture.

    Although his work evinces no antipsychiatric polemic or sentiment, the phe-
nomenological psychologist Louis Sass has reconceptualized schizophrenia
and its symbolic significance in no less radical a fashion. In his magnum opus,
*Madness and Modernism: Insanity in the Light of Modern Art, Literature and
Thought* (1992), as well as in numerous publications in psychological, philosophical, and literary journals, Sass has repeatedly highlighted the limitations
of conventional psychiatric, psychoanalytic, *and* antipsychiatric (including
what he calls 'avant-garde') accounts of schizophrenia. Working in the phenomenological tradition pioneered by Karl Jaspers, Eugene Minkowski,
Wolfgang Blankenburg, and Kimura Bin, Sass's work is driven by an ethical
imperative to reinstate the humanity of schizophrenia and 'to dissipate the

atmosphere of unutterable mystery and profundity' that surrounds it (Sass, 1994b, p. 9). His own model focuses 'on certain formal or structural aspects or pervasive infrastructures of experience' rather than the aetiological, somatic, or psychological explanation of symptoms (Sass, 2004b, p. 75, see also Sass, 2001, p. 266), and emphasizes exigent introspection, hyperreflexivity, ipseity disturbance, and other so-called negative symptoms as defining features of schizophrenia. Sass's work is distinctive on a number of grounds, but for the purposes of this book merits detailed analysis for two reasons. First, Sass's account of schizophrenia operates *outside* the logic of the sublime that prevails in clinical and antipsychiatric theory and so provides a vantage point from which to illuminate the operation of the schizophrenic sublime. Secondly, Sass claims that the phenomenology of schizophrenia offers special insight into the structures of *modern* subjectivity, an argument that will again help illuminate, if not challenge, the postmodern cultural theory discussed in the next chapter.

The first task of this chapter is to discuss the relationship between Sass's critique of psychiatry, psychoanalysis, and antipsychiatry, and my reading of the schizophrenic sublime. I then elaborate the theoretical and metatheoretical originality of his account of schizophrenia.[1] As I will argue, Sass's nuanced analysis resolutely resists repeating or reinforcing any association between schizophrenia and sublimity; rather than merely opposing or inverting the dominant paradigm, his model remains exterior to its logic. We then return to an issue foregrounded by the antipsychiatry movement, namely, schizophrenia's relationship to modern culture and subjectivity. Sass's argument—that there are strong affinities between madness, modernism, and modernity—is certainly persuasive, but his assertion of a contiguous relationship between modernism and postmodernism, modernity and postmodernity, is, I suggest, less so. Drawing on Zygmunt Bauman's sociological studies of the substantive structural differences between modernity and postmodernity (or 'liquid modernity'), in particular his analysis of the shift from a panoptic to a consumerist regime of the self, I will argue that the affinities Sass identifies between modernity and schizophrenia invite reassessment and reconceptualization for the postmodern era.

Dementia, regression, Dionysus: three tropes of madness

Sass begins his survey of theories of schizophrenia with the two accounts psychiatry advances of its prized object—the doctrine of 'the abyss' and the

---

[1] Sass does acknowledge the method's practical limitations and ongoing difficulties in establishing a psychiatric research programme applicable to large patient populations (Sass and Parnas, 2001, pp. 347–8).

paradigm of the 'broken brain' (Sass, 1992, pp. 16–19). The idea of the broken brain has been if not always the foremost then certainly the most enduring explanation of schizophrenia. Kraepelin's dementia praecox, as the name suggests, made mental deterioration the defining feature of the disease model of schizophrenia, and contemporary biological psychiatry continues to approach schizophrenia as a deficiency or decline in cognitive and neurological functioning.[2] As we saw in Chapter 1, Karl Jaspers was the earliest expositor of the doctrine of the abyss, the idea that schizophrenia is by definition beyond empathetic understanding. Both accounts attribute this 'ununderstandable' disorder an as yet inexplicable biological aetiology. Doubly incomprehensible, schizophrenia acquires a special status within this psychiatric classification: it is 'no longer psychologically understandable like the mood disorders, but not yet neuropathologically explicable like the dementias' (Barrett, 1998c, p. 476). Where Robert Barrett reads this 'fence perching' as evidence of the social construction of schizophrenia as a liminal category, Sass more persuasively argues that it renders the schizophrenic patient 'psychiatry's quintessential other— the patient whose essence is incomprehensibility itself' (Sass, 1987a, p. 4; 1992, p. 19). Sass does not dispute the idea that biological and genetic factors may well be influential in determining the onset and development of schizophrenia;[3] however, he strenuously opposes the 'interpretive nihilism' that results from defining schizophrenic symptoms in purely somatic terms or classifying them merely as bizarre (Sass, 1992, p. 7; 2004b, p. 73).

In his thoughtful and provoking article 'Taxonomy and Ontology in Psychiatry', Matthew Broome cites approvingly the anti-essentialist view that

[2] According to Sass, the 'deficit view of schizophrenia' promotes 'a condescending, sometimes denigrating attitude that sees schizophrenia, the prototypical form of madness, entirely in terms of the loss of higher or more quintessentially human capacities of mind and spirit' (Sass, 2000–2001b, p. 56). In his later work, Sass is particularly critical of this model as it applies to the so-called negative symptoms of, for example, flatness of affect, autism, and anhedonia. Viewing these symptoms exclusively in terms of a decline, deficit, or diminishment is not only 'mechanistic and reductionistic', it also fails to account for the presence of *additional* and altered forms of experience (Sass, 2003, p. 154; 2001).

[3] In his 'Epilogue: Schizophrenia and Modern Culture' Sass points out that 'After nearly a century of research, schizophrenia can still be said to be "a condition of obscure origins and no established aetiology, pathogenesis and pathology", without even any clear disease marker or laboratory test by which it can readily be identified. Currently available evidence is insufficient to allow us to do more than endorse, with a sense of real certainty, a few very general statements: for example, that *some* structural or physiological abnormalities of the brain are probably implicated in the pathogenesis of many (perhaps most) cases of schizophrenia (though not necessarily as a primary or sufficient cause); that many cases have a significant genetic component; and that some as yet unspecified psychological or social factors are important in the maintenance and shaping, and perhaps also in the etiology, of most—if not all—such illnesses' (Sass, 1992, pp. 356–7).

psychiatric classification should be first and foremost of 'practical, pragmatic, and heuristic value' adding that 'if it reveals anything important ontologically or epistemologically that is a remarkable coincidence and nosologically irrelevant' (Broome, 2007, p. 312). The question of whether schizophrenia and other mental disorders are natural kinds has been extensively analysed (see Bolton, 2008; Cooper, 2005, 2007; Hacking, 1999), but in the context of the current discussion the notion of essences highlights a surprising convergence between Sass's work and the psychiatry of which he is so critical. As Broome (2007, p. 310) argues:

> Contemporary phenomenological psychiatry and psychopathology, at least conceptually, share strong similarities with the realism of biological psychiatry. Both methods of investigation seek to find *the defining characteristic* of a mental illness. For phenomenology, this characteristic is some essential feature of subjective experience, whereas for biological psychiatry it may be a particular activation of neural circuitry or a discrete genetic polymorphism. Furthermore, the investigations of both fields may be complementary . . .

As we will see, in Sass's phenomenological account, schizophrenia does describe an essential or fundamental transformation in the self (Sass, 2007); however, as I hope to make clear, it is the question of understanding that sharply distinguishes Sass's work from mainstream psychiatry, as it is the issue of comprehensibility rather than essences which underlies schizophrenia's association with the sublime.

Incomprehensibility and interpretive nihilism are certainly not charges that could be levelled against the psychoanalytic approach to psychosis, but if anything, Sass subjects these interpretations of psychotic symptomatology to a critique even more stringent than that mounted against biological psychiatry. Psychoanalysts, Sass argues, have understood schizophrenia as the regression to or fixation at the earliest stages of psychic development, a state that is pre-Oedipal, pre-ego, and pre-civilization. This teleological narrative locates schizophrenia at or prior to the birth of subjectivity; it 'welcome[s] the schizophrenic back into the human fold, but only in the subordinate position of the child' (Sass, 1992, p. 20). If my analysis of schizophrenia as the sublime object of psychiatry shares much in common with *Madness and Modernism*'s account of psychiatry's doctrine of the abyss and broken brain, my reading of the status of schizophrenia in psychoanalytic discourse diverges significantly from Sass's 'regressive hypothesis'. In Chapter 2, I argued that psychoanalytic writers since Freud have produced schizophrenia as a sublime text. Severing the connection, essential to the treatment of neurosis, between the interpretation and alleviation of symptoms, psychoanalysts find meaning in schizophrenic delusions and hallucinations but suggest that the schizophrenic patient herself is beyond analytic reach. My close reading of key psychoanalytic accounts of psychosis—offered by Abraham, Jung, Freud, Lacan, and numerous commentators on the Schreber case—foregrounds texts which, from a literary and cultural studies perspective, have had their greatest influence beyond a strictly clinical context.[4] Sass, by contrast, mentions Freud only briefly and Lacan not at all; he concentrates instead on some of the most influential figures in American ego psychology and Kleinian analysis (Sass, 1992, pp. 412–3). It would appear, then, that our findings are not so much incompatible as incomparable.

In the absence of a close or sustained engagement with the foundational analyses of schizophrenia (in particular the work of Abraham and Jung), Sass overlooks the concerted effort made by early psychoanalysts to redefine schizophrenia as a psychoneurosis, efforts that predate the texts he suggests inaugurated the regressive hypothesis.[5] More surprising, considering the extraordinary breadth of material covered in *Madness and Modernism*, and the many references to Marguerite Sechehaye's analysis of Renee's *Autobiography of a Schizophrenic Girl*, is that Sass also neglects the much-celebrated work of another star on the psychoanalytic stage: Frieda Fromm-Reichmann. Fromm-Reichmann is highly regarded for her pioneering work at the Chestnut Lodge clinic in the 1930s and 1940s, and her belief, rare in America at that time, that psychoanalysis could have positive outcomes for people diagnosed with schizophrenia (Hornstein, 2000). In the 1960s and 1970s, Joanne Greenberg's best-selling autobiographical novel, *I Never Promised You a Rose Garden* (1964), together with its film adaptation (Page, 1977), gave a patient's-eye view of Fromm-Reichmann's psychotherapeutic practices and elevated her to an almost-celebrity status.[6] If, as Sass claims, one of the most troubling assumptions operative in

---

[4] For example, although it seems to have attracted little clinical attention, especially in America, Lacan's model of psychosis is a huge influence on Deleuze and Guattari's anti-Oedipal model of schizophrenia, and, as I will discuss in the next chapter, on models of postmodern 'schizophrenic' subjectivity.

[5] At first Sass suggests it is Freud's analysis of the Schreber case, but later he credits Victor Tausk's 1919 paper 'On the origin of the "influencing machine" in schizophrenia' (1950) as playing the decisive role in inaugurating the psychoanalytic approach to psychosis (Sass, 1992, pp. 20, 218).

[6] Hornstein writes that to the surprise of many, '*Rose Garden* gained a huge following and has been continuously in print for thirty-five years. It has sold 5.7 million copies, been translated into a dozen languages, and been transmuted into a movie, a pop song, and a cultural cliché. Mental patients hailed *Rose Garden*, psychiatrists denounced it, and it became the lightning rod for controversy about schizophrenia and its treatment. Eventually Joanne's and Frieda's identities were revealed, and they become one of those couples— like Freud and Dora . . . —that psychoanalysts revere like martyred saints' (Hornstein, 2000, p. xiv). *Rose Garden*'s psychological sophistication is also praised by Jeffrey Berman (1985).

the regressive hypothesis or 'primitivity interpretation' is that it seems 'inherently condescending' (Sass, 1987a, p. 7) and ultimately unhelpful in the treatment of schizophrenia, Fromm-Reichmann's work is surely a significant and influential exception to the rule.

Last but not least, Sass turns to the antipsychiatric and avant-garde celebration of schizophrenia as a joyous liberation from the codes and conventions of society, self, and rationality. The 'Dionysian' model of madness promoted by Laing, Foucault, Deleuze, and Guattari inverts the values of the psychoanalytic narrative by celebrating the loss of ego boundaries as the freedom of unfettered desire: 'The avant-gardists and antipsychiatrists have emphasized the positive side [of psychic "regression"]—excesses of passion, vitality, and imagination—yet they, no less than the traditional analysts, assume that the schizophrenic lacks the self-control, awareness of social convention, and reflexivity of "civilized" consciousness' (Sass, 1992, p. 22; see also 1987a, p. 8; 1996, pp. 73–5). Sass is justly critical of antipsychiatric romanticism and reads the 'Dionysian' discourse or behaviour of many psychotic patients 'not as expressions of a naturally overflowing vitality but as defenses *against* the devitalization and derealization' that is schizophrenia (Sass, 1992, p. 238, italics in the original). However, as we have seen in the preceding two chapters, the antipsychiatric valourization of the schizo is more complex than perhaps it first appears. Sass, clearly, is no Deleuze and Guattari enthusiast, but he is also not a close reader of *Anti-Oedipus*. For example, he argues that Deleuze and Guattari see madness as 'a spontaneous, natural, and pre-civil mode of being which comes to be oppressed or constrained by the forces of society and self-control' (Sass, 1992, p. 106), but in so doing overlooks their claim that schizophrenia is also capitalism's 'deepest tendency' (Deleuze and Guattari, 1982, p. 245). Sass's discussion of antipsychiatric and avant-garde models of schizophrenia draws attention to their metatheoretical connection to psychoanalysis, but does not investigate the antipsychiatric critique of psychiatric and psychoanalytic paradigms and practices, nor consider the sociopolitical aims and outcomes of their revisioning of madness. It is also the case that Sass overlooks some striking similarities between his own and Deleuze and Guattari's analysis of schizophrenia.[7]

[7] For example, as Deleuze makes particularly clear in 'Schizophrenia and Society', he and Guattari are opposed to models of schizophrenia that fixate on regression, deficiency, or dementia, and agree that 'the real difficulty is to give an account of schizophrenia as something with positive traits, and as such, not to reduce it to the lacunal or destructive traits it engenders in a person'. The idea that 'If schizophrenia seems like the sickness of today's society, we should not look to generalizations about our way of life, but to very precise mechanisms of a social, political, and economic nature' (Deleuze, 2006, pp. 23, 28) is also

Psychiatry is charged with 'interpretive nihilism', psychoanalysis with con-descension, the antipsychiatric avant-garde with the failure to account for the complexity of schizophrenic symptomatology and suffering.

> At the deepest level, then, all three of these models—psychiatric, psychoanalytic, and avant-gardist—share the assumption that schizophrenic pathology must involve a loss of what, in the West, has long been assumed to be the most essential characteristics of mind or subjectivity: the capacities for logic and abstract thinking, for self-reflection, and for the exercise of free will.

> (Sass, 1992, p. 23)

Sass identifies the common theoretical ground occupied by these discourses (schizophrenia as a loss of rationality) but does not inquire as to their meta-theoretical inter-relationship.[8] I have argued that these models articulate schizophrenia through the logic of the sublime, situating schizophrenia at the limits of psychological, rational, therapeutic, and empathetic understanding. Significantly, although the word is mentioned, the sublime does not appear in *Madness and Modernism* structurally or as a critical category. So, although Sass does not put it in these terms, I would argue that it is this idea of a sublime schizophrenia—radical in its essential unundersandability—that Sass seems to find wholly inadequate to the task of approaching schizophrenic experience. Without disregarding the psycho*pathology* of schizophrenia (psychic upheav-als and profound transformations in the understanding of self and world), Sass endeavours to understand the full gamut of psychotic experience in its clinical, as well as cultural, context.

Schizophrenia and hyperreflexivity

Madness and Modernism extends the central arguments of Sass's influential article 'Introspection, Schizophrenia and the Fragmentation of the Self', and lays the foundation for much of his subsequent work on the 'negative' symp-toms, delusions, self-disturbances, and creativity of schizophrenia. Analysing the full arc of psychotic experience—from the schizoid personality to the

---

clearly shared by Sass in his detailed analysis of the relationship between schizophrenia and specific mechanisms of modernity.

[8] Similarly, Robert Barrett, focusing on the themes of degeneration, disintegration, and division, has argued that although all three disciplines 'might like to have seen themselves as poles apart, their differences were superficial, for they reproduced, in their own respec-tive technical idioms, the same underlying construction of schizophrenia. This is a case of a deep cultural structure producing three apparently different surface forms' (Barrett, 1998b, p. 631). Building on the work of Sass and of Barrett, my analysis of the 'schizo-phrenic sublime' is an attempt to explore the nature and effects of this 'deep cultural structure'.

prodromal and acute phases of psychosis—Sass demonstrates 'that much of what has been passed off as primitive or deteriorated is far more complex and interesting—and self-aware—than is usually acknowledged' (Sass, 1992, p. 9). His central thesis is neatly summarized in the following question: 'What if madness, in at least some of its forms, were to derive from a heightening rather than a dimming of conscious awareness, and an alienation not from reason but from the emotions, instincts and the body?' (Sass, 1992, p. 4). The schizophrenic dissolution of self, he argues, is not the result of the disintegration of the ego; rather it is caused by an unabating and acute self-awareness. Schizophrenic experience, he argues, 'may be characterised less by fusion, spontaneity, and liberation of desire than by separation, restraint, and an exaggerated cerebralism and propensity for introspection' (Sass, 1992, p. 10). And if hyperreflexivity is schizophrenia's 'master theme' (Sass, 1992, p. 11), the paradox is central to its articulation:

> Schizophrenics can be hypersensitive to human contact but also indifferent. They can be pedantic or capricious, idle or diligent, irritable or filled with an all-encompassing yet somehow empty hilarity. They can experience a rushing flow of ideas or a total blocking; and their actions, thoughts and perceptions can seem rigidly ordered or controlled (exhibiting a 'morbid geometrism'), but at other times chaotic and formless. They will sometimes feel they can influence the whole universe, at other times as if they can't control even their own thoughts or their own limbs—or, in what is one of the supreme paradoxes of this condition, they may have both these experiences at the same moment.

> (Sass, 1992, p. 26; see also Sass, 1987a, p. 9; 1994b)

In his later work, Sass brings together the key themes of exaggerated cerebralism, exigent introspection, hyperreflexivity, and '"intrapsychic ataxia" (a separation of cognition and emotion)' (Sass, 1992, p. 109) into a more succinct definition of schizophrenia as 'a disorder of self-experience (an ipseity disturbance) involving hyperreflexivity and diminished self-affection (i.e. heightened awareness of aspects of experience that would normally remain tacit or presupposed and decline in the feeling of existing as a subject of awareness)' (Sass, 2001, p. 251, elaborated at 253; Sass and Parnas, 2003).

Four further features of Sass's phenomenological model are important to note. First, he repeatedly stresses the importance of so-called negative symptoms in defining schizophrenia and schizophrenia spectrum disorders, arguing that these 'are not, in fact, straightforward deficit states, but involve the presence of "positive" aberrations of various kinds' (Sass and Parnas, 2001, p. 350; see also Sass, 1996, 2000, 2003, 2004a). Instead of limiting his interpretive energies to 'decoding' the hallucinations and delusions of the acute phase, Sass advocates a holistic approach that foregrounds the less remarkable, but no less significant, dimensions of schizophrenic experience. Second, Sass is also keen to distance himself from the view, advanced by R.D. Laing among others, that schizophrenia is an intelligible or strategic response to, for example, unbearable interpersonal relationships. He states clearly that while he portrays schizophrenia as something of a 'metapathology' (Sass, 2000, p. 322)—a state of excessive self-reflexivity, self-consciousness, and self-alienation—this does not imply that schizophrenic symptoms are volitional or in any way willfully engaged (Sass, 1992, p. 240).[9] Sass further avoids another pitfall of empathetic inquiry: translating the seemingly ununderstandable into the perfectly intelligible.[10] Illuminating the strong affinities between modernism and schizophrenia—especially in such a detailed and sophisticated manner—runs the risk of equating one with the other; however, Sass never loses sight of the alienness and psychopathological severity of schizophrenia. Like Jaspers, he views the 'praecox feeling' as its defining feature, but suggests that the clinician's sense of alienation in fact gives him or her greater insight into the disorienting experience of schizophrenia's psychic upheavals.[11] Finally, and, from the perspective of this inquiry into schizophrenia's status in cultural as well as clinical contexts, perhaps most significantly, Sass explicitly brackets the question of schizophrenia's aetiology.[12] The claim that schizophrenia is a disorder of the self stands apart from and so cannot be easily contradicted by any hypothesis regarding its genetic, neurochemical, or environmental origins (Sass, 1992, p. 388; Parnas and Sass, 2001, p. 102).

In short, Sass does not simply question the findings and methodologies of the dominant theories of psychosis: he looks beyond psychiatric, psychoanalytic, and antipsychiatry metatheory to develop an original and compelling account of schizophrenia that does not have recourse to the logic of the sublime. Although there are moments in *Madness and Modernism* when Sass uses the language of the sublime, writing, for example, of an inner world 'marked

---

[9] 'For, what patients like those we have been considering cannot seem to control is self-control itself; what they cannot get distance from is their own endless need for distancing; what they cannot be conscious of is their own hypertrophied self-consciousness and its effect on their world' (Sass, 1987, p. 27).

[10] As an example, we might think of Morton Schatzman's (1973) essentially reductive claims about the aetiology and symbolic significance of Schreber's delusions.

[11] Sass notes that 'the observer's alienation may not, in fact, indicate a total failure of empathy: it may be a *shared* alienation, a feeling evoked by accurate intuitions of what the patient is actually going through. Could it be, then, that the dizzying abyss we feel in the presence of certain schizophrenic patients is connected with the *mise en abyme* into which they themselves are falling?' (Sass, 1992, p. 240)

[12] Aetiological issues are discussed in depth only in the epilogue and the appendix of *Madness and Modernism*.

by . . . the uncanniness of immense spaces and the enigmas of gleaming surfaces and brilliant light' (Sass, 1992, p. 5),[13] these are no indication of an
underlying belief in schizophrenia's fundamental incomprehensibility. This
point is worth emphasizing. The sublime, as I understand and am using the
term, directs our attention towards comprehensibility rather than ontology; it
is the idea of an essential mystery, rather than an essence per se, which is central to the operation of the disciplinary sublime in psychiatry. Against those
who would prefer that key aspects of schizophrenia *necessarily* remain inaccessible to interpretation (Read, 2003), Sass draws schizophrenic experience into
the fold of understandability. Against those who would argue that schizophrenia is a stage through which we all pass (Klein, 1952), or which can be dismissed as medicalized malingering (Szasz, 1976), Sass insists that it involves
significant, but not incomprehensible, transformations in the structure of
experience.[14]

Schizophrenia, modernism, and modernity

It is these transformations, Sass argues, that can illuminate central tendencies
within modernism. The interpretive strategy of *Madness and Modernism* is
carefully and clearly outlined: rather than establish a causal relationship
between madness and modernism, his analysis highlights their affinities and
points of convergence (Sass, 1992, pp. 9, 339). Sass's primary interest is in high
modernism, 'the most advanced art and literature of the twentieth century',
and he compares schizophrenia to a diverse range of literary, artistic, and
philosophical works united by their underlying interest in, or manifestation of,
forms of alienation and self-consciousness (Sass, 1992, pp. 9, 37). Modernism
is thus distinguished not only from realism, romanticism, and popular culture,
but also from modernity, here conceptualized as the material conditions of
existence. In an argument that can only be described as itself bizarre, Robert

---

[13] Here, it appears as though Sass is referring to Renee's description of the 'Land of Light'
(Renee, 1970, p. 44).

[14] A similar argument is mounted by medical anthropologist Janis Hunter Jenkins (2004),
who endeavours to show 'how the experiences of people with schizophrenia can be quintessentially extraordinary just as they can be exquisitely ordinary' (Jenkins and Barrett,
2004a, p. 11). Like Sass, she cautions that 'A single-minded focus on the similarities
between those who have schizophrenia and those who do not carries the risk of negating
what is so extraordinary about this illness, underestimating the intensity of suffering it
entails, and overlooking the resilience of those who grapple with it. But if the focus is
restricted to understanding differences between abnormal and normal, the risk is one of
devaluing the person with schizophrenia. Difference may lead to diminution and decomposition of the person into an object' (ibid.).

Barrett (1998c, p. 484) has taken Sass to task over the potentially negative effects of this comparison:

> Likening the 'schizophrenic' to modernism, itself such an odd fish, may have the effect of pasting another layer of bizarreness onto this cultural category. [. . .] For individuals defined as 'schizophrenic', it may not be helpful to be compared with a movement that is so bizarre and alienating as to make you believe your experiences were more bizarre than you first thought, or make you feel typecast as an alien.

As Sass rightly observes in his rejoinder to Barrett, the complexities of modernism—like schizophrenia—may *appear* difficult to comprehend but this does not mean that they are unknowable or without meaning. On the contrary, the depth and richness of modernist expression is such that schizophrenia is, if anything, 'valorized rather than denigrated by being compared with many of the difficult but highly valued products of modernist culture' (Sass, 1998, p. 500).

Madness and Modernism discusses many of the twentieth century's most esteemed writers and artists; however, Sass in this text and elsewhere accords pride of place to Daniel Paul Schreber and Antonin Artaud, whom he describes not as typical but exemplary modern madmen (Sass, 1992, p. 246; 1996).[15] The gender specificity here is telling and worthy of a brief detour. Women, in *Madness and Modernism*, are conspicuously few and far between;[16] the overwhelming majority of 'exemplary' modernists and schizophrenic patients are European men, as are the intensely creative schizoid and schizotypal intellectuals mentioned in his later work (Sass, 2000–2001b, p. 72). My point here is not to accuse Sass of bias or oversight; rather, it is to suggest that there may be affinities not just between schizophrenia and modernism, but also between schizophrenia, modernism, and masculinity as it has been conceptualized in the industrialized West. Metzl's (2009) powerful study of the racialization of schizophrenia in the civil rights era is clearly also apposite here. Sass states in the prologue to *Madness and Modernism* that in the history of madness 'Nearly

---

[15] I discussed Sass's analysis of the panoptic and solipsistic Schreber at length in Chapter 3. Artaud's autobiographical writing and his theatre of cruelty are at the forefront both of Sass's analysis of 'negative' symptoms and of creativity and schizophrenia. Analysing the writing of the early twentieth century's two most celebrated psychotic patients also serves a strategic function in so far as it enables him to refute explicitly the regressive and Dionysian models of madness and to demonstrate the superiority of his phenomenological model in accounting for the totality of their schizophrenic experience.

[16] Renee's *Autobiography* (1970) and Natalija's delusion of the influencing machine (Tausk, 1950) are the two most referenced examples of female schizophrenic experience; in the case of modernism, the writing of Virginia Woolf and Natalie Sarraute receive the most attention.

always insanity involves a shift from human to animal, from culture to nature, from thought to emotion, from maturity to the infantile and the archaic' (Sass, 1992, p. 4). Has it also involved a shift from 'masculine' to 'feminine'? And if so, how does Sass's model reverse this trend? In her hugely influential book *The Female Malady*, Elaine Showalter argues that traditionally women have been situated 'on the side of irrationality, silence, nature, and body, while men are situated on the side of reason, discourse, culture, and mind. [. . .] Thus, madness, even when experienced by men, is metaphorically and symbolically represented as feminine' (Showalter, 1987, pp. 3–4). In his analysis of the Schreber case, Sass explicitly raises the question of an opposition between the hyperreflexivity of schizophrenia and the 'feminine' experience of embodied subjectivity,[17] so is his claim in *Madness and Modernism* that schizophrenia is 'an alienation not from reason but from the emotions, instincts and the body' (Sass, 1992, p. 4), more suggestive than he perhaps allows? Although pursuing this line of inquiry is, unfortunately, beyond the scope of this chapter, as I have discussed elsewhere (Woods, in press) Sass's work clearly points towards new directions for research into the relationship between schizophrenia, gender, race, and postmodern cultural productions.

What is more central to this study of schizophrenia in clinical and cultural theory is Sass's discussion of postmodernism as a continuation of modernism, an intensification of the modernist interest in hyperreflexivity and self-alienation. Sass's references to postmodernism as a movement emphasize his view that it is merely a subtype of modernism, or, better still, a kind of hyper-modernism. Citing, among others, Jean-François Lyotard, Julia Kristeva, Frank Kermode, and Frederick Karl as advocates of the continuity thesis, Sass somewhat controversially identifies poststructuralist theorists Jacques Derrida and Paul de Man as exemplary postmodernists and, with the exception of Andy Warhol, does not discuss popular postmodernisms of any kind. His preference for post-romantic modernism over the 'further turn of the screw of self-consciousness called postmodernism' is clearly stated (Sass, 1992, p. 37).[18] Concentrating

---

[17] Sass interprets Schreber's delusional transvestism as a culturally determined way of working through the duality between subject and object: 'For Schreber, transformation into a woman implies losing in the competition of consciousness, ceding one's epistemological centrality and becoming a mere object defined by the other's sovereign awareness'. Sass continues: 'The experience of feminization was, in fact, Schreber's major antidote to the intellect, his palliative for the self-torturing mind. Though on one level a sign of persecution and defeat, it also had soothing and reassuring effects, allaying the restlessness and insidious self-undermining by his compulsive thinking and self-consciousness' (Sass, 1994b, pp. 123, 126).

[18] References to 'so-called' postmodernism, and to postmodernism as a distinct category, frequently appear in brackets or footnotes (for example Sass, 1987, p. 13; 1992, pp. 8, 29).

on aspects of postmodernism that extend or exaggerate modernism's anti-romanticism, Sass questions even the relevance of the temporal distinction, arguing that 'the stylistic features and aesthetic attitudes identified as post-modern (e.g. an emphatic self-referentiality, profound relativism and uncer-tainty, extreme irony, and tendencies towards fragmentation) have in fact been with us throughout the twentieth century' (Sass, 1992, p. 418). For Sass, schizophrenia illuminates the hyperreflexive and self-alienating tendencies in high modernism that are also present and, if anything, more pronounced in postmodernism.

Introducing a third piece in the puzzle—namely, an underlying material reality, or the context in which both schizophrenia and modernism are manifest—Sass in the epilogue of *Madness and Modernism* considers the issue of an association, affinity, and aetiological link between schizophrenia and modernity (see also Sass, 1994a).[19] Here, although he does not reference it directly, he extends the analyses undertaken in David Michael Levin's edited collection *Pathologies of the Modern Self* (Levin, 1987b). Levin's founding premise is one with which Sass would surely agree: the self is subject 'to afflic-tions that are specific manifestations of its historical situation', pathologies of individual will that 'are also pathologies collectively willed into being, pro-duced by our institutions, customs and practices' (Levin, 1987b, pp. 1, 16). Reflecting on the relationship between schizophrenia and modernity, Joel Kovel argues that it 'takes on especially severe, dehumanized proportions' in the technocratic West (Kovel, 1987, p. 334; see also Braun, 1995); James Glass that it testifies to 'the power of society in defining, enclosing, and terrorizing the self' (Glass, 1987, p. 406; 1993); and Levin asks:

> What if the truth in schizophrenia is one that, because of its distinctively greater vul-nerability to what is craziest in civilization, speaks to the needs of its time, and speaks very clearly, considering the pain, attempting to call attention, at this time and for us, to the terror of self-destructiveness and the horror of nihilism, which rage in reso-nance with one another like an epidemic in our civilization? What if schizophrenia is the *painful truth* about a world that our metaphysics both founds and reflects?
>
> (Levin, 1987a, p. 523, italics in the original)

Like Levin, Kovel, and Glass, Sass finds compelling evidence to suggest that 'whether considered from a historical or cross-cultural standpoint, modern Western civilization does seem to have a statistical association with schizophrenia,

---

On postmodernism as anti-romanticism see Sass, 1992, pp. 344, 39–40, 417–8; 1998, p. 499; 2000–2001a, p. 81.

[19] Sass includes postmodernity in his definition of modernity, an issue to which we will return.

or at least with its severely chronic or autistic forms' (Sass, 1992, p. 366; 1997, p. 217). Thematically linked through the master theme of hyperreflexivity, madness and modernism are also historically and materially entwined. Is this coincidence? Does modern culture make people mad, or do mad people make modern culture? Or should we view both madness and modernism as 'consequences or reflections' of modernity (Sass, 1992, p. 357)? Sass clearly favours the last of these four interpretive options. Drawing on the work of Anthony Giddens, Peter and Brigitte Berger, and above all Foucault, Sass argues that modernity precipitates huge changes in the structure of experience and self-knowledge. The increased 'bureaucratization, technologization, secularization, and rationalization' of society (Sass, 1997, p. 219); the production of the epistemological subject both as an object of knowledge and as constitutive of the world; the philosophical emphasis on 'disengagement and self-consciousness' and the psychologization of human experience—these are just some of the tendencies in modern civilization which are not simply reflected in the content of schizophrenic symptoms but contribute to the very appearance and the structure of the disorder itself (Sass, 1992, pp. 369–71).

We are at last in a position to pose to *Madness and Modernism* the key question with which the rest of this book is concerned: if, contra Sass, postmodernity is not simply the intensification of modernity, but an era marked by a new regime of the self, what can we say about the relationship between schizophrenia, postmodern culture, and society? If we agree with Sass that 'the psychotic person may at times live out, in exaggerated, almost literal fashion, the ontological and epistemological assumptions of his or her age' (Sass, 1997, p. 222), how might a 'postmodern schizophrenia' differ from a schizophrenic experience considered exemplary of modernity? In the next chapter I examine in more depth various accounts of the figure of 'the schizophrenic' as broadly representative of the postmodern subject; however, in order to think through how Sass's analysis might be brought to bear on the question of schizophrenia's symbolic relationship to the postmodern, we need first to examine in more detail the arguments in favour of identifying the shift from modernity to postmodernity as a fundamental change in the material conditions of existence.

The question of postmodernity

Postmodernity, as Barry Smart observes, is a term that generates controversy across a broad range of fields and disciplines and inspires reactions that are 'rarely sober, measured or thoughtful' (Smart, 1993, pp. 11–12). This is clearly not the place to survey comprehensively competing definitions of postmodernity, nor canvass the entire range of arguments for and against its existence. Sass, as we have seen, follows Anthony Giddens and others in emphasizing the lasting significance of the modern project: the idea that, as there has been no demonstrably significant shift in social and economic organization, postmodernity is, at most, something like 'modernity with bells on' (Gauntlett, 2002). The claim that there has been not only a significant, but also a radical, shift in late twentieth-century Western society has in my view been most convincingly argued by socialist, Marxist, and post-Marxist thinkers who use the concept of postmodernity to identify and interpret an economically and technologically distinct historical period. Fredric Jameson and Jean Baudrillard, whose work is the central focus of the next chapter, are among the leading advocates of the idea of a radically altered material and cultural reality, but they are supported in this argument by a diverse chorus of critical voices. Donna Haraway, for example, in her famous cyborg manifesto, points to new biotechnologies, proliferating communication systems, and an exploitative multinational home-work economy as key indicators that older hierarchical social structures have been replaced by the 'scary new networks' of the 'informatics of domination' (Haraway, 1985, p. 80). Gilles Deleuze states unequivocally that Foucault's disciplinary society has given way to control society characterized by 'ultrarapid forms of apparently freefloating control' that operate through a viral, decentralized logic (Deleuze, 2002, p. 318). David Harvey, the influential Marxist geographer, pinpoints 1972 as the year the world changed: flexible modes of capitalist accumulation and new social structures began decisively to transform the experience of space and time (Harvey, 1990, p. vii). The society of mass media, the spectacle and simulacra; the global village; an information age that is cybernetic, digital, and posthuman—these are only some of the ways postmodernity has been described. To focus on the issue at hand—namely, the question of how Sass's model of schizophrenia might illuminate a distinctively postmodern condition—I want to turn now to the work of one of the most famous sociologists of the postmodern, Zygmunt Bauman.

For Bauman, postmodernity refers not to the end of modernity but simply to 'particular features of the "world out there"'. 'We are', he suggests, 'as modern as ever, obsessively "modernizing" everything we can lay our hands on', but major shifts in social and economic organization justify speaking now of a new era (Bauman and Tester, 2001, pp. 96–8).[20] Bauman has published many analyses of the postmodern condition detailing the transition from 'solid' to 'liquid' modernity (Bauman, 1991, 1993, 1996, 2000, 2006). As Bauman explains, liquid modernity is at once continuous with solid modernity (as it is 'melting' and 'disembedding') and discontinuous with it (as there is 'no solidification of

---

[20] Bauman rejected the terms postmodernism and postmodernity because they were both fraught and all-too-fashionable.

the melted, no re-embedding') (Bauman and Tester, 2001, pp. 97–8). The distinction is not one between two substantively different states comprising radically dissimilar elements, but refers to the structure, process, and organization of society. In the era of globalization, the market, more so than the state, determines the pace, flexibility, and mutability of social life. 'We live today under conditions of *permanent revolution*', writes Bauman, and so 'constant change is . . . the supreme norm of behavior, advertised and promoted as the recipe of survival in the turbulent and no more predictable world' (ibid.). Liquid modernity's effects on the subject are many, but foremost among them is the loosening of the structures of community and hence of social identities. Bauman therefore suggests that:

> Perhaps instead of talking about identities, inherited or acquired, it would be more in keeping with the realities of the globalising world to speak of *identification*, a never-ending, always incomplete, unfinished and open-ended activity in which we all, by necessity or by choice, are engaged.

> (Bauman, 2001, p. 129, italics in the original)

Boundaries, in liquid modernity, are dissolved as quickly as they are resurrected; anxieties are aroused and assuaged in an ever-accelerating cycle; identities are easily adopted and discarded; there is, in short, no possibility of a fixed or stable self.

To look more precisely at Bauman's account of the mechanisms of subject formation, we can concentrate on his *Work, Consumerism and the New Poor* (2005). According to Bauman, the industrialization and rapid expansion of capitalist production in the nineteenth century were predicated on a 'supreme regulatory principle', that of the work ethic (Bauman, 2005, p. 37). This ethic promoted the value of work as 'a noble and ennobling activity' (Bauman, 2005, p. 5), and preached the virtues of life-long planning and commitment, of saving as opposed to spending, of choosing the dignity of labour over the short-term pleasures of consumption. Industrialists, clergymen, government officials, and military officers encouraged modern men (more so than women) to view work as the most important aspect of their lives: the centre of psychic and social orientation (Bauman, 2005, p. 17). However, at the centre of modernity, Bauman finds a paradox: 'The work ethic called people to *choose* a life devoted to labour; but a life devoted to labour meant no choice, inaccessibility of choice and prohibition of choice' (Bauman, 2005, p. 19, italics in the original). And at the heart of this paradox, Bauman, like Sass and Foucault, finds that truly modern mechanism: the panopticon.

For all three thinkers, the panopticon is the key to understanding how 'the individualized, self-scrutinizing, interiorized subject of modern Western culture' came into being (Sass, 1997, p. 206). Foucault famously interpreted the structure of Jeremy Bentham's panopticon as a symbol for the operation of modern disciplinary power. The inmates in the cells of the panopticon are permanently vulnerable to the watchful gaze of those in the central tower, an arrangement that fosters in them a form of self-scrutiny which functions regardless of whether or not they are in fact being watched. As Sass puts it:

> The panoptical arrangement makes individuals feel constantly exposed to an external, normalising gaze, therefore subjecting them to the dictates of an authority that must ultimately be internalised. Foucault sees this arrangement as the essential manifesta- tion of modern power relationships instantiated in many institutions and social prac- tices. It fosters forms of disciplinary self-control that eradicate spontaneity, increase inwardness and isolation, and instil the inner divisions of a relentlessly self-monitoring mode of consciousness.

(Sass, 1997, p. 206; 1992, pp. 251–8)

As I discussed in Chapter 2, Sass argues that schizophrenia can be seen both as an exaggeration of and an escape from the relentless self-monitoring inspired by modern institutions (Sass, 1992, p. 372). So it is the panoptic Schreber who reveals not the symbolic structures of modernity (an argument made by Eric Santner), but the very structure of its consciousness: 'madness, at least in Schreber's case, turned out to be one of the most extreme exemplars *of* this civilization—a simulacrum of the modern world in the most private recesses of the soul' (Sass, 1992, p. 373, italics in the original).

For Bauman, however, the key point to emphasize is that by imposing 'one, uniform pattern of regular and predictable behaviour upon a variegated and essentially unruly population of inmates' (Bauman, 2005, p. 14), panoptic power ultimately functions to eliminate choice. It is the issue of choice, and its panoptic regulation, that he claims underlies the twentieth century's most radical sociological upheaval. Bauman argues that society is no longer regu- lated through the panoptical logic of the work ethic but organized around an aesthetic of consumption. Whether we call it liquid, late-, second-, or postmo- dernity, society today addresses, engages, and constructs its members prima- rily as consumers, and 'to embrace the modality of the consumer means first and foremost falling in love with choice' (Bauman, 2005, pp. 24, 30). The cycle of creating, fulfilling, recreating, and re-fulfilling desire is crucial to the suc- cessful operation of a consumer society. Reducing the lag between the satisfac- tion of desire and its reactivation 'is best achieved if the consumers cannot hold their attention nor focus their desire on any object for long; if they are impatient, impetuous and restive, and above all easily excitable and equally susceptible to losing interest' (Bauman, 2005, p. 25). 'The everyday world of the postmodern habitat is', as Dennis Smith observes in his commentary on the work of Bauman, 'episodic, haphazard, inconsistent and contingent' (Smith, 1999, p. 158). Consequently, consumers have little incentive to be interested in life-long ambitions, commitments, or even identities: everything is embraced lightly, partially, and provisionally, to be replaced or displaced as fashion and circumstance dictate.

One of the most salient features of consumer society on this analysis is 'the retreat of the panoptical techniques of domination' (Bauman and Tester, 2001, p. 90):

> The kind of drill in which the panoptical institutions excelled is hardly suitable for the training of consumers. Those institutions were good at training people in routine, monotonous behaviour, and reached that effect through the limitation or complete elimination of choice; but it is precisely the absence of routine and the state of constant choice that are the virtues (indeed, the 'role prerequisites') of a consumer.
>
> (Bauman, 2005, pp. 24–5, 29)

Whereas the work ethic required people to choose a lack of choice (work was the only conscionable option), consumer society functions to maximize and valourize choice and has no need of disciplinary mechanisms that would reinstate norms or limits. According to Bauman, it is not the panopticon but the synopticon, which supplies the 'pattern of existence' in consumer society (Smith, 1999, p. 153). As Mathiesen (1997, p. 219) explains, the synopticon refers to 'a situation where a large number focuses on something in common which is condensed'. Instead of the few watching the many in an environment of surveillance and control, the many watch the few: consumers are trained by a celebrity elite whose every move is documented by the mass media (Bauman, 2005, pp. 52–4). Whereas the panopticon is a repressive mechanism—curtailing choice, commanding adherence to the work ethic—the synopticon, as Tony Blackshaw notes, 'needs no coercion' and functions simply to promote 'new' and 'cool' ways of living a life obedient only to desire (Blackshaw, 2005, p. 129).

Bauman is right, I think, to associate postmodernity with a synoptic regime, but his claim that 'Whatever else the present stage in the history of modernity is, it is also, perhaps above all, *post-Panoptical*', seems to fly in the face of empirical fact (Bauman, 2000, p. 11).[21] Whether travelling, shopping, banking, driving, internet-surfing, or simply meandering through public space, 'Now more than ever, we are under surveillance' (Levin et al., 2002, p. 10). Postmodernity sees not the decline of panopticism but its radical proliferation, privatization, and decentralization; as David Lyon suggests, surveillance and 'surveillance technologies are vitally implicated in the processes of postmodernity' and are crucial, not peripheral, to the smooth functioning of consumer

---

[21] Indeed, surveillance studies has emerged as a new trans-disciplinary academic field, complete with a peer-reviewed online journal *Surveillance and Society*.

society (Lyon, 2003, p. 165). In his article, 'The Kindler, Gentler Gaze of Big Brother: Reality TV in the Era of Digital Capitalism', Mark Andrejevic makes a compelling argument regarding the role of surveillance-based reality television in 'training viewers and consumers for their role in an "interactive" economy' (Andrejevic, 2002, p. 251). Surveillance, as it appears on shows like *Big Brother*, to name but the most obvious, is not, as in George Orwell's day, associated with totalitarian control but with sensation, fun, and self-expression. The kind of subjectivity 'consonant with an emerging online economy' is one that 'equates submission to comprehensive surveillance with self-expression and self-knowledge' (Andrejevic, 2002, p. 253). Observation is no longer menacing but entertaining (Weibel, 2002, p. 215). To the postmodern consumer/viewer eager to prove their authentic and honest selves, 'the persistent gaze of the camera provides one way of guaranteeing that "realness"' (Andrejevic, 2002, p. 266). What we are witnessing, according to Slavoj Žižek (2002, p. 225),

> . . . is the tragi-comic reversal of the Bentham-Orwellian notion of the Panopticon-society in which we are (potentially) 'observed always' and have no place to hide from the omnipresent gaze of the Power: today anxiety seems to arise from the prospect of NOT being exposed to the Other's gaze all the time, so that the subject needs the camera's gaze as a kind of ontological guarantee of his/her being.

Foucault's modern panopticon, according to Sass, 'fosters forms of disciplinary self-control that eradicate spontaneity, increase inwardness and isolation, and instil the inner divisions of a relentlessly self-monitoring mode of consciousness' (Sass, 1997; 1992, pp. 251–8). Its postmodern equivalent replaces self-control with self-expression. Here, self-consciousness might not tend towards inwardness and isolation, but be the very precondition for an inter-subjectively meaningful being. Postmodern panopticism does not address its subjects as people of depth and conscience, nor inculcate a duty to conform to the norm; rather it fosters performativity, individualism, and the pursuit of happiness through consumption. In this sense, then, postmodern consumer society does not so much abandon the panoptic regime as harness its production of self-monitoring subjects to different ends.

This idea of a seismic shift in the structure and regulatory principles of modernity resonates with most if not all of the major accounts of postmodernity, and thus provides strong grounds from which to inquire as to parallel transformations at the level of ontology (see also Lee, 2000, p. x). Here, we re-engage Sass's argument in *Madness and Modernism*: if schizophrenia 'installs the public world in the most private recesses of the soul' (Sass, 1992, p. 106, italics in the original), how might it reflect such upheavals in the social realm? Bearing in mind that these changes in no way signal a return to pre-modern, pre-industrial modes of life, we should expect an affinity between schizophrenia

and postmodernity to continue, if not intensify the affinity between schizophrenia and modernity. Sass's comment here is brief but suggestive:

> Certain theorists who see Western societies as having moved to a stage of *post*moder-
> nity emphasize a somewhat different set of developments [from the rationality and
> reflexivity promoted by modern institutions], among them: the waning of affect, the
> dissolution of the sense of separate selfhood, the loss of any sense of the real, and the
> saturation by images and simulacra detaching from all grounding outside themselves;
> these, obviously, are more than a little reminiscent of certain schizoid and schizo-
> phrenic tendencies, and it is not difficult to imagine that such general cultural devel-
> opments might also influence the modes of experience characteristic of such
> individuals.

(Sass, 1992, p. 372)[22]

In order to explore the relationship between schizophrenia and postmodernity in the light of *Madness and Modernism* we need to introduce a third term
back into the equation, namely, postmodernism. Sass, as we know, identifies
a resemblance between high modernism, a movement renowned for its icono-
clasm, elitism, and intellectualism, and schizophrenia, the century's most
severe psychopathology, suggesting both can be seen as 'consequences or
reflections' of modernity. Implicit here and hence unremarked are two further
correlations between schizophrenic phenomenology and high modernism as
they appear in his analysis: both are *extreme* or *exceptional* cases (opposed to the
'normalcy' of mass or popular culture), and both articulate and reinvigorate
models of psychic depth.

Postmodernism is credited with collapsing the boundary between high art
and low art, or between high modernism and popular culture; extending, as it
were, high modernist techniques, thematic concerns, and aesthetic strategies
into the commercially driven realm of mass culture. It is also—in the work of
Bauman and many others—associated with a decentring of subjectivity, articulated either as the loss of 'masterful', meaningful, autonomous human self, or
the recognition that such an experience of selfhood was only ever a fiction. If
schizophrenia has an affinity with postmodernism, we might hypothesize two
things: (i) that the phenomenology of schizophrenia will resonate across a
larger number of cultural sites, but (ii) that it will no longer speak resound-
ingly of psychic depth. Exigent introspection, or 'the desperate attempt to
locate a self as solid as a thing', will still lead 'to the feeling of having no self,
no still point at the center of a turning world' (Sass, 1987a, pp. 23–4) but in

---

22 Here Sass references Jameson's 'Postmodernism and Consumer Society' but somewhat
surprisingly does not engage Jameson's claim—to be discussed in the next chapter—that
the figure of 'the schizophrenic' is the exemplary postmodern subject.

postmodernity, I am suggesting, perhaps the experience of having no solid self is not only more commonplace, but actually what consumer society encourages in its subjects. In turning now to postmodern cultural theory, we can see the figure of 'the schizophrenic' recast from being the apotheosis of modern subjectivity to the quotidian, prototypical postmodern subject.

Chapter 6

Postmodern schizophrenia

Postmodern cultural theory of the late twentieth century has used the term schizophrenia to ends far removed from the clinical diagnosis of individual suffering. By the early 1980s, *Anti-Oedipus* and the antipsychiatry movement had introduced new and politically charged models of schizophrenia to the academic establishment, greatly extending its symbolic capacities and potential. Since then, virtually every aspect of late twentieth-century aesthetic and cultural production—including visual art, literature, television, cinema, architecture, and music—as well as the generalized subjective experience of postmodernity, has been understood through its lens. This chapter is specifically concerned with the major theoretical works identifying the figure of 'the schizophrenic' as representative or typical of the postmodern subject. Although this argument is advanced in an array of different contexts, across a range of disciplines, my analysis concentrates on key texts by Jean Baudrillard, Fredric Jameson, David Harvey, Mark Currie, John Johnston, and Steven Frosh. If, as Robert Barrett suggests, 'People categorized as "schizophrenic" have long been entrusted with this duty of symbolizing society, its structural elements, its definition of personhood, its contradictions [and] its paradoxes' (1998c, p. 484), what is distinctive about these theorists' claim that schizophrenia can be used, however (il)legitimately, to interpret specific aspects of postmodernity? And how can this be understood within the context of the accounts of schizophrenia discussed so far in this book?

We saw in the previous chapter that Louis Sass's phenomenological approach to schizophrenia situated it outside the logic of the sublime that I have argued underscores psychiatric, psychoanalytic, antipsychiatric, and even anti-Oedipal accounts of the disorder. Attentive throughout to phenomenological detail, Sass discusses specific alterations in the schizophrenic experience of self and world, drawing on clinical and cultural examples to show that schizophrenia both is and is not within the realms of empathetic understanding. By contrast, in mobilizing a comparatively two-dimensional model of schizophrenia to stand for a *general* mode of Western late twentieth-century subjectivity, postmodern cultural theorists return to the sublime, inaugurating a fourth mode of schizophrenic sublimity I call the paradoxical sublime.

The idea of the paradoxical sublime is inspired by literary theorist Linda Hutcheon's analysis of paradoxical postmodernism, which she describes as a 'postmodernism of complicity and critique, of reflexivity and historicity, that at once inscribes and subverts the conventions and ideologies of the dominant cultural and social forces of the twentieth-century western world' (Hutcheon, 1989, p. 11). To operate paradoxically is, according to Hutcheon, to exploit and undermine, 'to install and then subvert'. It is this propensity to 'use and abuse' critical and aesthetic concepts and strategies which is for Hutcheon the most prominent feature of postmodern cultural productions (Hutcheon, 1988, p. 101). My suggestion here is that the schizophrenic sublime is similarly 'used and abused' by postmodern cultural theorists. As I will argue, the efficacy of the topos of schizophrenia in postmodern cultural theory depends upon its sublime status in psychiatric, psychoanalytic, and especially antipsychiatric discourse. However, using schizophrenia so capaciously redefines the disorder as quotidian—that is, as no longer pathological, because it is illustrative of contemporary subjectivity per se. This renders the term virtually empty, (over) inflates its symbolic capacity at the expense of its phenomenological and psychological specificity, and consequently conceals some of its more troubling implications. Postmodern theorists therefore do not challenge or deconstruct schizophrenia's sublime status; theirs is not the repudiation but the inflation and subsequent deliquescence of the schizophrenic sublime.

Worth noting from the outset are two effects of the paradoxical sublime as it operates in postmodern cultural theory. First, it pathologizes instead of merely describing the decentring of subjectivity and the so-called end of subjective depth. The Western self is, as Clifford Geertz has suggested, conceptualized '"as a bounded, unique, more or less integrated motivational and cognitive universe, a dynamic centre of awareness, emotion, judgment, and action organized into a distinctive whole and set contrastively both against other such wholes and against its social and natural background"' (quoted in Sass, 1992, p. 215; see also Fabrega, 1989; Rose, 1996). 'Postmodern schizophrenia' declares an end to this humanist model of the self. A second consequence of the paradoxical sublime is that it repositions the marginal *as* central; the apotheosis as the average; the pathological as normal, even ubiquitous.[1] In so

----

[1] Alain Ehrenberg's *The Weariness of the Self* offers an interesting parallel to the argument I will present in this chapter. Despite significant differences (not least of which is that Ehrenberg's book-length study remains centrally focused on the changing clinical fortunes of depression), Ehrenberg, like Jameson, Baudrillard, and other theorists of 'postmodern schizophrenia', uses a concept once understood to designate 'the exceptional' to interpret the *general* structure of subjectivity in the 'emancipatory' era of post-1968 liberal individualism: 'In the sixteenth century, melancholia was the elective illness of the

doing, does the topos of schizophrenia in postmodern cultural theory actually illuminate or interpret the experience of postmodernity? Can it help us to investigate, rather than simply describe, what it is to be, in Bauman's terminology, 'a liquid modern'?

These questions will be brought to bear first on Jean Baudrillard's *The Ecstasy of Communication* (1988) and then Fredric Jameson's 'Postmodernism, or the Cultural Logic of Late Capitalism' (1984b), an essay that arguably did more than any other to popularize the idea of schizophrenia as the representative form of postmodern subjectivity. Critics have for the most part followed Jameson in rejecting as 'morbid' any association between his model of 'schizophrenia' and its clinical analogues, but as with Deleuze and Guattari's model of schizophrenia-as-process, a close reading of his argument demonstrates the opposite. Concentrating on the three texts that most directly inform Jameson's account—Lacan's work on psychosis (1966, 1993), Renee's *Autobiography of a Schizophrenic Girl* (1970), and *Anti-Oedipus* (1982) itself[2]—I will look at what

---

exceptional man, of he who had nothing above him. During the Romantic period, it stood at the crossroads of creative genius and madness. Today, it is the situation of every individual in Western society. I want to provide a glimpse of this history while showing that contemporary depression is the marriage between the traditional melancholia of the exceptional person and the modern egalitarian idea that anyone can be exceptional . . . . [I approach depression] as an attitude, a mindset heavy with multiple social practices and representations of ourselves in a society in which values associated with autonomy (e.g. personal choice, self-ownership, individual initiative) have been generalized . . . . Thus, depression brings together all the tensions of the modern individual' (Ehrenberg, 2010, p. xxx).

[2] Curiously, there is no reference to Joseph Gabel's *False Consciousness* (1976) in Jameson's *Postmodernism, or the Cultural Logic of Late Capitalism*, or, as I have already noted, in *Anti-Oedipus*. Whether this book-length study of schizophrenia and false consciousness was simply unknown to Jameson, or represented precisely the kind of Marxist–psychiatric scholarship he sought to distance himself from, is difficult to judge. Certainly Gabel's Minkowski-influenced account of the phenomenology of schizophrenia (emphasizing morbid rationalism, the collapse of affect, a sense of social alienation, and a breakdown in the experience of lived time) is highly relevant to Jameson's Lacanian-inspired account of the temporal and linguistic collapse of subjectivity in 'postmodern schizophrenia'. Indeed, although he does not reference Jameson, Deleuze, or Guattari specifically here, Alastair Morgan suggests that post-1960s 'Schizophrenia no longer comes to be read as the incarnation of a generalized loss of life in terms of reification [Gabel's position], but is mapped on to the speeded-up nature of modern life in general. The instability of identity, the fluidity and speeding up of sensory inputs and perceptions, the inability to form lasting relationships; schizophrenia as psychosis becomes a mirror of the postmodern in a reversal of Gabel's original socio-pathological parallelism' (Morgan, 2010, p. 184). A more comprehensive study of *False Consciousness* in connection with *Anti-Oedipus* and *Postmodernism, or the Cultural Logic of Late Capitalism* is clearly warranted.

must be downplayed, side-stepped, or even repressed in order for this meta-phor to function, and argue that it is Jameson's analysis that most clearly dem-onstrates what I have described as the paradoxical operation of the schizophrenic sublime. Following Jameson's lead—albeit with significant variations—David Harvey (1990), Mark Currie (1998), John Johnston (1990), and Stephen Frosh (1991) have all used schizophrenia as a heuristic device to explore the experience of postmodernity. In the final part of this chapter I consider the strengths and limitations of these various deployments of schizo-phrenia. Re-engaging Sass's analysis of schizophrenia and modernity, I argue that they are more suggestive than has previously been acknowledged, but suffer also from the very problems they diagnose.

Introducing the figure of 'the postmodern schizophrenic'

Edited by Hal Foster and first published in 1983, *The Anti-aesthetic* (1983) was one of the earliest collections of essays on postmodern culture and has remained among the most influential. In it, the postmodern subject is diagnosed as schizophrenic in two successive seminal articles: Fredric Jameson's 'Postmodernism and Consumer Society' and Jean Baudrillard's 'The Ecstasy of Communication'. Baudrillard's essay was expanded and re-published as a slim Semiotext(e) Foreign Agents monograph in 1988. Jameson's analysis of the postmodern was extended in his 1984 *New Left Review* article 'Postmodernism, or the Cultural Logic of Late Capitalism', which in turn became the first chap-ter of his 1991 book of the same name. Jameson would come to be hailed as 'theorist supreme of the postmodern' (Hardt and Weeks, 2000, pp. 1–2); Baudrillard as its prophet and high priest (Bailey, 2006). Writing in the after-math of *Anti-Oedipus*, Jameson and Baudrillard both proposed new ways of conceptualizing the association between capitalism and schizophrenia, identi-fying the figure of 'the schizophrenic' not as the revolutionary but the casualty of late capitalist postmodernity. Postmodern schizophrenia is defined not as rebellious, counter-cultural, transcendent, or even bizarre, but as a historically specific form of subjective disintegration, a final flattening of psychic depth. The trope functions to pathologize contemporary subjectivity and implicitly to reinforce the idea that it is hermeneutically inaccessible, that the heap of frag-ments conceals no latent meaning. What works against this emerging view of the sublimity of postmodern schizophrenia is simply that it characterizes *all* contemporary subjects: no longer exceptional—or even the clue to the 'true' operation of desire—schizophrenia is the universal fate of the postmodern masses.

We live, according to Baudrillard, in an age characterized by the promiscuous proliferation of networks of communication. It is an era of surfaces without depth; an era of immanence in which transcendence is no longer possible; an era of obscenity:

> Obscenity begins when there is no more spectacle, no more stage, no more theatre, no more illusion, when every-thing becomes immediately transparent, visible, exposed in the raw and inexorable light of information and communication.
>
> *We no longer partake of the drama of alienation, but are in the ecstasy of communication.*
> [...]
>
> It is no longer the obscenity of the hidden, the repressed, the obscure, but that of the visible, the all-too-visible, the more-visible-than-visible; it is the obscenity of that which no longer contains a secret and is entirely soluble in information and communication.

(Baudrillard, 1988, pp. 21–2, italics in the original)

Writing at the dawn of the digital age and before the rapid rise of mobile and internet technologies, Baudrillard's emphasis on the epoch-defining significance of information and its circulation is prescient.[3] In Baudrillard's highly mediatized West, the flow and form of communication constitute the whole of social space, collapsing any notion of interior and exterior. The network encompasses everything and conceals nothing; it abolishes representation, Baudrillard argues, because there is no longer a space or even a distinction between sign and referent. Earlier scenes or sites of representation—the mirror, the theatre, the stage, the public and private sphere—no longer have any meaning as we exist not 'as playwrights or actors but as terminals of multiple networks' (Baudrillard, 1988, p. 16).

Baudrillard, like Deleuze and Guattari before him, turns to 'metaphors drawn from pathology' to explain the impact of obscene communication on the subject (who is, again, assigned the masculine pronoun):

> If hysteria was the pathology of the exacerbated staging of the subject—of the theatrical and operational conversion of the body—and if paranoia was the pathology of organization—of the structuring of a rigid and jealous world—then today we have entered into a new form of schizophrenia—with the emergence of an immanent promiscuity and the perpetual interconnection of all information and communication networks. No more hysteria, or projective paranoia as such, but a state of terror which

---

[3] Although, ironically, it could also be said to be 50 years too late. In 1937 a feature article in *Harper's Magazine* had already 'declared that Americans lived in an "Age of Schizophrenia", a "dazzling world of bright light and swift movement and flashing communications in which the man of flesh and blood makes it impossible to make a home"' (quoted in Metzl, 2009, p. 37).

> is characteristic of the schizophrenic, an over-proximity of all things, a foul promiscu-
> ity of all things which beleaguer and penetrate him, meeting with no resistance, and no
> halo, no aura, not even the aura of his own body protects him. In spite of himself the
> schizophrenic is open to everything and lives in the most extreme confusion. He is the
> obscene victim of the world's obscenity. The schizophrenic is not, as generally claimed,
> characterized by his loss of touch with reality, but by the absolute proximity to and
> total instantaneousness with things, this overexposure to the transparency of the
> world. Stripped of a stage and crossed over without the least obstacle, the schizo-
> phrenic cannot produce the very limits of being. He becomes a pure screen, a pure
> absorption and resorption surface of the influent networks.

> (Baudrillard, 1988, pp. 26–7)

Baudrillard may draw his metaphors from psychology, but he does so only
to proclaim the end of the psyche itself. Emptied out, flattened into two dimensions and existing in a state of 'total instantaneousness', 'the schizophrenic' is
a non-self connected to and constituted by decentralized networks; a screen
across which the binary code of information simply flickers. Baudrillard's
vision is one of final reification—the schizophrenic-as-terminal effectively
signals the termination of subjectivity. The ecstasy of communication further
results in a postmodern transubstantiation: flesh becomes code, and the body
dematerializes into information. It is the sublime dissolution of the self—
engulfed by the world, 'the schizophrenic' 'cannot produce the very limits of
being'—but also the dissolution of self within the sublime, within a seemingly
infinite, decentred network of information that itself defies representation. In
one fell swoop, the masses are portrayed as pathologically passive, and the
prognosis is not good: there is, it would appear, no way of reconstituting the
self through, in spite of or in opposition to, the inexorable flow of information
and communication.

If, as I have argued, the effect of Baudrillard's analysis is to produce a paradoxically sublime schizophrenia, the question remains 'Why schizophrenia?'
Baudrillard does not refer to specific psychiatric, psychoanalytic, antipsychiatric,
or even autobiographical accounts of psychosis in his description of the
subject-as-terminal, nor can his 'schizophrenic' screen be said to exhibit anything remotely resembling a specifically psychotic symptom. Yet it would be
disingenuous to suggest, especially in the light of his claim to uncover a history
of pathology, that this use of the term is arbitrary or incidental, or that it is
merely a more sophisticated synonym for madness.

Baudrillard's admittedly brief excursion into the territory of deterritorialized
desire could not be said to comprise a considered engagement, let alone
critique, of Deleuze and Guattari's analysis of capitalism and schizophrenia,
but it is not difficult to spot *Anti-Oedipus* lurking in the background of *The
Ecstasy of Communication*. Like Deleuze and Guattari's schizo, Baudrillard's

'schizophrenic' is no longer possessed of psychic depth or interiority. 'He' is constituted by the fluxes of the world, only here there is no celebration of the free flow of desire because being plugged into postmodernity induces a state of paralysis, 'terror' and 'extreme confusion' more akin to that suffered by the 'immense transfixed hippopotamus'. Indeed, if explained in anti-Oedipal terminology, Baudrillard's 'schizophrenic-as-terminal' is a full body without organs: 'the unproductive, the sterile, the unengendered, the unconsumable' (Deleuze and Guattari, 1982, p. 8).[4] *The Ecstasy of Communication* can further be seen to invert Lacan's model of a sublime schizophrenia. Baudrillard repeats Lacan's idea that psychosis is a problem in the symbolic register, but implies that schizophrenia results from an *over-proximity* to communication, an *immersion* in information, rather than expulsion from the phallic system of signification. Where for Judith Butler and Slavoj Žižek schizophrenia marks the limits of subjectivity,[5] for Baudrillard schizophrenia is a state of blank terror caused by an excess of signifiers, and an inability to differentiate or distance self from world. It is the sublime dissolution of subjectivity into 'the smooth and functional surface of communication' (Baudrillard, 1988, p. 12).

Schizophrenia and 'The Cultural Logic of Late Capitalism'

If *Anti-Oedipus* was the first and most polemical analysis to link capitalism and schizophrenia, Fredric Jameson's 'Postmodernism, or the Cultural Logic of Late Capitalism', allegedly the most cited article of the 1980s (Kellner, 1989, p. 2), served emphatically to recode and popularize that link as paradigmatically postmodern. Although it owes a clear, if again unacknowledged, debt to Deleuze and Guattari's model of 'ideal or heroic schizophrenia' (Jameson, 1991, p. 154), Jameson's loosely Lacanian account of postmodern schizophrenia does not follow these earlier theorists in positing its transcendent potential. Rather, like Baudrillard, he suggests the figure of 'the schizophrenic' is both product *and* symptom of late capitalism, and as such has no way of surmounting the late capitalist predicament. As with *Anti-Oedipus*, the overwhelming majority of critics have accepted Jameson's reassurance that he is not offering 'some culture-and-personality diagnosis of our society' in the mode of

---

4 Deleuze and Guattari describe this state of catatonic immobility as belonging to 'the realm of antiproduction': 'In order to resist organ-machines, the body without organs presents its smooth, slippery, opaque, taut surface as a barrier. [. . .] In order to resist using words composed of articulated phonetic units, it utters only gasps and cries that are sheer unarticulated blocks of sound' (Deleuze and Guattari, 1982, pp. 8–9).

5 Exiled to a 'psychotic abyss outside the symbolic domain,' 'the schizophrenic' designates that which is beyond the intelligible (Lacan, quoted in Žižek 1999, p. 273; see also 'Arguing with the Real' in Butler, 1993).

Christopher Lasch (1978),[6] and have consequently refused or failed to inquire into the relationship between postmodern schizophrenia and its clinical antecedents and inspirations. These dominant readings strike me as highly selective and somewhat counterintuitive, ignoring as they do Jameson's references to clinical literature and the centrality accorded to schizophrenia in his overall argument. By contrast, my analysis of 'The Cultural Logic of Late Capitalism' seeks to redress this scholarly oversight by concentrating on what is absent from or omitted in the translation of clinical condition into cultural theory. Cognizant of the dangers of over-reading Jameson's model of postmodern schizophrenia, I will endeavour to demonstrate that its complex engagement with clinical accounts of schizophrenia is more suggestive than Jameson and his critics have perhaps allowed, in that it also, like Baudrillard's work, begins the operation of the paradoxical sublime.

With this end in mind, the first step must be to consider schizophrenia's role within Jameson's analysis of postmodernism as the cultural dominant of the late twentieth century. According to Jameson, the case for the existence of postmodernism depends upon 'the hypothesis of some radical break . . . generally traced back to the end of the 1950s or early 1960s' (Jameson, 1991, p. 1). The break in question is the emergence of a new form of capitalism most strongly associated with the rise of multinational corporations, but including also:

> The new international division of labor, a vertiginous new dynamic in international banking and the stock exchanges (including the enormous Second and Third World debt), new forms of media interrelationship (very much including transportation systems such as containerization), computers and automation, the flight of production to advanced Third World areas, along with all the more familiar social consequences, including the crisis of traditional labor, the emergence of yuppies, and gentrification on a now-global scale.

> (Jameson, 1991, p. xix)

Following Marxist economist Ernest Mandel, Jameson argues that late capitalism is the 'purest' form of capitalism because its 'prodigious expansion of capital into hitherto uncommodified areas' (Jameson, 1991, pp. 36, 4) signals the total interpenetration of commerce and culture. Whereas Deleuze and Guattari appeared disinterested in the empirical analysis of historically specific forms of capitalism,[7] Jameson's periodizing hypothesis treats postmodernism

---

[6] Jameson states that 'there are . . . far more damaging things to be said about our social system than are available through the use of psychological categories' (Jameson, 1991, p. 26). However, as I will endeavour to show, he certainly uses schizophrenia to damaging effect.

[7] *Anti-Oedipus* posits three historical periods or phases—primitive territorial, despotic, and capitalist—but does not distinguish different forms of capitalism.

not only as the cultural manifestation of the specific technological and socio-logical upheavals of late capitalism, but as 'the internal and superstructural expression of a whole new wave of American military and economic domina-tion throughout the world' (Jameson, 1991, p. 5).[8]

For Jameson, like Baudrillard, postmodernism is characterized above all by a loss of depth. The eclipse of parody by pastiche, the loss of the historical referent, the flattening of space into surfaces, the rise of simulacra, and the abandonment of theoretical depth models are all symptomatic of 'a new kind of flatness or depthlessness, a new kind of superficiality' that he identifies as 'perhaps the supreme formal feature' of the postmodern (Jameson, 1984b, p. 9). If we follow the trajectory of Jameson's argument closely, it is clear that this aesthetic and interpretive depthlessness registers a related mutation in lived experience: the waning of affect and the decentring of subjectivity. Referring primarily to examples in visual art (Van Gogh and Munch as the exemplars of high modernism, Andy Warhol in the postmodern dock) Jameson argues that the 'great modernist thematics of alienation, anomie, solitude, social fragmen-tation and isolation' no longer resonate in the postmodern era (Jameson, 1991, p. 11). Existential angst and psychic complexities have dissolved into free-floating feelings: depersonalized, discrete emotional intensities; isolated moments of euphoria, exhilaration, and disorientation. Whereas 'anxiety is a hermeneutic emotion, expressing an underlying nightmare state of the world', moments of affective intensity should not be misconstrued as meaningful responses to postmodernity because they bear no relation to context (Jameson, quoted in Stephanson, 1988, p. 4). The scream—a cry from the abyss of the soul—is replaced by the hallucinogenic high, the flash of panic, the fleeting euphoria, the twinge of fear, the moment of exhilaration. As emotional narra-tive disintegrates into emotionally charged moments, the waning of affect points to a profound change in the experience of subjectivity:

> The notorious burn-out and self-destruction cases of the ending 1960s [*sic*], and the great dominant experiences of drugs and schizophrenia—these would seem to have little enough in common anymore, either with the hysterics and neurotics of Freud's own day, or with those canonical experiences of radical isolation and solitude, anomie, private revolt, Van Gogh-type madness, which dominated the period of high modern-ism. This shift in the dynamics of cultural pathology can be characterized as one in which the alienation of the subject is displaced by the fragmentation of the subject.
>
> (Jameson, 1991, p. 14)

---

8 Consequently, 'every position on postmodernism in culture—whether apologia or stig-matization—is also at one and the same time, and *necessarily* an implicitly or explicitly political stance on the nature of multinational capitalism today' (Jameson, 1991, p. 3).

The transition from the modern self—a bounded ego or psyche projecting outwards the drama of inner feeling—to a fragmented, decentred postmodern subject is troped negatively as the collapse of subjective boundaries, the abolition of depth, the evacuation not only of anxiety but also of all individual feeling.

The decentred subject is for Jameson the causal link between late capitalism and the postmodern aesthetic: the 'disappearance of the individual subject' results in the impossibility of individual style and the rise of an aesthetics of fragmentation (pastiche), the 'waning of the great high modernism thematics of time or temporality', and the consequent weakening of historicity (Jameson, 1991, p. 16). Jameson's portrait of the decentred subject so far resembles that of fellow Marxist literary critic Terry Eagleton: a 'dispersed, decentered network of libidinal attachments, emptied of ethical substance and psychical interiority, the ephemeral function of this or that act of consumption, media experience, sexual relationship, trend or fashion' (Eagleton, 1985, p. 71). Why, then, does Jameson go one step further in describing the decentred subject as schizophrenic? Is it to draw attention to the fact that late capitalism precipitates not a shift but a *crisis* in subjectivity? Does it, despite Jameson's explicit disavowal of any association with the 'morbid' psychiatric reality of schizophrenia, function not only to diagnose, but also to pathologize, the postmodern self, as most critics seem to suggest? Or is there something more subtle at work here?

For Jameson, identity is a function of language; a coherent sense of self is created and sustained through the temporal organization of linguistic signifiers. On his account, schizophrenia is the disintegration of this 'objective mirage of signification', such that 'when the links of that signifying chain snap, then we have schizophrenia in the form of a rubble of distinct and unrelated signifiers'. 'If we are unable to unify the past, present and future of the sentence', Jameson argues, 'then we are similarly unable to unify the past, present and future of our own biographical experience or psychic life. With the breakdown of the signifying chain, therefore, the schizophrenic is reduced to an experience of pure material signifiers, or in other words of a series of pure and unrelated presents in time' (Jameson, 1991, p. 26). Schizophrenia is a form of 'linguistic malfunction' that produces a temporal crisis: history and the future collapse into the perpetual present. If the modernist self projected outwards the anxiety of the age, 'the postmodern schizophrenic' is reduced to perceiving and representing the world in fragments, moments and isolated intensities. As John O'Neill observes 'action, project, and orientation collapse in the literal, nauseous, and real present' (O'Neill, 1989, p. 148; see also Jameson, 1991, p. 27).

To capture this experience, Jameson quotes a long passage from *Autobiography of a Schizophrenic Girl* (in which Renee, using the language of the sublime, describes 'the first appearance of those elements which were always present in later sensations of unreality: illimitable vastness, brilliant light, and the gloss and smoothness of material things' (Renee, 1970, pp. 21–2, quoted by Jameson, 1991, p. 27). We will return to the issue of schizophrenic phenomenology later in the chapter; here, it is sufficient to note that this choice of example works *against* Jameson's claim that 'postmodern schizophrenia' bears no relationship to any form of psychiatric disorder. Jameson's references to a Lacanian view of psychosis further undermine this claim and are bedevilled by contradiction. 'I found Lacan's account of schizophrenia useful', he writes, 'not because I have any way of knowing whether it has clinical accuracy but because—as description rather than diagnosis—it seems to me to be a suggestive aesthetic model' (Jameson, 1991, p. 26). In a footnote, Jameson then directs the reader to Lacan's analysis of Schreber in *Écrits*, with the rider that 'Most of us have received this classical view of psychosis by way of Deleuze and Guattari's *Anti-Oedipus*' (Jameson, 1991, p. 420). Yet there is nothing 'classical' about Deleuze and Guattari's portrayal of the process of schizophrenia, nor can *Anti-Oedipus* possibly be understood as a wholehearted endorsement of the Lacanian model of psychosis. So what *is* the relationship between Jameson's account of schizophrenia, as outlined earlier, and Lacan's 'On a Question Preliminary to any Possible Treatment of Psychosis', and where, in turn, do Deleuze and Guattari fit in?

Lacan's conviction that the 'drama' of psychosis is situated 'in man's [*sic*] relation to the signifier' (Lacan, 1966, p. 214) underscores Jameson's construction of schizophrenia as a crisis in the symbolic register, as a problem of language and not fantasy, of a self already conceptualized as operating independently of others. In an echo of his reluctance to investigate the precipitating factors in the decentring of subjectivity, Jameson states: 'I must omit the familial or more orthodox psychoanalytic background to this situation', or what is for Lacan 'paternal authority now considered as a linguistic function' (Jameson, 1991, p. 26). As I discussed at length in Chapter 2, Lacan posited that 'the defect that gives psychosis its essential condition' and structure is 'the foreclosure of the Name-of-the-Father in the place of the Other, and in the failure of the paternal metaphor' (Lacan, 1966, p. 215). How then should we interpret Jameson's omission of this 'essential' point; his refusal to see the schizophrenic's linguistic crisis as the crisis of a symbolic order structured by the phallus?

Without elaborating on its consequences, Stephen Frosh highlights succinctly one of the key problems of this account: 'What is gained . . . is a set of enticing metaphors; what is lost is the specificity of the original concept. Here, that means a failure to explore the nature of the Lacanian psychotic' (Frosh, 1991, p. 160). Jacqueline Rose is more targeted in her critique: 'Jameson bypasses that traumatic point of sexual differentiation at which the psychotic delusion seizes the subject', a move that allows him to present the breakdown of the signifying chain 'exclusively in terms of the perpetual intensity of the signifier' (Rose, 1988, p. 242). She goes on to argue that 'if one puts back the "Name-of-the-Father" into the account of psychotic breakdown then—without celebrating the form of that disturbance—it nonetheless becomes impossible to invoke it without recognizing the far-reaching implications in the field of sexuality of this crisis of naming itself' (Rose, 1988, p. 243). Jameson's omission certainly has implications for a feminist (re)appraisal of the causes and consequences of the 'postmodern schizophrenic's' disruption of phallic discourse, but my more immediate concern is with the way Jameson both draws on and disavows schizophrenia's status as sublime. It is clear that in the wake of a strong counter-cultural antipsychiatry movement, and the publication of the exuberant post-Marxist *Anti-Oedipus*, schizophrenia was very much on the agenda of cultural theory in the late 1970s and very early 1980s. Jameson's return to Lacan must be read first and foremost as a return to the realm of psychopathology; a rejection of the 'ideal schizophrenia' proposed by Deleuze and Guattari (Jameson, 2002, p. 194) in favour of the idea of an irreparably dysfunctional psychic structure. Jameson follows Lacan in suggesting what is in effect a sublime schizophrenia: it is an ontology of dispersal from which it appears impossible to rehabilitate the monad of modernism; it is a state of such extreme psychic disintegration that no representation—whether conscious or phantasmagoric—is possible except in isolated fragments; and consequently, it is a subjective mode resolutely impervious to any hermeneutic analysis, whether psychological, psychoanalytic, or otherwise. However—and this is crucial—because schizophrenia is the fate wrought by late capitalism on all, because, in Rose's words, 'it becomes precisely the drama of all . . . subjects' (Rose, 1988, p. 243), schizophrenia is extended across the whole of social space and loses its distinctiveness, its reference to specific psychopathology, its capacity to designate difference.

Jameson uses clinical, autobiographical, and philosophical accounts of schizophrenia which emphasize its sublimity, but by calling upon schizophrenia to describe (as well as to designate as hermeneutically inaccessible) the dissolution of modernist subjectivity as a ubiquitous condition, he renders paradoxical the schizophrenic sublime. The idea that schizophrenia in 'The Cultural Logic of Late Capitalism' is paradoxically sublime finds further support in Jameson's discussion of the postmodern 'technological' sublime.

For Jameson, as Lawrence Grossberg notes, the disintegration of subjectivity functions as the pivotal link between the material conditions of postmodernity and the postmodern aesthetic: 'Textual fragmentation is a sign of the real fragmentation of our subjectivity; which is itself a sign of the intentional (both ideological and material) fragmentation of space in multinational capitalism' (Grossberg, 1988, pp. 173–4). 'Postmodern hyperspace', as Jameson calls it,

> ... has finally succeeded in transcending the capacities of the individual body to locate itself, to organize its immediate surroundings perceptually, and cognitively to map its position in a mappable external world. It may now be suggested that this alarming disjunction point between the body and its built environment ... can itself stand as the symbol and analogon of that even sharper dilemma which is the incapacity of our minds, at least as present, to map the great global multinational and decentered communicational network in which we find ourselves caught as individual subjects.

> (Jameson, 1991, p. 44)

Physical disorientation in a media-saturated metropolis reflects a more profound spatial disorientation: the dissolution of subjectivity in the 'impossible totality' of late capitalism itself (Jameson, 1991, p. 37); 'schizophrenia' through exposure to what Jameson variously calls the 'camp', 'hysterical', 'postmodern', or 'technological' sublime. If every diagnosis is a prognosis, this is dire indeed. In what reads as a variation on Baudrillard's thesis, we are, it seems, 'schizophrenic' because it is impossible to achieve critical distance from the global system in which we are immersed; trapped in the perpetual present of the global flow of capitalism, and dazzled by the materiality of the signifier in isolation, it is impossible to undertake the project of 'cognitive mapping' that Jameson identifies as the solution both to subjective re-orientation and the current representational crisis.[9]

Beyond Jameson

Jameson's and Baudrillard's vision of a postmodern subject 'schizophrenized' by late capitalist postmodernity has enjoyed a wide circulation and exerted considerable influence within postmodern literary and cultural theory. Marxist geographer David Harvey, for whom the postmodern condition is synonymous with the time–space compression effected by flexible modes of capital accumulation, endorses Jameson's account of schizophrenia as an essentially

---

[9] Jameson defines cognitive mapping as 'the coordination of existential data (the empirical position of the subject) with unlived, abstract conceptions of the geographic totality'. In the spatial and social confusion of postmodernity, it is the means by which 'we may again begin to grasp our positioning as individual and collective subjects and regain a capacity to act and struggle' (Jameson, 1991, pp. 51, 54).

accurate portrait of postmodern ontology. Although he criticizes Jameson for downplaying the potential terror of the schizophrenic state of unreality,[10] Harvey agrees that the experience of a perpetual present is a direct conse- quence of a 'general speed-up in the turnover time of capital', which accentu- ates the 'volatility and ephemerality of fashions, products, production techniques, labour processes, ideas and ideologies, values and established prac- tices' (Harvey, 1990, pp. 351, 285, see also 291). Mark Currie has also used schizophrenia—as discussed by Jameson, Harvey, Deleuze, and Guattari—to explain time compression in consumer society. According to Currie, the tem- poral structure of cultural narratives is indexed to the commodity cycle of late capitalism: the rapidity with which events are consigned to the past, only to be reinstalled in the present, mirrors the short shelf-life of the commodity as dictated by the rapid turnover of capital. The moment of consumer choice is a suspension of narrative in time, and closely resembles the temporal and linguistic fragmentation of schizophrenia. Currie sees 'the schizophrenic',

> ... as an interpreter whose disorder is to multiply and destabilise meanings, to experi- ence the world spatially as a theatre of signs and discourses which cannot exclude each other and which constitute a babble of voices: to experience selfhood not as an ordered narrative but as multiple identification amongst the babble of discourses. The schizo- phrenic is not so much nature's poststructuralist sociologist as *the product* of a schiz- oid culture which seems to aspire to the collapse of linear meaning into the compressed time of a perpetual present.
>
> (Currie, 1998, p. 103, my italics)

In a now-familiar generalization, he goes on to suggest that 'There may then be a sense in which we are all moving towards a schizophrenic mode of cul- tural experience, as our minds change in response to space–time compression' (Currie, 1998, p. 103).

This is certainly a view shared by Robbie Goh, who argues that 'cultural schizophrenia in this sense is an inability for the everyday subject to step out- side of and separate himself or herself from the totalizing and disorienting processes of capitalist flows (not merely of money, but also of related tech- nologies, timing, images and aspects)' (Goh, 2008). John Johnston, in his 'Ideology, Representation, Schizophrenia: Toward a Theory of the Postmodern Subject', gives a useful overview of how such a change might be experienced:

> Although the 'schiz' proclivity for discontinuous inscription and a textuality of surfaces problematizes the formation of typical themes, he or she will admit to a continuing

---

[10] Harvey (1990, p. 351) accuses Jameson of 'making it all seem like a well-controlled LSD trip rather than a succession of states of guilt, lethargy, and helplessness coupled with anguished and sometimes tempestuous dislocation'.

fascination with the logic of the simulacrum, with networks and circuitry, both infor-
mational and physical (as in the highway as semiotic system), with the body as site or
screen, with space, sights, and sounds (not the modernist place), with speed-ups and
slow-downs (not modernist simultaneity), with dispersions, dispossessions, becom-
ings (not modernist archetypal recurrences and recenterings). Further, the 'schiz' has
remarked that others find his or her behaviour a source of fascination, especially the
looping and syncoped state of consciousness, the Lacanian 'fadings' and, above all,
affects in extremis: either flat and toneless, or hallucinatory and delirious. (To these
observers, neurotic styles of behavior now appear 'campy' and humorous.)

(Johnston, 1990, p. 90)

Johnston's description is exemplary of postmodern theory's tendency
both to normalize schizophrenia and pathologize 'normal' subjectivity as radically decentred and spoken by the 'tongues of consumerism' (Finlay, 1989,
p. 45).

Harvey, Currie, Johnston, and others[11] follow Jameson in emphasizing the
links between schizophrenia and the general subjective experience of contemporary capitalism—effecting, as I have already suggested, an inflation of the
schizophrenic sublime wherein the pathological becomes representative and
its potency as a marker of difference is neutralized. Of course, the suggestion
that the figure of 'the schizophrenic' is representative of all postmodern subjects has also attracted significant criticism from within cultural theory. Harvey
cautions that the Deleuzoguattarian 'hyper-rhetoric', which extrapolates revolutionary agency from the experiences of people with severe mental illness 'can
dissolve into the most alarming irresponsibility' (Harvey, 1990, p. 351; see also
Glass, 1993). Currie, noting that 'there are few postmodern thinkers who
believe in the idea of an inner life or a private domain of subjectivity', suggests
that the claim that postmodern consumer culture has a schizophrenic effect
upon the subject 'should be understood less in the spirit of an analogy between
the mind and the world than as a dismantling of the boundary between them'
(Currie, 1998, p. 102). Two of the strongest critiques mounted against 'postmodern colonists of the imagery of psychosis' (Frosh, 1991, p. 132) have come
from Stephen Frosh and Anthony Elliott in their books on psychoanalytic and
social theory. Although broadly sympathetic to the idea that schizophrenia
does in some sense register or reflect aspects of postmodern culture, both
remain wary of the loss of 'critical clarity' that comes with 'brandishing clinical

---

[11] See my discussion in the previous chapter of essays collected in *Pathologies of the Modern
Self* (Levin, 1987b). See also the edited collection *Pathology and the Postmodern: Mental
Illness as Discourse and Experience* (Fee, 2000), and analogous accounts of the 'multiphre-
nia' (Gergen, 1991) and 'telephrenia' (Gottschalk, 2000) of the self.

terms as if they were weapons' (Frosh, 1991, p. 5). As Frosh (1991, p. 128) reminds us:

> Remembering how to maintain the boundaries of a metaphor, commenting on psychotic discourse without ennobling it, knowing the difference between signifier, signified and real: these are tasks of a theory which are constantly under pressure when the object of that theory is the subversive theorisation implicit in psychotic thought.

Postmodern theorists, Frosh argues, fail to account for the specificity of the psychotic process, for differences in class, race, and gender, and for differences in the underlying social processes involved in subject formation (Frosh, 1991, p. 5). As a consequence, the idea of schizophrenic subjectivity cannot account 'for resistance, revolution, or even just some forms of sanity' (Frosh, 1991, p. 149), and we must instead look to imagination, fantasy, and libidinal intensity to understand the impact of postmodernism on subjectivity (Elliott, 1996).

These criticisms—important as they are—address the structural limitations of the analogy but not its detail, as they could easily extend to the appropriation of any psychiatric concept. Staying for the moment within the framework of cultural theory, we can see that although Jameson and Baudrillard use schizophrenia explicitly to draw attention to psychic and linguistic dysfunction, implicitly their models point to a further crisis in embodiment. Whether this is symptomatic of a significant conceptual blind spot in the work of these first-world white male intellectuals, or, on a more generous reading, is an unacknowledged but nonetheless suggestive dimension of their theories of schizophrenic subjectivity, the 'postmodern schizophrenic' appears in their work as a disembodied subject.[12] Whereas Avital Ronell (1989, p. 109) has argued persuasively that 'the schizophrenic gives us exemplary access to the fundamental shifts in affectivity and corporeal organization produced and commanded by technology, in part because the schizophrenic inhabits these other territorialities', Baudrillard's 'pure screen' seems to exist independent of any fleshy reality, as does Jameson's syntactically fragmented 'schizophrenic'. For all of Jameson's discussion of the quantifiable material markers of this new epoch, arguably its most basic material reference point is absent. Jameson does concede that postmodern hyperspace 'stands as something like an imperative to grow new organs, to expand our sensorium and our body to some new, as yet unimaginable, perhaps ultimately impossible, dimensions' (Jameson, 1991,

---

[12] Kathleen Kirby (1996, p. 51) makes a similar point, arguing that these theorists construe schizophrenia as a temporal rather than spatial disorder: 'While nominally a dysfunction of time, schizophrenia equally represents a dysfunction of space: a failure to adhere to an external reality, to arbitrate the distinction between inside and outside, and to hold the surrounding world together in a meaningful totality. The perception of such a subject would be an unmediated barrage of disordered stimuli whose immediate presence assaults the surface of the exposed subject'.

p. 39). However, although gesturing towards the importance of the body in navigating physical space, he overlooks its importance to subjective orientation in historical and cultural space, much less its role in constituting sexual and racial identities. For Jameson, it is class consciousness, rather than corporeality, which is essential to the cognitive mapping of the postmodern, but implicitly his model of schizophrenia stands as an urgent imperative to reconceptualize embodiment rather than somehow do away with it altogether.

The limitations of these accounts of postmodern ontology should be clear by now. Unable to account for difference of any kind, 'the schizophrenic' as representative casualty of the postmodern is disembodied and deprived of agency (Woods, 2002), a spectre of depthlessness that perhaps says more about the pessimism of cultural theory than it does about the experience of postmodernity. In the remainder of this chapter, however, I want to argue that despite these limitations, the analyses advanced by Jameson, Baudrillard, and others actually lay the foundation for a more nuanced account of the symbolic relationship between schizophrenia and postmodernity. The problem, as I see it, is that a two-dimensional model of schizophrenia is deployed to diagnose the postmodern subject as two-dimensional. Revisiting Jameson's claims in the light of Sass's analysis of schizophrenic phenomenology allows us to develop a richer, more complex account of a specifically postmodern schizophrenia.

The postmodern *stimmung*

Jameson turns to Renee's *Autobiography of a Schizophrenic Girl* to describe the schizophrenic experience engendered by the postmodern:

> I remember very well the day it happened. We were staying in the country and I had gone for a walk as I did now and then. Suddenly, as I was passing the school, I heard a German song; the children were having a singing lesson. I stopped to listen, and at that instant a strange feeling came over me, a feeling hard to analyse but akin to something I was to know too well later—a disturbing sense of unreality. It seemed to me that I no longer recognized the school, it had become as large as a barracks; the singing children were prisoners, compelled to sing. It was as though the school and the children's song were set apart from the rest of the world. At the same time my eye encountered a field of wheat whose limits I could not see. The song of the children imprisoned in the smooth stone school-barracks filled me with such anxiety that I broke into sobs. I ran home to our garden and began to play 'to make things seem as they usually were', that is, to return to reality. It was the first appearance of those elements which were always present in later sensations of unreality: illimitable vastness, brilliant light, and the gloss and smoothness of material things.

> (Renee (1970, p. 21) quoted by Jameson, 1991, p. 27)[13]

....

[13] Renee (1970, p. 22) continues: 'I have no explanation for what happened, or why. But it was during this same period that I learned my father had a mistress and that he made my

I have already noted that the choice of a clinical example—rather than, say, an artistic portrayal of 'unreality'—works against Jameson's clinical agnosticism. His claim that the affective intensity 'here described in the negative terms of anxiety and loss of reality', could be imagined 'just as well ... in the positive terms of euphoria' (Jameson, 1991, pp. 27–8), also appears as a somewhat unconvincing attempt to negate the detail as well as the significance of his chosen example (Taylor, 1987, p. 67). Pelagia Goulimari has argued that because he 'has eyes only for the unlimited wheat field' Jameson fails to recognize the importance of history within Renee's biographical narrative. Encompassed within a clearly articulated personal history ('I remember well the day it happened') is, according to Goulimari, 'a genuine historical experience', a sudden flashback to a time of war, 'barracks' and 'prisoners' (Goulimari, 2004).[14] More obviously, the fact that Renee's is an autobiographical account of her *first* schizophrenic break—an encounter with the sublime that would recur in 'later sensations of unreality'—suggests that memory and the capacity for coherent self-representation survive in schizophrenia; that the self is not reduced to the irredeemable state of psychic and temporal fragmentation Jameson diagnoses; that schizophrenia does not so much annihilate but alter the self.

But what of the experience itself? Here, we can turn to Sass's illuminating discussion in *Madness and Modernism* of *Autobiography of a Schizophrenic Girl*. According to Sass, Renee's description of her first experience of unreality is an exemplary account of the *stimmung*, or the aura of strangeness that signals and precedes the psychotic break.[15] The beginning of this phase—the *trema*—is likened to an 'anticipatory stage fright':

> At these moments the patient will be suspicious and restless, often filled with anticipation or dread. Normal emotions like joy and sadness will be absent, the mood veering

mother cry. This revelation bowled me over because I heard my mother say that if my father left her, she would kill herself'. Needless to say, the psychosexual significance of this scene goes unremarked in Jameson's analysis.

[14] Goulimari is here drawing on Deleuze and Guattari's account of the suprapersonal (historical, political, religious, racial) significance of schizophrenic delusions. Unfortunately, she has her history wrong. *Autobiography of a Schizophrenic Girl* was published in 1951. Although it is unclear how much time elapsed between the events described in the book and its publication, Renee is at least in her early 20s by the end of the narrative, and says that she had her first experience of unreality (quoted earlier) at the age of 5. If her delusions register any impressions of the Second World War, they are clairvoyant rather than historical.

[15] Following Giorgio de Chirico and Friedrich Nietzsche, Sass uses the 'untranslatable' German term *stimmung* to refer to this change in the subject's experience of the world (rather than the subject's response to this change) (Sass, 1992, pp. 44–5, 424; see also 1988).

instead between anxiety and a kind of electric exaltation. Generally the person has a sense of having lost contact with things, or of everything having undergone some subtle, all-encompassing change. Reality seems to be unveiled as never before, and the visual world looks peculiar and eerie—weirdly beautiful, tantalizingly significant, or perhaps horrifying in some insidious but ineffable way.

(Sass, 1992, pp. 47, 44)

The *trema* in turn inspires in patients an intense scrutiny of the world he calls the 'truth-taking stare'. Sass continues, describing this state in terms that evoke the sublime:

This is a strange and enigmatic atmosphere, a mood that infuses everything yet eludes description almost completely. [. . .] Still, everything is totally and uncannily transformed: the fabric of space seems subtly changed; the feeling of reality is either heightened, pulsing with a mysterious, unnameable force, or else oddly diminished or undermined—or, paradoxically, things may seem (as one patient put it) both 'unreal and extra-real' at the same time.

(Sass, 1992, p. 44)

The *trema*, accompanied by the truth-taking stare, has three aspects: 'Unreality, where the world is devoid of feeling or authenticity; Mere Being, where the sheer fact of existence defies speech and understanding; Fragmentation, where details or parts overwhelm the synthetic whole' (Sass, 1992, p. 50). It is succeeded by the *apophany*, a state in which the previously de-realized world is suddenly and peculiarly saturated with meaning, a state in which signifiers appear ominously opaque, pointing not to any particular or specific meaning but 'to the sheer presence of meaningfulness itself' (Sass, 1992, p. 53).

I have quoted Sass's description of the schizophrenic *stimmung* at length because it seems to me to supply the phenomenological detail lacking from 'The Cultural Logic of Late Capitalism'. Sass's description of the *trema* and *apophany* correlates with Jameson's analysis of *Autobiography of a Schizophrenic Girl*:

First the breakdown of temporality suddenly releases this present of time from all the activities and intentionalities that might focus it and make it a space of praxis; thereby isolated, that present suddenly engulfs the subject with undescribable vividness, a materiality of perception properly overwhelming, which effectively dramatizes the power of the material—or better still, the literal—signifier in isolation. This present of the world or material signifier comes before the subject with heightened intensity, bearing a mysterious charge of affect, here described in the negative terms of anxiety and loss of reality, but which one could just as well imagine in the positive terms of euphoria, the high, the intoxicatory or hallucinogenic intensity.

(Jameson, 1991, pp. 27–8)

These sublime moments of schizophrenic dissolution can be understood, according to Jameson, as 'unconscious points of contact with that equally unfigurable and unimaginable thing, the multinational apparatus, the great suprapersonal system of late capitalist technology' (Jameson, 1988, p. 73). This schizophrenic experience of the postmodern is *not* one of hallucinations, delusions, or even the so-called negative symptoms of autism and anhedonia. Nor does it reverberate with complexity and psychic depth: for Jameson, the 'great modernist thematics of alienation, anomie, solitude, social fragmentation and isolation' bear no relationship to the enigmatic experience of '"intensities"' and 'pure material Signifiers', 'incomprehensible yet mesmerizing fragment[s] of language' (Jameson, 1991, pp. 11, 6, 28, 27).

Jameson's description of 'the schizophrenic's' perception of the mysterious affective charge and dazzling materiality of the isolated signifier supports Bauman's analysis of the consumer as seduced by the superficial allure of the commodity, as 'impatient, impetuous and restive', devoted to a perpetual cycle of desire–satiation–dissatisfaction, and relentlessly pursuing new and pleasurable sensations (Bauman, 2005, p. 25). It also resonates with Baudrillard's description of the ecstasy of communication and the hyper-real; a world deluged by information and images, sound bytes and slogans. The social space envisaged alluded to by these theorists is immediately recognizable in typically postmodern 'non-spaces' where individual identity and narrative are suspended: the bright lights and commodity overload of the shopping centre; the rapid flow of the freeway; the advertising-saturated domestic spectacle of television (Morse, 1990). From the neon-flooded metropolis to the plasticized environs of the international airport, postmodernity, 'pulsing with a mysterious, unnameable force', produces in its subjects the paradoxical experience of the hyper-real 'as both "unreal and extra-real" at the same time' (Sass, 1992, p. 44).

Approaching Jameson's model of schizophrenia through Sass's analysis of the *stimmung* adds to it a dimension of phenomenological and psychological sophistication, bringing us closer, I would argue, to a more nuanced account of certain (but by no means all) experiences of postmodernity. But can Jameson's model in turn enable us to rethink Sass's claims in *Madness and Modernism*? If schizophrenia 'proper' can be seen as the psychic internalization of panoptic modernity, could its *preliminary* stages paradoxically illuminate a more general experience of *post*modernity? Despite their many differences, the arguments of Jameson and Sass can be fruitfully drawn together in the idea of the postmodern *stimmung*; a model of schizophrenic experience, I suggest, that can help us to interpret the effects on particular subjects of a specifically *post*modern world. The next chapter explores this idea further by looking at the portrayal of 'schizophrenic' subjectivity in Bret Easton Ellis's 1999 novel *Glamorama*.

Chapter 7

Glamorama, postmodernity, and the schizophrenic sublime

What might a 'postmodern schizophrenia', or a postmodern *stimmung*, look like, and how might it feel?

As we saw in the previous chapter, cultural theorists like Baudrillard and Jameson used the concept of schizophrenia to try and describe something we could call a phenomenology of the postmodern. Schizophrenia, they suggest, offers us an insight into the effects of late capitalism on the subjective experience of time, 'emptied' interiority, (dis)embodiment and the (im)possibility of purposeful action. The limitations of this model—and its paradoxical dependency on the clinical accounts of schizophrenia from which it is so emphatically distinguished—have already been well canvassed. The aim of this chapter is to put phenomenological flesh on the bones, as it were, of cultural theory's suggestive but relatively two-dimensional account of 'postmodern schizophrenia'. To do this, we must venture beyond verisimilitude. Turning here to the clinical case history, or even the autobiographical account, would be to mis-read cultural theory as making interventions in clinical reality. As we have seen, cultural theory uses the concept of 'schizophrenia' as a trope, a metaphor, a symbol. Where better, then, to tease out its complexities than in the imagined worlds of literary fiction?

Using a literary text to unpack theoretical models of schizophrenia continues a strong tradition within psychoanalytic and cultural theory. As we saw in Chapter 2, it was not only the substance but also the much-lauded 'literariness' of Schreber's autobiography which made it the focus of psychoanalytic theories of psychosis and in turn instrumental to the operation of the textual sublime. Freud and Lacan frequently turn to classical myth and other fictions to substantiate as well as to illustrate their theories, and, as has been well documented, their work inspired a broader psychoanalytic interest and indeed investment in literature.[1] Avant-garde and antipsychiatric thinkers have also discovered in fictional texts powerful articulations of schizophrenic experience.

---

[1] Some of the most interesting analyses of the importance of literature to psychoanalysis are *Literature and Psychoanalysis: The Question of Reading, Otherwise* (Felman, 1982),

Deleuze and Guattari, for example, repeatedly point their readers to the operation of the desiring machines in Samuel Beckett's plays and develop from
Antonin Artaud's poetry the concept of a body without organs. Jameson draws
on the highly literary *Autobiography of a Schizophrenic Girl* to capture 'postmodern schizophrenia' at the experiential level, turning then to the language
of poet Bob Perelman to illustrate 'schizophrenic disjunction or écriture' at the
level of the aesthetic (Jameson, 1991, p. 28). However, by far the most comprehensive and ambitious analysis of schizophrenia through literature, and of
literature through schizophrenia, is Sass's *Madness and Modernism: Insanity in
the Light of Modern Art, Literature and Thought*. The 'interpretive strategy' and
central project of *Madness and Modernism* is to compare schizophrenia and
the 'sensibility and structures of consciousness found in the most advanced art
and literature of the twentieth century' (Sass, 1992, p. 8). In addition to referring to a wealth of literary examples, Sass writes in praise of the literary quality
of autobiography, suggesting Renee's *Autobiography of a Schizophrenic Girl*, for
example, offers some of the 'best descriptions' of the schizophrenic *stimmung*
because it is both psychologically interesting and aesthetically significant (Sass,
1992, p. 46).

This chapter will endeavour to show that if not the best, then certainly the
most complex and compelling, descriptions of the postmodern *stimmung* are
to be found in Bret Easton Ellis's *fin-de-millénaire* novel *Glamorama* (2000).[2]
Ellis is widely regarded as one of the foremost literary voices of his generation
(Beckett, 1999). A Brat Pack writer whose 'blank fiction' resonates with 'the
spirit of the age' (Annesley, 1998, p. 5), he is the infamous author of *American
Psycho* (1991), a novel judged to be so obscene that for years it was sold in
Australia in plastic wrap despite widespread critical acclaim. *Glamorama*, his
fourth novel, was popularly regarded as a failure, as this review in *The New
York Times* makes emphatically clear:

> *Glamorama*, as anyone can see, is a bloated, stultifyingly repetitive, overhyped book
> about an entire gang of fabulously good-looking and expensively dressed sociopaths
> who torture and dismember both women and men—and lots of them. [. . .] Ellis's
> satirical message is, essentially, a one-liner, and hardly an original one at that—celeb-
> rity culture is vapid, yes, and?—and isn't remotely worth the endless pages in which
> his vacuous and inconsequential characters talk vacuously and inconsequentially
> about vacuous and inconsequential things.
>
> (Mendelsohn, 1999; see also Blount, 1999; Richardson, 1999)

'Lacan: An Ethics of Speech' (de Certeau, 1983), *Freud's Literary Culture* (Frankland, 2000)
and *Literature in Psychoanalysis: A Reader* (Vine, 2005).

[2] This quotation and all future quotations in this chapter are reproduced from *Glamorama*
(Ellis, 2000). All page references will appear in parentheses after the quotation.

Glamorama's academic critics have, by contrast, embarked on a more robust engagement with the aesthetics and politics of the vacuous and the inconsequential. With its excess of pop cultural references, and its playfulness, ambiguity, superficiality, and self-consciousness, *Glamorama* epitomizes a postmodern aesthetic while taking as its narrative focus the effects on the subject of the technology, media networks, and politics of postmodernity. Enriching the imaginative possibilities of twenty-first-century violence, it serves as an 'apocalyptic pretext . . . crying out for a translation into a proper terrorist text' (Petersen, 2005, p. 144); enriching the imaginative capabilities of twenty-first-century fiction, it introduces 'what appears to be an unprecedented form of double-voiced first-person narrative' (Nielsen, 2006, p. 20; see also Heinze, 2008; Nielsen, 2004; Punter, 2003). With Sheli Ayers, we might say that *Glamorama*'s protagonist, Victor, and the 'enchanted panorama' he inhabits 'are symptomatic of a cultural condition' (Ayers, 2000, p. 3); but a stronger and I think more persuasive line of argument sees *Glamorama*—at the level of textuality, narrative, structure, theme, pace, indeed, in any and all of its literary dimensions—bring to life the 'postmodern schizophrenia' we have been analyzing across the last two chapters.

In *Madness and Modernism*, as in cultural theory more broadly, literature is certainly not attributed the same status as sociological or psychiatric research; its function as fiction is to illuminate, rather than to provide empirical or conclusive confirmation of a particular idea. Following Sass's suggestion that as 'the town criers of modern consciousness, schizophrenics are in a dual relationship with modernity, existing not just as a product *of* but also as reaction *against* the prevailing social order' (Sass, 1992, p. 372), the first part of this chapter aims to show how *Glamorama* presents Victor as exemplifying a specifically *post*modern consciousness. In part two I continue this project by drawing on the interdisciplinary discourse of Schreber studies. If Schreber has been repeatedly heralded as embodying a specifically *modern* schizophrenia, can we, using the same interpretive frameworks, consider Victor his fictional *post*modern equivalent? The third and final part of this chapter moves beyond an analysis of the events recounted in the narrative to the logic of the text itself. In calling upon 'postmodern schizophrenia' to interpret postmodernity, does this literary text, like its theoretical counterparts, also call upon schizophrenia's association with the sublime? Does it import not only the detail of cultural theory's model of schizophrenia, but the metatheoretical baggage that goes with it?

The town crier of postmodern consciousness

Written predominantly in the first person and present tense, from the perspective of New York's latest 'It-Boy' (140), *Glamorama* tells the story of a group of white, American model-slash-actors whose star status provides cover for terrorist operations. Overflowing with references to the celebrities, labels, locales, brands, music, and media of the 1990s, the book is a dizzying portrayal of the depthlessness and detritus of postmodern consumer culture. Its setting is the perpetual present of the celebrity modelling circuit—the 'apex of consumer society' (McInerney, 1998, p. 36)—where the unrelenting imperative to be hip prescribes a constant shift to the next commodified incarnation of cool. '"Out is in. In is out"', Victor proclaims, and '"If you need this defined for you, maybe you're in the wrong world"' (15). Fashion as a system exploits the fact 'that an infinite number of signifiers can be attached to an infinite number of signifieds' (Marshall, 1997, p. 11), and in *Glamorama* this semiotic freedom is taken to new and gruesome extremes: 'I finish reading an article about new mascaras (Shattered and Roach are the season's most popular) and hip lipsticks (Frostbite, Asphyxia, Bruise) and glam nail polish (Plaque, Mildew) and I'm thinking, genuinely, Wow, progress'(168). The elite world of high fashion here functions as a synecdoche of what Zygmunt Bauman calls liquid modernity: it both stands in for and epitomizes a culture fixated on the flow of aestheticized commodities. Ellis is also careful to capture stylistically its reliance on superficiality, excess, flux, and repetition. The pop references that clutter and date the novel constitute a 'dazzling textuality', which 'produces a kind of reality-vertigo-effect on the reader' (Ettler, 1999) but also evoke the logic and rapid pace of the cycle of consumption. As John Conley (2009, p. 120) observes, 'it is not only that Ellis writes *about* capitalism, but that Ellis literally writes a world made of money, for his grammar and syntax are formed in its image; Ellis is truly a writer of capitalism because it is capitalism that his sentences exemplify'. We can go so far as to argue, via Jameson, that *Glamorama*'s pop-cultural signifiers are signs of an 'absolutely fragmented and anarchic social reality'; 'broken pieces of language', which 'litter the commodity landscape', literary and literal, 'of a postmodernist late capitalism in full crisis' (Jameson, 1984a, p. 201).[3]

---

[3] Ellis's most striking presentation of this 'absolutely fragmented and anarchic social reality' is the grisly tableau created by a bombed aircraft: 'cell phones and laptops and Ray-Ban sunglasses and baseball caps and pairs of Rollerblades tied together and camcorders and mangled guitars and hundreds of CD's and fashion magazines (including the *YouthQuake* with Victor Ward on the cover) and entire wardrobes of Calvin Klein and Armani and Ralph Lauren hang from burning trees and there's a teddy bear soaked with blood and a Bible and various Nintendo games along with rolls of toilet paper and shoulder bags and engagement rings and pens and belts whipped off waists and Prada purses still clasped and boxes of Calvin Klein boxer-briefs and so many clothes from the Gap contaminated with blood and other body fluids and everything reeks of aviation fuel' (440–1).

Ellis has described *Glamorama*'s narrator—the all-American *YouthQuake* cover boy—not as a postmodern everyman but as the epitome of everything that is 'annoying and repellent' about men of his generation (Ellis quoted in Blume, 1999).[4] A model struggling to be an actor, singer, and night club entrepreneur, Victor is presented early on as a 'Nobody, up-and-comer, star, has been. Not necessarily in that order' (139). His modus operandi is the cultivation of cool and his maxim "'The better you look, the more you see'" (27, 56, 254). Victor is dedicated to the pursuit of pleasure, fame, and sensation and he therefore continuously adapts and remoulds himself according to the vagaries, fluctuations, and contradictions of fashion:

'The 90s are honest, straightforward. Let's reflect that', I say, moving around. 'I want something unconsciously classic. I want no distinctions between exterior and interior, formal and casual, wet and dry, black and white, full and empty—oh my god, get me a cold compress'. (50)

Through his encyclopaedic knowledge of pop music statistics and A-list celebrities Victor speaks a 'brain-dead bricolage' (Young, 1999), and, as this MTV interview suggests, appears to have no knowledge of life beyond *Entertainment Tonight*:

MTV (after polite laughter): 'No. What *really* makes you mad? What really gets you angry?'
ME (long pause, thinking): 'Well, recently, missing DJs, badly behaved bartenders, certain gossipy male models, the media's treatment of celebs . . . um . . .'
MTV: 'We were thinking more along the lines of the war in Bosnia or the AIDS epidemic or domestic terrorism. How about the current political situation?'
ME (long pause, tiny voice): 'Sloppy Rollerbladers? . . . The words "dot com"? . . .'
MTV (long pause): 'Anything else?'
ME (realizing something, relieved): 'A mulatto, an albino, a mosquito, my libido'.
MTV (long pause): 'Did you . . . understand the question?' (141–2, ellipses in the original)

Even in a scene hardly renowned for intellectual profundity, Victor is accused by his girlfriend of being particularly blank: "'Everyone knows a fuck of a lot more than you do and *it's not cute*'" (158, italics in the original).[5] Ayers (2000) has argued that 'despite (or perhaps because of) his vacuity, Victor emerges as a privileged knower. His ability to grasp things by their surface appearance and his mastery of fashion and pop-culture codes enable him to operate in this textual world'. But Victor's vacuity is also his vulnerability: he has 'adapted

[4] Victor Ward is a minor character in Ellis's 1987 novel *The Rules of Attraction*.
[5] It is not difficult to identify similarities here between *Glamorama* and Ben Stiller's 2001 film *Zoolander*; indeed, Ellis reportedly brought legal action against Stiller for copyright infringement in a case that was settled out of court.

well' to life as a terrorist precisely because he thinks 'that the Gaza Strip is a particularly lascivious move an erotic dancer makes' and 'that the PLO recorded the singles "Don't Bring me Down" and "Evil Woman"' (314, 315).

The novel opens as Victor's life begins to disintegrate. Accepting the mysterious offer of an expenses-paid trip to Europe to locate his ex-girlfriend, Jamie Fields, Victor finds himself the newest recruit in a kind of 'Prada Meinhof' gang (Houen, 2004, p. 427). Spatial and temporal co-ordinates are scrambled by the sudden appearance of a film crew recording and directing Victor's 'performance'. No explanation is offered, Victor just accepts constantly changing scripts, foreign cinematographers, acting coaching, and special effects as his new reality. After planting a bomb on the Paris Metro, for example, he dispassionately observes: 'Various shots of people blown apart, extras and stuntmen thrown off the lightweight steel car and onto the tracks. Shot of body parts— legs and arms and hands, most of them real—skidding across the platform' (319). As the violence escalates and another, unrelated crew appears to film the explosions, Victor becomes increasingly incapable of mapping his multiplying filmic realities, and the reader is tethered to his confusion. Scenes start being shot without him and continue beyond their scripted parameters (311); plots conflict (315, 329); the first film crew abandons the project only to become part of an explosion filmed by the second (350); and finally, Victor's narrative voice collapses with the inclusion of 'objectively' narrated scenes (from 304) and the intrusion of an unidentified narrative voice (from 340). *Glamorama* is not, however, a realist novel about the making of a terrorist action film; too much occurs 'off-camera' for the presence of these film crews to provide a complete, or adequate, rationale for the terrorist activities. This is the novel's interpretive impasse: no one has yet attempted to examine—much less explain—Ellis's literary aesthetics or terrorist thematics in the context of these puzzling contradictions.

The most persuasive interpretation of these logical disjunctures in the text is, I will argue, to see them as manifestations of an experience that closely resembles the 'postmodern schizophrenia' we have explored in previous chapters. Although he is not concerned with psychiatric verisimilitude and never uses the term explicitly, Ellis imparts to Victor a range of 'symptoms' consonant with the kind of states described as 'schizophrenic' in cultural theory, 'symptoms' linked aetiologically to specific aspects of postmodernity. In his article 'Broadcasting and Schizophrenia', John Peters (2010, p. 134) argues that the mass media creates a structural resemblance between celebrity and psychotic discourse:

> Celebrities engage in institutionally sanctioned forms of excess: money, sex, drugs and styles of communication. Broadcast celebrities are ritually permitted to carry on

schizophrenic discourse. (The mentally ill, Goffman argued, lack just this permission.) Celebrities are trained to monitor every single gesture they make as if it were rife with potential significance, to address sound and image machines in jumbled 'takes' that can be edited later, and to speak to absent strangers as if they were friends.

Victor's celebrity identity, and in turn his 'schizophrenic discourse', is a function of surfaces rather than an expression of psychic depth: overexposed to the sensory stimuli of postmodernity and immersed in its perpetual present, he is irreconcilably fragmented, subject to affective fluxes and incapable of meaningful self-definition. Positing terrorism as if not an inevitable, then certainly a logical, extension of the cult of celebrity,[6] *Glamorama* maps the intensification of Victor's psychosis against his increasing proximity to the networks of power in late capitalist postmodernity.

There is, from the outset, however, a clearly delusional dimension to Victor's perceptual machinery. *Glamorama* opens with Victor fuming about the presence of specks on the walls of his soon-to-be-opened club:

'Specks, man, look at these fuckers. They glow. They're *glowing*, JD', I whisper. 'Jesus, they're everywhere'. Suddenly I notice an entire new patch and yelp, gaping. 'And I think they're *spreading*. I don't think that patch was here before!' I swallow, then croak in a rush. 'My mouth is incredibly dry because of this—could someone get me an Arizona diet iced tea in a bottle, *not* a can?' (6)

As no one else present is able to confirm their existence, Victor appears to be attaching a special significance (if not malevolent intent) to something only he perceives. The specks suggest that Victor lives in 'a pixelated and infinitely transformable universe' (Ayers, 2000, p. 7), but they also evoke the schizophrenic *stimmung*—a perception of the world as simultaneously meaningful but devoid of meaning, affectless but highly charged, fragmented but overwhelming in its totality. '[I]ncomprehensible yet mesmerizing', the world appears before the subject with a 'hallucinogenic intensity' (Jameson, 1991, pp. 27–8) suggestive of the sublime, but what is a particularly postmodern about this experience, according to Jameson, is its everydayness. Victor sees not just the luminous specks, but also the entire fabric of social life, as simultaneously overloaded with meaning and as fleeting, trivial, transparent. It is a

---

6 As one character explains: "'How did [terrorist leader Bobby Hughes] recruit people? . . . It was only models . . . and famous models. . . . He wasn't interested in anyone else. . . . He would use the fact that as a model all you do all day is stand around and do what other people tell you to do. . . . He preyed on that . . . and we listened . . . and it was an analogy that made sense . . . in the end . . . when he asked . . . things of us . . . and it wasn't hard to recruit people . . . everyone wanted to be around us . . . everyone wanted to be movie stars . . . and in the end, basically, everyone was a sociopath . . . and all the girls' hair was chignoned . . . and the Who was always playing somewhere . . .'" (309, ellipses in the original).

mode of experience that Ellis presents not as a radical deviation from the accepted norm, but rather as the exaggeration or intensification of a wider experience of postmodernity's perpetual present.

As the narrative, and the *stimmung*, progresses, Victor's perceptual faculties become increasingly distorted and his symbolic order a chaos of broken pieces of reality. Virtually all spaces are freezing (from 15); confetti appears everywhere (from 88); an unseen man whistles 'The Sunny Side of the Street' (from 114); flies cluster everywhere despite the cold (from 172); his limbs start periodically falling asleep (from 303); finally, the smell of shit begins to overwhelm his fly-filled and freezing celebrity haunts (from 316). These are not clues but a deluge of seemingly random signs, a 'rubble of distinct and unrelated signifiers' (Jameson, 1991, p. 26) whose ominous opacity complements their vivid affective charge.[7] Victor, like the schizophrenic screen in Baudrillard's *The Ecstasy of Communication*, suffers from an 'over-proximity of all things'; things that invade his field of vision, his thoughts, ears, nostrils and appendages, and from which 'not even the aura of his own body protects him' (Baudrillard, 1988, pp. 26–7). Victor's fragmented but highly charged corporeality—along with the intensity of his own physical reactions (tears, vomit, laughter, insomnia, numbness, and panic)—here also recalls Deleuze and Guattari's account of the 'bands of intensity, potentials, thresholds, and gradients', which constitute for the schizo 'A harrowing, emotionally overwhelming experience, which brings [him] as close as possible to matter, to a burning, living centre of matter' (Deleuze and Guattari, 1982, p. 19).[8]

Victor's subjective disintegration does not, however, result from his proximity to the 'burning, living center of matter', but from his immersion in the technological sublime, the 'impossible totality' of late capitalism (Jameson, 1991, p. 37). Deleuze and Guattari argue that 'all delirium possesses a world-historical, political, and racial content' (Deleuze and Guattari, 1982, pp. 274, 88, see also 352, 362, 365), and Victor's 'postmodern schizophrenia' speaks of an era of simulation, surveillance, and digital mass media; a consumer culture

---

[7] John Conley (2009) offers an extended reading of one of these signifiers in his article on poverty in *American Psycho* and *Glamorama*. Noting that the olfactory is frequently missing from the Ellisian world, he argues that the smell of shit is one of the novel's most 'insistent' tropes and that it points among other things to the underlying putrescence of celebrity culture. This is a compelling and even seductive argument, but one which seems to overdetermine the meaning of one signifier while ignoring the less suggestive but no less insistent tropes identified above.

[8] In a perverse 'literalisation' or materialization of Deleuze and Guattari's concept of the 'body-without-organs', Victor later watches helpless and hysterical as his ex-girlfriend Chloe's organs liquefy and gush out of her vagina.

notable for the speed and mobility of capital; a world in which fashion and violence can become indistinguishable, as:

> The catwalks seemed longer, the paparazzi were both more and less frantic, girls were wearing bones, bird skulls, human teeth, bloody smocks, they held fluorescent water pistols, there was serious buzz, there was zero buzz, it was the epitome of hype, it was wildly trivial (408).

The 'industries' of fashion and terror both operate out of the logic of the simulacrum, where the manipulation of the image can proceed indefinitely:

> Lips are digitally thickened, freckles are removed, an ax is placed in someone's outstretched hand, a BMW becomes a Jaguar which becomes a Mercedes which becomes a broom which becomes a frog which becomes a mop which becomes a poster of Jenny McCarthy (357).

And its effects are not merely aesthetic: '"You can move planets with this . . . You can shape lives. The photograph is only the beginning. [. . .] Were you there or were you not? It all depends on who you ask, and even that really doesn't matter anymore"' (358). If, as Žižek (2002, p. 225) claims, the camera's gaze today provides for each of us an 'ontological guarantee' it is one which has, in *Glamorama*, long since expired.[9]

Like fashion, the terrorist violence of *Glamorama* operates without identifiable logic or structure; it is 'crazy, viral [and] mediationless' because 'it never passes via the mediation of meaning' (Baudrillard, 1993, p. 70). The model–terrorists take to extremes the deterritorializing logic of the schizo; however, their anti-Oedipal agency does not threaten but *reinvigorates* the late capitalist system: 'We're at a dinner party . . . and it's all rather subdued since a small percentage of the invited guests were blown up in the Ritz yesterday. For comfort, people went shopping, which is understandable even if they bought things a little too enthusiastically' (360). Ellis, with Jameson and Baudrillard, seems unconvinced that the 'schizophrenic' emptying out of subjectivity serves any politically emancipatory purpose; it is, rather, precipitated by and in the service of capitalist power structures.

Ontologically insecure, addicted to tranquilizing drugs, and bereft of an intellectual arsenal, Victor's feeble grip on reality loosens steadily as his involvement in violence increases. Andy Warhol is said to have quipped, 'If it gets too intense, just pretend it's a movie'. It is advice Victor heeds. As I have suggested,

---

9 In his analysis of *Glamorama*, Walter Benn Michaels argues that as terrorism eclipses national and ideological forms of conflict, it signals a move from politics and belief to biopolitics and being. If the 'discourse of terrorism' is the 'discourse of the replacement of ideology by ontology' (2003, p. 111), clearly it both registers and heightens the ontological insecurity of an image-addicted era.

there are sufficient narrative inconsistencies to make it clear that *Glamorama* is not a realist novel about the making of a terrorist action film. The presence of successive film crews shooting some but not all of the scenes of terrorism and torture can be more persuasively interpreted as a postmodern *stimmung* extending into full-blown psychosis. The appearance of the entire cinematic apparatus—from the technicians to their technical equipment—is not simply narcissistic wish-fulfilment but a delusional projection of Victor's consciousness of himself as a star. These complex and contradictory delusions of grandeur in turn function to insulate Victor from the reality of his actions: 'I'm smiling, confused, weirded out at how focused Bentley seems and shocked at how gruesome and inauthentic the waxwork looks' (283). 'The shock, the sirens, the hundred wounded—it's all so familiar. The director is relying on a really top-notch editor to put the footage together' (306). The more wide-ranging the terrorist conspiracies, the more extreme the violence, the greater the number of film crews required to account for it, and the more inconsistent and desperate Victor's delusional system becomes. Gaps and fissures appear; cinematic logic is exceeded; the real re-enters the picture:

> The actor doesn't know anything. He memorized a different script. He's not delivering the performance that Bobby wants. He was miscast. He was wrong for this part. It's all over. Bobby instructs Bruce to pour acid on the actor's hands. Pain floods his face as he gazes at me, crying, and then his leg is sawed off. (359)

If Victor looks to the film crews to explain his ultraviolent, hyperreal world, it is clear that any security they offer can only be fleeting; his is not a stable delusional structure but one that is partial, provisional, and perpetually in flux.

A postmodern Schreber?

Victor is not a modernist monad but every inch a postmodern subject; he is an endlessly adaptive, even malleable, sensation-seeking 'tissue of quotations' (Barthes, 1977, p. 146) and more than fits the symptomatological profile for 'postmodern schizophrenia'. One way of interpreting Victor's first-person narrative as specifically postmodern is, as I have demonstrated, to read him as an embodiment of the 'schizophrenic' subjectivity described by cultural theorists. There is, however, another interpretive possibility, and that is to draw on the interdisciplinary discourse of Schreber studies. *Memoirs of My Nervous Illness* has become something of a privileged urtext in schizophrenia discourse. Setting to one side the psychoanalytic accounts of Schreber's psychosis, there are three distinct ways in which his delusional cosmology has been read as quintessentially modern: it is seen to offer insight into modern disciplinary power, to reveal the structures of modern consciousness, and to symbolize a hidden history of modernity. Each of these ways of interpreting *Memoirs* can, I suggest, be fruitfully engaged in the analysis of *Glamorama*. Although I am wary of overstating the comparison between Schreber and Victor, if the contemporary societal condition is, as is widely claimed, one which calls into question the status of the real and declares an end to subjective depth, the move from an autobiographical to a fictional text and from the genius of a Judge to the vacuity of a model–terrorist is itself already suggestive of a shift from modernity to postmodernity. If that is the case, and Schreber can be seen as the 'canary in the mine shaft' (Gilman, 1996, p. 16) of *fin-de-siècle* modernity, is Victor the It-Boy of schizophrenizing *fin-de-millénaire* postmodernity?

As we saw in Chapter 2, Louis Sass and Eric Santner have both found in Schreber's schizophrenic symptomatology the effects of modern forms of disciplinary power. Instead of casting Schreber's father Moritz as the sadistic villain in a psychosexual drama, Sass argues that:

> The techniques recommended by Moritz Schreber can, in fact, be said to involve the two great bulwarks of the modern disciplinary order of power/knowledge described by Foucault: namely, 'exercise', whose goal is the creation of docile bodies; and 'the examination', whose purpose is the monitoring—ultimately, the self-monitoring—of action and thought.

> (Sass, 1994b, p. 112)

Santner's analysis of disciplinary power extends from the family to medico-pedagogy and biological psychiatry:

> One might say, then, that the chronic state of emergency generating the bizarre array of symptoms and delusions described in *Memoirs* was inaugurated by . . . the disciplinary power to which Schreber had been exposed since early childhood and to which he was exposed again, through a different form, in the psychiatric institutions of Flechsig and Weber; Schreber's soul murder becomes, from this perspective, a sustained traumatization induced by exposure to, as it were, *fathers who knew too much.*

> (Santner, 1996, p. 86, italics in the original)

In *Glamorama* we find the problem of paternal and paternalistic power/knowledge is explicitly that of American late capitalist postmodernity. Mapped against Victor's ontological unravelling is the shadowy rise of his father, Samuel Johnson, who plans to leave the US Senate in a bid for the presidency. To his horror, Victor discovers that his father is involved with terrorist leader Bobby Hughes (423), and the novel's two endings, to which we will turn in a moment, plot two responses to this revelation. In the first, Victor reclaims the patronymic surname Johnson and gives his father's election campaign full terrorist backing (452); in the second, when Victor Ward sees footage revealing his father to be the mastermind of all the horrors that have taken place, he has to 'hold a hand over [his] mouth to stop the screaming' (475).

Jameson has argued that the postmodern culture so painstakingly documented by Ellis 'is the internal and superstructural expression of a whole new wave of American military and economic domination throughout the world' (Jameson, 1991, p. 5; see also Stephenson, 2007). Baudrillard goes further in suggesting that as the only superpower, America 'has fomented all this violence which is endemic throughout the world, and hence that (unwittingly) terroristic imagination which dwells in all of us' (Baudrillard, 2002, p. 4). Is this model–terrorist's 'schizophrenia' the result of his exposure to the very structures of late-capitalist culture through a 'father who knew too much'? And is it an exposure that he, like Schreber, can *only* process through psychosis? True to the undecidability of the novel, Victor's throwaway description of his father as a mere 'contrivance . . . [a] plot device' (36) also suggests this is nothing more than a satirically Oedipal twist on the conspiracy-theory worldview.[10] However, if Samuel Johnson is the Name-of-the-Father foreclosed by Victor Ward, he and the socio-symbolic order he authorizes make a dramatic reappearance in the Real of his 'schizophrenic' experience.

One of the effects of modern disciplinary power is, according to Foucault, the regulation of subjects through the promotion of an inner panopticism. Sass explains that:

> The panoptical arrangement makes individuals feel constantly exposed to an external, normalising gaze, therefore subjecting them to the dictates of an authority that must ultimately be internalized. Foucault sees this arrangement as the essential manifestation of modern power relationships instantiated in many institutions and social practices. It fosters forms of disciplinary self-control that eradicate spontaneity, increase inwardness and isolation, and instil the inner divisions of a relentlessly self-monitoring mode of consciousness.

> (Sass, 1997, p. 206; see also Sass, 1992, pp. 251–8)

For Sass, Schreber's schizophrenia can be read as the intensification of this 'relentlessly self-monitoring' mode of modern consciousness. In Chapter 5 I argued that postmodern institutions promote a substantively different panoptic regime: consumer society encourages self-scrutiny not to homogenize and discipline its subjects, but to make them better consumers. Self-control is in the service of self-expression, and, to re-engage Bauman's analysis, under a synoptic arrangement, the lives of a celebrity elite provide the template for how others should feel and act as well as what they should buy. *Glamorama*

---

[10] Or, in Jamesonian parlance, a degraded attempt at cognitive mapping (Jameson, 1991, p. 38; 1988, p. 356).

registers this paradigm shift in the panoptic regime of the self on multiple levels. Victor's use of filmic language ('Stills from Chloe's loft' (39), 'But someone's calling "Cut!"' (94), 'I'm undergoing a slow-motion hidden freak-out' (145)) emphasize that he interprets himself, as a star, through the (actual and imagined) cinematic gaze, just as he interprets his world as a filmic text. This propensity is gradually concretized until he is surrounded by the actors, extras, and cinematographers who, for the rest of the novel, shadow his every move. Whereas Schreber's persecuting God demanded that he continually prove his rationality, the film crews relentlessly demand of Victor a performance, an outward display of emotions, a stereotyped presentation of lines. Manifestations of a postmodern panopticism, the film crews attend only to surfaces, not to psychic complexity, but do so in a way that is as persistent as it is pernicious.

Schreber's suffering has been, as we know, repeatedly read as a symbolic revelation of the history of modernity. According to Santner, 'To traverse, with Schreber, the fantasy space of *his* own private Germany . . . is to encounter European modernity from the perspective of those figures in whom modern European society "secreted" its disavowed knowledge of chronic structural crisis and disequilibrium' (Santner, 1996, p. 144). For Santner, Schreber's history of modernity, precisely because it is 'secret history', invites a hermeneutical response, a probing of its depths and symbolic possibilities. By contrast, the 'obscenity' of *Glamorama*'s postmodernity is, to borrow again from Baudrillard, 'no longer the obscenity of the hidden, the repressed, the obscure, but that of the visible, the all-too-visible, the more-visible-than-visible; it is the obscenity of that which no longer contains a secret and is entirely soluble in information and communication' (Baudrillard, 1988, p. 22). *Glamorama*'s YouthQuake cover boy is not only 'more-visible-than-visible', but he is also meant to be the epitome of all that is desirable. In this narrative, disciplinary power no longer concentrates its 'schizophrenizing' operation in the domestic sphere, the psychiatric clinic, or even the court room, but in the synoptic celebrity-obsessed mass media, the world of simulacra in which Victor has a leading role. Victor's schizophrenia does not therefore encode 'the drama of alienation' but flagrantly dramatizes the 'ecstasy of communication' (Baudrillard, 1988, p. 22).

Glamorama and the schizophrenic sublime

So far I have argued that *Glamorama* exemplifies cultural theory's model of postmodern schizophrenia and that Victor, like Schreber, can be seen to 'live out, in exaggerated, almost literal fashion, the ontological and epistemological assumptions of his . . . age' (Sass, 1997, p. 222). We can now consider the issue of how, in its presentation of schizophrenia, this literary text, like its theoretical counterparts, negotiates the schizophrenic sublime. I do not wish to imply here that the sublime must necessarily be found in the structure of all representations of schizophrenia: as Sass's model of schizophrenia amply demonstrates, it is of course possible to think outside the parameters of psychiatric metatheory. Ellis, I will argue, does not. On the contrary, far from rendering the schizophrenic sublime defunct, or even paradoxical, *Glamorama* returns to the tropes of late nineteenth-century psychiatry, mobilizing a model of schizophrenia as something that is in essence unknowable, that is beyond comprehension, and that has at its core a kernel of unreason resistant to interpretation.

From the outset, what we might think of as Victor's 'schizophrenic symptoms'— his visual, tactile, olfactory, and auditory hallucinations (the specks, confetti, flies, and freezing feeling; the smell of shit; 'The Sunny Side of the Street') and his delusional structures (the contradictory filmic plots)—function as inscrutable signifiers. That they can be symbolically linked to postmodernity, and seen as the expression of a synoptic postmodern consciousness, does not diminish their status as 'uninterpretable' but suggests that uninterpretability is very precisely a postmodern phenomenon. Here, instead of undertaking the hermeneutic investigation of psychic secrets, '*We'll slide down the surface of things*' (144, 145, 146, 150, 152, 154, 157, 164, italics in the original). Victor's observation, or more precisely, his quotation of the U2 song 'Even Better Than the Real Thing', alerts us to the futility of searching for meaning that might well be inaccessible, if indeed it is present at all. Throughout this chapter I have drawn attention to *Glamorama*'s opacity, its contradictions, and its diegetic dysfunctionality. As the narrative progresses, the realities of this 'postmodern schizophrenia' multiply to the point where mapping this textual labyrinth becomes impossible. *Glamorama*'s final chapters seem to play, provocatively, upon the reader's disorientation. Will the mystery of Victor's 'schizophrenic' experience be resolved, its aetiology clearly established, its parameters clearly drawn? Or will it remain impenetrable?

In a telling scene, at the height of the terrorist plotting, Victor is briefly reunited with his ex-girlfriend Chloe and attempts to explain why he fled New York:

> 'I thought it'd solve everything if I . . . just left', I tell her. 'I was just . . . directionless, y'know, baby?'
> 'Because?'
> A sigh. 'Because where I was going . . .' I stop, my throat tightens.
> 'Yeah?' she whispers. 'Because where you were going . . .' she coaxes.
> I breathe in and then I'm reduced.
> 'There was no one there', I whisper back. (409, ellipses in the original)

This is both a lie (Victor is sent to Europe by the mysterious Mr Palakon) and a rare moment of insight. Victor's introspection leads him to realize that there is 'no one there', and this idea of a non-self is manifested in the text in the dominant motif of identity confusion. Victor is *consistently* accosted by people who swear that they have seen him in places he swears he was not.[11] The question, raised early on, is whether he is the victim of amnesia, deception, mistaken identity, insidious hoax, or diabolical fantasy. Or, if there is 'no *one* there' is it in fact because there are two (or more?) Victors there, as the novel's two contradictory endings clearly imply?[12]

In the first ending, Victor re-establishes himself in New York as Victor Johnson, the successful son of a presidential candidate. Although still accosted by flies, cold, and confetti, he has taken up a leadership role within the terrorist network and seems better equipped to cope with its vicissitudes.[13] In the second ending, the film crew flies Victor Ward to Milan, where he is effectively imprisoned—psychotic, terrified, and killing time—in a hotel room. Desperate, he calls his sister in Washington:

'Sally, it's really me, please—' I gasp.
'It's for you', I hear her say.
  The sound of the phone being passed to someone else.
  'Hello?' a voice asks.
  I don't say anything, just listen intently.
'Hello?' the voice asks again. 'This is Victor Johnson', the voice says. 'Who is this?'
  Silence.
'It'd be really cool if you stopped bothering my sister', the voice says.
'Okay?'
  Silence.
  'Goodbye', the voice says.
  A click.
  I'm disconnected. (476)

This trans-Atlantic phone call does not conform to the clichéd notion of a split personality, Jekyll-and-Hyde type madness; it is a climactic moment of

---

[11] And, it should be noted, the confusion is not just visual. It reaches a climax in the scene quoted earlier, when although Victor has not left Paris in months, Chloe tells him that they conceived a child days ago in New York.

[12] Ellis toys with the reader in a scene where the terrorists' reliance upon digital image manipulation is revealed. The files are variously titled Victor and '"Victor"', suggesting that there is still a meaningful distinction between original and imitation, until upon closer inspection it becomes clear that there is no correlation between the use of scare quotes and the images we assume to be surveillance of the 'real' Victor.

[13] Take for example this exchange with his newly appointed 'guru and spiritual advisor': 'Don't fear the reaper, Victor,' Deepak says, walking away. I'm nodding mindlessly, a vacant grin pasted on my face, until I turn around and mutter to myself, 'I *am* the fucking reaper, Deepak . . .' (445–6).

ontological rupture that emphatically reinforces the sublimity of Victor's 'schizophrenia'. So although Hendrik Skov Nielsen argues that 'the double takes over not just the identity and life of Victor Ward but the narration of the narrative, which itself becomes doubled and double-voiced' (Nielsen, 2006, pp. 24–5), I am inclined to agree with David Punter (Punter, 2003, p. 72) that this 'uncanny doubling' is in fact 'an uncanny awareness of multiplicity', for in postmodernity 'two lives, as it were, are not enough'. Victor's psychic splitting cannot be safely contained by the trope of the double, much as we might wish it, if only because there are no limits to his digital or cinematic incarnations. As much as Nielsen (Nielsen, 2006, p. 26) would like to propose that the double subsumes and destroys the narrator on the thematic level, in the narrated universe *and* as 'the enunciator of "I"', his argument rests on the capacity to distinguish the 'real' or primary Victor from his double, which is, in the logic of *Glamorama*, impossible (see also Helyer, 2009, p. 295). Just as both or even all Victors are equally (un)real, so the two 'endings' are equally (im)plausible and neither offers any solution to the mystery of this experience.

The last, short chapter of *Glamorama* is the novel's aesthetic high point and its most unambiguous presentation of the sublime. Self and image merge in the final dissolution of subjectivity:

> I'm drinking a glass of water in the empty hotel bar at the Principe di Savoia and staring at the mural behind the bar and in the mural there is a giant mountain, a vast field spread out below it where villagers are celebrating in a field of long grass that blankets the mountain dotted with tall white flowers, and in the sky above the mountain it's morning and the sun is spreading itself across the mural's frame, burning over the small cliffs and the low-hanging clouds that encircle the mountain's peak, and a bridge strung across a pass through the mountain will take you to any point beyond that you need to arrive at, because behind that mountain is a highway and along that highway are billboards with answers on them—who, what, where, when, why—and I'm falling forward but also moving up toward the mountain, my shadow looming against its jagged peaks, and I'm surging forward, ascending, sailing through dark clouds, rising up, a fiery wind propelling me, and soon it's night and the stars hang in the sky above the mountain, revolving as they burn.
>
> The stars are real.
>
> The future is that mountain. (481)[14]

---

[14] The final sentence refers back to an earlier conversation between Victor and his father:
'I'm staking out new territory, Dad.'
'Which is?'
I stare straight ahead. 'The future.' (77)
It also uncannily recalls a schizophrenic patient's description of the alternation of space and time: 'The past is the precipice. The future is the mountain' (quoted in Sass, 1992, p. 160).

These three sentences reverberate with ambiguity. First the mural of a pastoral scene—significantly, a far cry from the postmodern digital mediascape—extends beyond its frame, and then Victor becomes absorbed into the space and time of the image. It is a posthumanist but neoromantic scene: a surrender of the last vestiges of subjectivity into the realm of the sublime. Victor's 'schizophrenic' self-dissolution reads as though he is relinquishing the struggle over his image existence. He transcends the landscape of advertising ('billboards with answers on them') into one uncontaminated by the commodified clutter and violence of postmodernity. Here, are we no longer on the celebrity modelling circuit but back in the territory of Kraepelin's 'mental shipwrecks' (Kraepelin, 1981, p. 275) left as readers with Jaspers's sense of 'a gulf which defies description' (Jaspers, 1972, p. 447)?

In Chapter 2 I argued that Schreber can be said to have suffered at the threshold of the sublime: forever forced to reassert his powers of reason to an invasive and persecutory God. *Glamorama*'s final scene can be read as Victor's response to the same predicament: only here he gives up the struggle and is completely subsumed by the sublime encounter, transcending ego and Oedipus, language and embodiment, time, and consciousness. *Glamorama* puts a postmodern spin on psychiatry's sublime object by suggesting that the delusions and self-dissolution of 'postmodern schizophrenia' are not psychic secrets awaiting decryption, but revelations of a self evacuated of psychic depth. If *Memoirs* is a modern text *about* a modern schizophrenia, *Glamorama*'s 'undecidability' and hermeneutic inaccessibility mark it as a postmodern text that reproduces a 'postmodern schizophrenia' at the level of its textual logic. Here, in the arena of contemporary literature, in a text that makes no explicit reference to clinical theory, the schizophrenic sublime appears with surprising force where we might least expect to find it.

Conclusion

Ten years or so after the publication of *Glamorama*, the American professor of communication studies John Durham Peters has declared an end to our intellectual fascination with schizophrenia:

> Madness, especially schizophrenia, was once at the center of the intellectual agenda. A wide range of mid-20th-century thinkers . . . followed Sigmund Freud and Karl Jaspers in seeing psychopathology as the key to understanding modernity—and communication. The antipsychiatry movement of the 1960s and the general replacement of the talking cure with psychopharmacological treatment in the past couple of decades have shifted intellectual fascination largely away from schizophrenia. So perhaps have changing practices of communication. (Peters, 2010, p. 137)

For Peters (2010, p. 138), the symptoms of schizophrenia were a 'fit' with the technologies and modes of address, the 'nonverbal codes and simulated sociability' of radio and television. Communication throughout the twentieth century depended for its intelligibility on the distinction between two forms of address—the impersonal discourse of broadcasting and the personal discourse of telephony; the public speech of a pluralized self with the private speech of a unitary self (Peters, 2010, p. 131)—and in schizophrenia these distinctions are collapsed. The 'twilight of broadcasting', then, also signals an end to schizophrenia's intellectual allure, not because its symptoms have nothing in common with new and emerging communication technologies, but rather because what was once considered pathological is now an unremarkable feature of the everyday:

> The divide between interpersonal and mediated communication is blurring. No longer is speaking into the air considered appropriate for broadcasting but tragic (or comic) for interpersonal relationships. People now 'broadcast themselves' on YouTube and accumulate 'friends' in social networking sites. They walk around in public, talking animatedly to an invisible partner and nobody thinks they are crazy. Anyone with a music player can simulate the radiohead experience of having voices and sounds emanating from the center of their skull. The new regime seems messier and more pragmatic; less delusional but more socially stunted. Who needs telepathy when you have texting? Or thought broadcasting when you have Twitter? [. . .] What was once mad or uncanny is now routine: hearing disembodied voices and speaking to nobody in particular . . . (Peters, 2010, p. 138)

Peters's argument here resonates with a claim we have already examined in some detail, namely, that 'schizophrenia' can speak of and to the everyday experiences of postmodernity.

But what if ours is no longer a postmodern era? Did America's response to the attacks of 11 September 2001 mark 'the complete triumph of postmodernism' (Michaels, 2003, p. 113), or did the event and its aftermath make the postmodern impossible? Will global recession finish off whatever vestiges of the postmodern remained in the first years of the twenty-first century?

These questions are too broad to engage with fully in the final moments of a book, but that does not make them unimportant. Models of postmodern 'cultural schizophrenia' still enjoy a certain critical currency (see for example Goh, 2008), but will it be the case that changes in the structures of communication extinguish our 'intellectual fascination' with schizophrenia, as Peters suggests? And might this perhaps be mirrored by an attendant decline in 'clinical fascination' with the concept of schizophrenia, at least amongst those who believe that the label itself is not helpful to the analysis or treatment of severe mental distress? It is, perhaps, too soon to tell.

Without attempting to predict the future trajectory of our fascination, what I have sought to do in this book is to show how schizophrenia has enthralled and eluded theorists throughout the twentieth century. I have navigated the wide, varied, and conflict-ridden terrains of clinical and cultural theory using the concept of the schizophrenic sublime to interpret the connections between heterogeneous discourses and to identify the points of divergence between theoretical positions. The sublime places its emphasis on the (in)comprehensibility of schizophrenia—its status as un/knowable, un/interpretable, un/intelligible—and on the role it plays in sustaining a particular disciplinary field. So, as psychiatry's sublime object, a disorder whose cardinal feature is its opacity, schizophrenia has been the key site of disciplinary expansion. Psychoanalysis transformed this unknowable object into an untreatable text open to endless reinterpretation. Cultural theory's appropriation of schizophrenia began as an intervention in clinical theory and practice, and became a radical reappraisal of schizophrenia's role in explaining non-pathological modes of enlightened, deterritorialized, modern, and postmodern subjectivity. Tracing an arc from modern psychiatry to postmodern cultural theory, we have moved from a clinical discourse, which unambiguously constructs schizophrenia as its sublime object, to a cultural discourse which renders diffuse or paradoxical the schizophrenic sublime. Psychoanalytic, antipsychiatric, and anti-Oedipal accounts of schizophrenia can be situated at various points along this progression, and, as we have seen, Louis Sass's work offers a vantage point outside the sublime from which to examine in more detail the idea, fully realized in Ellis's novel, that schizophrenia can illuminate the experience of postmodernity.

Of course, this is by no means the only story to be told about schizophrenia in the twentieth century, nor would all the theorists I have discussed even see themselves as protagonists in the same narrative. The texts analysed here—psychiatric textbooks, psychoanalytic seminars, antipsychiatric tracts, and theoretical works—are key sites in the discursive construction of schizophrenia, and in identifying the operation of the schizophrenic sublime in clinical and cultural theory, I have not attempted to account for its appearance beyond the textual sphere. Embodied, interpersonal encounters between individuals—to take just one example—clearly have an enormously important role to play in the definition and management of schizophrenia, whether in the contexts of psychiatric and psychoanalytic therapy, mental health services, advocacy and support groups, or simply in day-to-day life. The question of whether the concept of a schizophrenic sublime would be of any value in understanding institutional and interpersonal exchanges is therefore still an open one, but I certainly do not wish to advance any a priori claims to this effect. Remaining resolutely in the textual sphere, my intent has been to offer a historical analysis of schizophrenia's representation that it is hoped will enrich our understanding of how such striking experience could come to be associated with not one but up to 100% of the population.

I want to conclude, then, by identifying two further areas of inquiry suggested by this analysis—two broad discursive fields in which the idea of the schizophrenic sublime might be constructively put to work. First, as *Memoirs of My Nervous Illness* has shown, autobiographies and biographies have occupied a privileged position in theoretical analyses of schizophrenia, and are an obvious starting point for considering if, and if so how, the sublime is called upon to describe schizophrenic experience by those it has affected most intimately. Perhaps surprisingly, given the prevalence of the disorder, and the wealth of more general 'madness' memoirs, in-depth autobiographical accounts of schizophrenia are relatively few and far between. Elaine Showalter (Showalter, 1987, p. 204) has identified the three 'best-known studies of the inner life of the schizophrenic' as Renee's *Autobiography of a Schizophrenic Girl* (1970), Greenberg's *I Never Promised You a Rose Garden* (1964) and Barbara O'Brien's *Operators and Things: The Inner Life of a Schizophrenic* (1960)—texts that certainly reward detailed examination (Woods, 2007). Anne Deveson's *Tell Me I'm Here* (1991), Lori Schiller's *The Quiet Room: A Journey Out of the Torment of Madness* (Schiller and Bennett, 1994), Richard McLean's *Recovered Not Cured: A Journey Through Schizophrenia* (McLean, 2003), Jonathan Caouette's film *Tarnation* (2003), Kurt Snyder's *Me, Myself and Them*

(Snyder et al., 2007), Elyn Saks's *The Centre Cannot Hold* (2007), and Paul Fearne's *Diary of a Schizophrenic* (2010) are among the most interesting recent publications. Against the background of the rising interest in narrative medicine (Charon, 2008), phenomenological psychiatry, and qualitative studies of the subjective experience of mental distress (Davidson, 2003; Geekie and Read, 2009; Lysaker and Lysaker, 2008;), looking beyond book-length autobiographies to other forms of biographical writing, such as *Schizophrenia Bulletin*'s 'First Person Accounts' is, in my view, an even more pressing task (Estroff, 2004; Geanellos, 2005; Hayne and Yonge, 1997). No comprehensive analysis of the relationship between autobiographical and biographical accounts of schizophrenia and clinical and cultural models of the disorder has yet been undertaken, but an examination of the extent to which these works engage, incorporate, or disavow the association between schizophrenia and the sublime could certainly bring metatheoretical focus to such a project.

The second textual arena to which I would like to draw attention comes more within the purview of cultural studies, sociology, history, and medical anthropology. How have clinical accounts of schizophrenia been taken up in the discourse of patient support groups, in mental health policy, in the promotion of psychopharmaceuticals, and in media depictions of psychotic experience? Is the sublime here in operation, or do representations of schizophrenia in these contexts adhere to a different logic? What are the key areas of contestation, and how have these in turn influenced biographical and even theoretical accounts of schizophrenic experience? The capacity of often very partisan and passionate accounts of schizophrenia to impact strongly upon public perceptions was most clearly demonstrated during the antipsychiatry movement of the 1960s and 1970s, but challenges to biological psychiatry from within and beyond the profession (Bracken, 2003; Crossley, 2006; Johnstone, 2000; Lewis, 2000; Laugharne, April 2002, 2004;), as well as powerful studies of the role of culture in the experience of schizophrenia (Jenkins and Barrett, 2004b) invite a reassessment of the relationship between clinical and non-clinical discourses of schizophrenia for contemporary times.

To what extent, then, do generically and culturally specific portrayals of schizophrenia reproduce, extend, or challenge the clinical picture of the disorder? Do they articulate schizophrenia through the vocabulary of the sublime, and if so, how? And can they in turn reveal shifts in the history of representing post/modern subjectivity more generally? These are the questions I suggest could inform the analysis of representations of schizophrenia in the two discursive contexts just outlined. The value, as I see it, of the kind of analysis I have undertaken throughout this book lies in focusing attention on the relationships between competing models of the disorder while leaving open the question of which has the strongest claim on the truth of schizophrenic experience. As we have seen, cultural theorists have been compelled, whether directly or indirectly, to negotiate schizophrenia's status as sublime within psychiatric and psychoanalytic discourse, to stake a claim if not at the level of clinical theory then certainly at the level of psychological metatheory. So let me finish with a question: If the category of the sublime provides a constructive framework through which to analyse the connections between clinical and cultural theory, can it in turn illuminate the way in which other thinkers—artists, literary critics, bureaucrats, journalists, advertisers, and patients themselves—use clinical accounts of schizophrenia?

References

Abbott, A. (2010). Schizophrenia: The drug deadlock. *Nature,* **468:** 158–9.

Abi-Rached, J. & Rose, N. (2010). The birth of the neuromolecular gaze. *History of the Human Sciences,* **23:** 11–36.

Abraham, K. (1972). The psycho-sexual differences between hysteria and dementia praecox. *The Selected Papers of Karl Abraham.* London: Maresfield Library.

Aldhous, P. (2009). Psychiatry's civil war. *New Scientist* [Online]. Available: http://www.newscientist.com/article/mg20427381.300-psychiatrys-civil-war.html [Accessed 20 February 2010].

Aldhous, P. (2010). Psychiatry's draft new 'bible' goes online. *New Scientist* [Online]. Available: http://www.newscientist.com/article/dn18508-psychiatrys-draft-new-bible-goes-online.html?full=true [Accessed 20 February 2010].

American Psychiatric Association (2000). *Diagnostic and Statistical Manual of Mental Disorders.* Washington: American Psychiatric Association.

Andreasen, N. (2004). *Brave New Brain: Conquering Mental Illness in the Era of the Genome.* Oxford: Oxford University Press.

Andrejevic, M. (2002). The kinder, gentler gaze of big brother: Reality TV in the era of digital capitalism. *New Media and Society,* **4:** 251–70.

Angermeyera, M. C., Holzingerb, A., & Matschingerc, H. (2009). Mental health literacy and attitude towards people with mental illness: A trend analysis based on population surveys in the eastern part of Germany. *European Psychiatry,* **24:** 225–32.

Annesley, J. (1998). *Blank Fictions: Consumerism, Culture and the Contemporary American Novel.* London: Pluto Press.

Appignanesi, L. (2008). *Mad, Bad and Sad: A History of Women and the Mind Doctors from 1800 to the Present.* London: Virago.

Artaud, A. (1976). *The Selected Writings of Antonin Artaud.* New York: Farrar, Straus and Giroux.

Ayers, S. (2000). *Glamorama* vanitas: Bret Easton Ellis' postmodern allegory. *Postmodern Culture,* **11.**

Bailey, J. (2006). Postmodernism and the disappearance of the real (lecture). *Postmodernism.* Parkville: University of Melbourne.

Baker, C., Crawford, P., Brown, B. J., Lipsedge, M., & Carter, R. (2010). *Madness in Post-1945 British and American Fiction.* London: Palgrave Macmillan.

Barham, P. (1993). *Schizophrenia and Human Value: Chronic Schizophrenia, Science and Society.* London: Free Association Books.

Barrett, R. J. (1996). *The Psychiatric Team and the Social Definition of Schizophrenia.* Cambridge: Cambridge University Press.

Barrett, R. J. (1998a). Conceptual foundations of schizophrenia: I. Degeneration. *Australian and New Zealand Journal of Psychiatry, 32:* 617–26.

Barrett, R. J. (1998b). Conceptual foundations of schizophrenia: II. Disintegration and division. *Australian and New Zealand Journal of Psychiatry, 32:* 627–34.

Barrett, R. J. (1998c). The 'schizophrenic' and the liminal persona in modern society. *Culture, Medicine and Psychiatry, 22:* 465–94.

Barthes, R. (1977). The death of the author. *Image, Music, Text.* London: Fontana.

Baudrillard, J. (1983). The ecstasy of communication. In: Foster, H. (ed.) *The Anti-Aesthetic: Essays on Postmodern Culture.* New York: The New Press.

Baudrillard, J. (1988). *The Ecstasy of Communication.* New York: Semiotext(e), Columbia University.

Baudrillard, J. (1993). *The Transparency of Evil: Essays on Extreme Phenomena.* London: Verso.

Baudrillard, J. (2002). *The Spirit of Terrorism and Requiem for the Twin Towers.* London: Verso.

Bauman, Z. (1991). *Modernity and Ambivalence.* Cambridge: Polity.

Bauman, Z. (1993). *Intimations of Postmodernity.* London: Routledge.

Bauman, Z. (1996). *Postmodernity and Its Discontents.* Cambridge: Polity.

Bauman, Z. (2000). *Liquid Modernity.* Cambridge: Polity.

Bauman, Z. (2001). Identity in the globalising world. *Social Anthropology, 9:* 121–9.

Bauman, Z. (2005). *Work, Consumerism and the New Poor.* Maidenhead: Open University Press.

Bauman, Z. (2006). *Liquid Life.* Cambridge: Polity.

Bauman, Z. & Tester, K. (2001). *Conversations with Zygmunt Bauman.* Cambridge: Polity Press.

Bebbington, P. & McGuffin, P. (eds.) (1988). *Schizophrenia: The Major Issues.* Oxford: Heinemann Medical Books.

Beckett, A. (1999). Leader of the Bret pack. *The Guardian,* Saturday January 9.

Beer, G. (1996). Forging the missing link: Interdisciplinary stories. *Open fields: Science in cultural encounter.* Oxford: Clarendon Press.

Bentall, R. P. (ed.) (1990). *Reconstructing Schizophrenia.* London: Routledge.

Bentall, R. P. (2004). *Madness Explained: Psychosis and Human Nature.* London: Penguin.

Bentall, R. P. (2009). *Doctoring the Mind: Is Our Current Treatment of Mental Illness Really Any Good?* New York: New York University Press.

Bentall, R. P., Jackson, H. F., & Pilgrim, D. (1988a). Abandoning the concept of 'schizophrenia': Some implications of validity arguments for psychological research into psychotic phenomena. *British Journal of Clinical Psychology, 27:* 303–24.

Bentall, R. P., Jackson, H. F., & Pilgrim, D. (1988b). The concept of schizophrenia is dead: Long live the concept of schizophrenia? *British Journal of Clinical Psychology, 27:* 329–31.

Berman, J. (1985). *The Talking Cure: Literary Representations of Psychoanalysis.* New York: New York University Press.

Berrios, G. E. & Hauser, R. (1995). Kraepelin: Clinical section, part 2. In: Berrios, G. E. & Porter, R. (eds.) *A History of Clinical Psychiatry: The Origin and History of Psychiatric Disorders.* London: Athlone.

Berrios, G. E., Luque, R., & Villagrán, J. M. (2003). Schizophrenia: A conceptual history. *International Journal of Psychology and Psychological Therapy*, 3: 111–40.

Blackshaw, T. (2005). *Zygmunt Bauman*. London and New York: Routledge.

Bleakley, A. & Bligh, J. (2009). Who can resist Foucault? *Journal of Medicine and Philosophy*, 34: 368–83.

Bleuler, E. (1950). *Dementia Praecox or the Group of Schizophrenias*. New York: International Universities Press.

Blount, J. (1999). *Glam Slam* [Online]. Available: http://www.flagpole.com/Issues/02.17.99/lit.html [Accessed 23 February 2003].

Blume, H. (1999). Portrait of the artist as a social satirist [Online]. *Atlantic Unbound*. Available: http://www.theatlantic.com/unbound/bookauth/ba990210.htm [Accessed 24 February 2003].

Bogue, R. (1989). *Deleuze and Guattari*. London: Routledge.

Bolton, D. (2008). *What is Mental Disorder? An Essay in Philosophy, Science, and Values*. Oxford: Oxford University Press.

Bortle, S. (Spring 2001). R. D. Laing as negative thinker. *Janus Head*, 4.

Boyers, R. & Orrill, R. (eds.) (1972). *Laing and Anti-psychiatry*. London: Penguin.

Boyle, M. (1990). *Schizophrenia—A Scientific Delusion?* London: Routledge.

Bracken, P. J. (2003). Postmodernism and psychiatry. *Current Opinion in Psychiatry*, 16: 673–7.

Bracken, P. & Thomas, P. (2005). Postpsychiatry: Mental Health in a Postmodern World. Oxford: Oxford University Press.

Bracken, P. & Thomas, P. (2010a). From Szasz to Foucault: On the role of critical psychiatry. *Philosophy, Psychiatry, & Psychology*, 17: 219–28.

Bracken, P. & Thomas, P. (2010b). Is private (contract-based) practice an answer to the problems of psychiatry? *Philosophy, Psychiatry, & Psychology*, 17: 241–5.

Bracken, P., Khalfa, J., & Thomas, P. (2007). Recent translations of Foucault on mental health. *Current Opinion in Psychiatry*, 20: 605–8.

Braidotti, R. (2005). Schizophrenia. In: Parr, A. (ed.) *The Deleuze Dictionary*. Edinburgh: Edinburgh University Press.

Braun, J. (1995). Schizophrenia: A transcultural view. In: Braun, J. (ed.) *Social Pathology in Comparative Perspective: The Nature and Psychology of Civil Society*. Westport, Connecticut: Praeger.

Breggin, P. R. (1991). *Toxic Psychiatry: Why Therapy, Empathy, and Love Must Replace the Drugs, Electroshock, and Biochemical Theories of the 'New Psychiatry'*. New York: St Martins Press.

Broome, M. R. (2007). Taxonomy and ontology in psychiatry: A survey of recent literature. *Philosophy, Psychiatry, and Psychology*, 13: 303–19.

Buchanan, I. (2008). *Deleuze and Guattari's* Anti-Oedipus: *A Reader's Guide*. London: Continuum.

Buchanan, R. W., Kreyenbuhl, J., Kelly, D. L., Noel, J. M., Boggs, D. L., Fischer, B. A., Himelhoch, S., Fang, B., Peterson, E., Aquino, P. R., & Keller, W. (2010). The 2009 schizophrenia port psychopharmacological treatment recommendations and summary statements. *Schizophrenia Bulletin*, 36: 71–93.

Burke, E. (1987). *A Philosophical Enquiry into the Origin of Our Ideas of the Sublime and Beautiful*. Oxford: Basil Blackwell.

Burston, D. (1996). *The Wing of Madness: The Life and Work of R. D. Laing*. Cambridge, MA: Harvard University Press.

Burston, D. (Spring 2001a). R. D. Laing and the politics of diagnosis. *Janus Head,* **4**.

Burston, D. (Spring 2001b). Special issue: The legacy of R. D. Laing (editorial). *Janus Head,* **4**.

Busfield, J. (1996). *Men, Women and Madness: Understanding Gender and Mental Disorder*. London: Macmillan.

Butler, J. (1993). *Bodies that Matter: On the Discursive Limits of Sex*. London and New York: Routledge.

Canetti, E. (1962). *Crowds and Power*. London: Victor Gollancz.

Caouette, J. (dir.) (2003). *Tarnation*. USA: Wellspring.

Carpenter, W. T. (2009). Anticipating DSM-V: Should psychosis risk become a diagnostic class? *Schizophrenia Bulletin,* **35**: 841–3.

Castle, D. J. (2000). Women and schizophrenia: An epidemiological perspective. In: Castle, D. J., McGrath, J., & Kulkarni, J. (eds.) *Women and Schizophrenia*. Cambridge: Cambridge University Press.

Charon, R. (2008). *Narrative Medicine: Honoring the Stories of Illness*. New York: Oxford University Press.

Cheetham, M. A. (1995). Moments of discipline: Derrida, Kant, and the genealogy of the sublime. In: Rajan, T. & Clark, D. L. (eds.) *Intersections: Nineteenth-Century Philosophy and Contemporary Theory*. Albany: State University of New York Press.

Chesler, P. (1972). *Women and Madness*. New York: Allen Lane.

Chung, M. C., Fulford, K. W. M. B., & Graham, G. (eds.) (2007). *Reconceiving Schizophrenia*. Oxford: Oxford University Press.

Colebrook, C. (2002). *Understanding Deleuze*. Crows Nest, NSW: Allen and Unwin.

Colebrook, C. (2006). *Deleuze: A Guide for the Perplexed*. London and New York: Continuum.

Conley, J. (2009). The poverty of Bret Easton Ellis. *Arizona Quarterly,* **65**: 117–37.

Cooper, D. (1970). *Psychiatry and Anti-psychiatry*. St Albans: Paladin.

Cooper, R. (2004). What is wrong with the DSM? *History of Psychiatry,* **15**: 5–25.

Cooper, R. (2005). *Classifying Madness: A Philosophical Examination of the Diagnostic and Statistical Manual of Mental Disorders*. Dordrecht: Springer.

Cooper, R. (2007). *Psychiatry and Philosophy of Science*. Durham: Acumen.

COPE Initiative. (2010). *Campaign for the Abolition of the Schizophrenia Label* [Online]. University of Manchester. Available: http://www.caslcampaign.com/ [Accessed 23 October 2009].

Craddock, N. (2010). Robust empirical data and clinical utility: The only drivers of change, commentary on . . . the classification of mental disorder. *Advances in Psychiatric Treatment,* **16**: 20–2.

Craddock, N. & Owen, M. J. (2005). The beginning of the end for the Kraepelinian dichotomy. *British Journal of Psychiatry,* **186**: 364–66.

Craddock, N. & Owen, M. J. (2007). Rethinking psychosis: The disadvantages of a dichotomous classification now outweigh the advantages. *World Psychiatry,* **6**: 84–91.

Craddock, N. & Owen, M. J. (2010a). Data and clinical utility should be the drivers of changes to psychiatric classification. *British Journal of Psychiatry,* **197**: 158–9.

Craddock, N. & Owen, M. J. (2010b). The kraepelinian dichotomy—going, going . . . But still not gone. *British Journal of Psychiatry,* **196**: 92–5.

Craddock, N., O'Donovan, M. C., & Owen, M. J. (2009). Psychosis genetics: Modeling the relationship between schizophrenia, bipolar disorder, and mixed (or 'Schizoaffective') psychoses. *Schizophrenia Bulletin,* **35**: 482–90.

Craig, T. K. J. (2008). Recovery: Say what you mean and mean what you say. *Journal of Mental Health,* **17**: 125–8.

Crapanzano, V. (1998). 'Lacking now is only the leading idea, that is—we, the rays, have no thoughts': Interlocutory collapse in Daniel Paul Schreber's *Memoirs of My Nervous Illness. Critical Inquiry,* **24**: 737–68.

Cresswell, M. (2008). Szasz and his interlocutors: Reconsidering Thomas Szasz's 'myth of mental illness' thesis. *Journal for the Theory of Social Behaviour,* **38**: 23–44.

Crichton, P. (2000). 'A profound duplicity of life': Uses and misuses of 'schizophrenia' in popular culture and professional diagnosis. *Times Literary Supplement,* March 31.

Crossley, N. (1998). Transforming the mental health field: The early history of the national association for mental health. *Sociology of Health and Illness,* **20**: 458–88.

Crossley, N. (1999). Fish, field, habitus and madness: The first wave mental health users movement in Great Britain. *British Journal of Sociology,* **50**: 647–70.

Crossley, N. (2002). Repertoires of contention and tactical diversity in the UK psychiatric survivors movement: The question of appropriation. *Social Movement Studies,* **1**: 47–71.

Crossley, N. (2004). Not being mentally ill: Social movements, system survivors and the oppositional habitus. *Anthropology & Medicine,* **11**: 161–80.

Crossley, N. (2005). How social movements move: From first to second wave developments in the UK field of psychiatric contention. *Social Movement Studies,* **4**: 21–48.

Crossley, N. (2006). *Contesting Psychiatry: Social Movements in Mental Health*. Oxford and New York: Routledge.

Crossley, N. & Crossley, M. (2001). 'Patient' voices, social movements and the habitus: how psychiatric survivors 'speak out'. *Social Science and Medicine,* **52**: 1477–89.

Crow, T. J. (1985). The two syndrome concept: Origins and current status. *Schizophrenia Bulletin,* **11**: 471–88.

Crow, T. J. (1995). A continuum of psychosis, one human gene, and not much else—the case for homogeneity. *Schizophrenia Research,* **17**: 135–45.

Crow, T. J. (2008). The emperors of the schizophrenia polygene have no clothes. *Psychological Medicine,* **38**: 1681–5.

Currie, M. (1998). *Postmodern Narrative Theory*. London: Macmillan.

Cuthbert, B. N. & Insel, T. R. (2010). Toward new approaches to psychotic disorders: The NIMH research domain criteria project. *Schizophrenia Bulletin,* **36**: 1061–2.

Cutting, G. (1994). Foucault and the history of madness. In: Cutting, G. (ed.) *The Cambridge Companion to Foucault*. Cambridge: Cambridge University Press.

Davidson, L. (2003). *Living Outside Mental Illness: Qualitative Studies of Recovery in Schizophrenia*. New York: New York University Press.

Davidson, L. (2010). PORT through a recovery lens. *Schizophrenia Bulletin,* **36**: 107–8.

de Certeau, M. (1983). Lacan: An ethics of speech. *Representations,* **3**: 21–39.

de Certeau, M. (1988). The institution of rot. In: Allison, D. B., de Oliveira, P., Roberts, M. S. & Weiss, A. S. (eds.) *Psychosis and Sexual Identity: Towards a Post-Analytic View of the Schreber Case*. Albany: State University of New York Press.

Deleuze, G. (1990). Letter to a harsh critic. *Negotiations 1972–1990*. New York: Columbia University Press.

Deleuze, G. (2002). Postscript on control societies. In: Levin, T. Y., Frohne, U., & Weibel, P. (eds.) *Ctrl [space]: Rhetorics of Surveillance from Bentham to Big Brother*. Cambridge, Massachusetts: The MIT Press.

Deleuze, G. (2006). *Two Regimes of Madness: Texts and Interviews 1975–1995*. New York: Semiotext(e).

Deleuze, G. & Guattari, F. (1982). *Anti-Oedipus: Capitalism and Schizophrenia*. New York: Viking Press.

Deleuze, G. & Guattari, F. (1987). *A Thousand Plateaus: Capitalism and Schizophrenia*. Minneapolis: University of Minnesota Press.

Deleuze, G. & Guattari, F. (1990). Gilles Deleuze and Félix Guattari on *Anti-Oedipus* (conversation with Catherine Backès-Clément, l'arc 49 (1972)). *Negotiations 1972–1990*. New York: Columbia University Press.

Derrida, J. (1978). Cogito and the history of madness. *Writing and Difference*. London: Routledge & Kegan Paul.

Derrida, J. (1987). *The Truth in Painting*. Chicago: University of Chicago Press.

Derrida, J. (1998). 'To do justice to Freud': The history of madness in the age of psychoanalysis. *Resistances of Psychoanalysis*. Stanford: Stanford University Press.

Deveson, A. (1991). *Tell Me I'm Here*. Melbourne: Penguin.

Dixon, L. B., Dickerson, F., Bellack, A. S., Bennett, M., Dickinson, D., Goldberg, R. W., Lehman, A., Tenhula, W. N., Calmes, C., Pasillas, R. M., Peer, J., & Kreyenbuhl, J. (2010). The 2009 schizophrenia PORT psychosocial treatment recommendations and summary statements. *Schizophrenia Bulletin*, **36**: 48–70.

Dobbs, D. (2010). The making of a troubled mind. *Nature*, **468**: 154–7.

Donnelly, M. (1992). *The Politics of Mental Health in Italy*. London: Routledge.

Due, R. (2007). *Deleuze*. Cambridge: Polity Press.

Dupont, J. (1988). Ferenczi's 'madness'. *Contemporary Psychoanalysis*, **24**: 250–61.

Eagleton, T. (1985). Capitalism, modernism and postmodernism. *New Left Review*, **152**: 60–73.

Eagleton, T. (1990). *The Ideology of the Aesthetic*. Oxford: Basil Blackwell.

Editor. (2010). Combating schizophrenia. *Nature*, **468**: 133–4.

Ehrenberg, A. (2010). *The Weariness of the Self: Diagnosing the History of Depression in the Contemporary Age*. Montreal: McGill-Queen's University Press.

Elliott, A. (1996). *Subject to Ourselves: Social Theory, Psychoanalysis and Postmodernity*. Cambridge: Polity Press.

Elliott, A. (2002). The dislocating world of postmodernism. *Psychoanalytic Theory: An Introduction*. 2nd ed. Oxford: Blackwell.

Ellis, B. E. (1987). *The Rules of Attraction*. New York: Vintage Books.

Ellis, B. E. (1991). *American Psycho*. London: Picador.

Ellis, B. E. (2000). *Glamorama*. London: Picador.

Engstrom, E. J. (1995). Kraepelin: Social section. In: Berrios, G. E. & Porter, R. (eds.) *A History of Clinical Psychiatry: The Origin and History of Psychiatric Disorders.* London: Athlone.

Engstrom, E. J. & Weber, M. M. (2007). Making Kraepelin history: A great instauration? *History of Psychiatry,* **18**: 267–73.

Esquirol, J. E. D. (1965). *Mental Maladies, A Treatise on Insanity.* New York: Hafner.

Estroff, S. E. (1989). Self, identity, and subjective experiences of schizophrenia: In search of the subject. *Schizophrenia Bulletin,* **15**: 189–96.

Estroff, S. E. (2004). Subject/subjectivities in dispute: The poetics, politics, and performance of first-person narratives of people with schizophrenia. In: Jenkins, J. H. & Barrett, R. J. (eds.) *Schizophrenia, Culture, and Subjectivity: The Edge of Experience.* Cambridge: Cambridge University Press.

Ettler, J. (1999). Rebels without a cause. *Australian Book Review,* 213.

Evans, D. (1996). *An Introductory Dictionary of Lacanian Psychoanalysis.* London and New York: Routledge.

Fabrega, H. (1989). The self and schizophrenia: A cultural perspective. *Schizophrenia Bulletin,* **15**: 277–90.

Farmer, A. E., McGuffin, P., & Bebbington, P. (1988). The phenomena of schizophrenia. In: Bebbington, P. & McGuffin, P. (eds.) *Schizophrenia: The Major Issues.* Oxford: Heinemann Medical Books.

Farrell, J. (1996). *Freud's Paranoid Quest: Psychoanalysis and Modern Suspicion.* New York: New York University Press.

Fatemi, S. H. & Folsom, T. D. (2009). The neurodevelopmental hypothesis of schizophrenia revisited. *Schizophrenia Bulletin,* **35**: 528–48.

Fearne, P. (2010). *Diary of a schizophrenic.* Brentwood, Essex: chipmunkapublishing.

Fee, D. (ed.) (2000). *Pathology and the Postmodern: Mental Illness as Discourse and Experience.* London: Sage.

Felman, S. (ed.) (1982). *Literature and Psychoanalysis: The Question of Reading, Otherwise.* Baltimore: Johns Hopkins University Press.

Felman, S. (1985). *Writing and Madness: Literature/Philosophy/Psychoanalysis.* Ithaca: Cornell University Press.

Ferns, P., Barker, P., Beresford, P., Scott Blackman, P., Bracken, P., Christie, Y., Crepaz-Keay, D., Fernando, S., Gabriel, J., Henry, W. L., Kalathil, J., Keating, F., Moore, P., Stanley, J., Summerfield, D., Timimi, S., Vernon, P., Vige, M., Clear, P., Thompson, S., Gradwell, S., Martin, C., & Kollie, A. (2010). Poor research or an attack on black people? Letter from mental health campaigners on the alleged 'epidemic' of schizophrenia among British African Caribbean groups. *The Guardian* [Online]. Available: http://www.guardian.co.uk/society/2010/feb/03/mental-health-bme-schizophrenia-letter [Accessed 11 February 2010].

Fine, R. (1979). *A History of Psychoanalysis.* New York: Columbia University Press.

Fink, B. (1997). *A Clinical Introduction to Lacanian Psychoanalysis: Theory and Technique.* Cambridge, Massachusetts: Harvard University Press.

Finlay, M. (1989). Post-modernising psychoanalysis/psychoanalysing post-modernity. *Free Associations,* **16**: 43–80.

Foster, H. (ed.) (1983). *The Anti-Aesthetic: Essays on Postmodern Culture.* Port Townsend, Washington: Bay Press.

Foucault, M. (1970). *The Order of Things: An Archaeology of the Human Sciences.* New York: Random House.

Foucault, M. (1976). *Mental Illness and Psychology.* New York: Harper & Row.

Foucault, M. (1977). *Discipline and Punish: The Birth of the Prison.* London: Allen Lane.

Foucault, M. (1993). *Madness and Civilization: A History of Insanity in the Age of Reason.* London: Routledge.

Foucault, M. (1996). Madness, absence of an oeuvre. In: Lechte, J. (ed.) *Writing and Psychoanalysis.* London: Arnold.

Foucault, M. (2008). *Psychiatric Power.* New York: Macmillan.

Foucault, M. (2009). *History of Madness.* Abingdon: Routledge.

Fraguas, D. & Breathnach, C. S. (2009). Problems with retrospective studies of the presence of schizophrenia. *History of Psychiatry,* **20**: 61–71.

Frances, A. (2010). Opening Pandora's box: The 19 worst suggestions for DSM-5. *Psychiatric Times* [Online], 27. Available: http://www.psychiatrictimes.com/display/article/10168/1522341 [Accessed 20 February 2010].

Frank, M. (2001). The world as will and representation: Deleuze's and Guattari's critique of capitalism as schizo-analysis and schizo-discourse. In: Genosko, G. (ed.) *Deleuze and Guattari: Critical Assessments of Leading Philosophers.* London and New York: Routledge.

Frankland, G. (2000). *Freud's literary culture.* New York: Cambridge University Press.

Freud, S. (1963a). Lecture XXVI the libido theory and narcissism. In: Strachey, J. (ed.) *The Standard Edition of the Complete Psychological Works of Sigmund Freud.* London: The Hogarth Press and the Psycho-Analytic Institute.

Freud, S. (1963b). Lecture XXVII transference. In: Strachey, J. (ed.) *The Standard Edition of the Complete Psychological Works of Sigmund Freud.* London: The Hogarth Press and the Institute of Psycho-Analysis.

Freud, S. (1981). Psycho-analytic notes on an autobiographical account of a case of paranoia (dementia paranoides). In: Strachey, J. (ed.) *The Standard Edition of the Complete Psychological Works of Sigmund Freud.* London: The Hogarth Press and the Institute of Psycho-Analysis.

Freud, S. (1985a). Letter of December 6 1896. In: Masson, J. M. (ed.) *The Complete Letters of Sigmund Freud to Wilhelm Fliess 1887–1904.* Cambridge, Massachusetts: The Belknap Press of Harvard University Press.

Freud, S. (1985b). Letter of May 30 1986. In: Masson, J. M. (ed.) *The Complete Letters of Sigmund Freud to Wilhelm Fliess 1887–1904.* Cambridge, Massachusetts: The Belknap Press of Harvard University Press.

Freud, S. (1995). An autobiographical study (1925). In: Gay, P. (ed.) *The Freud Reader.* London: Vintage.

Freud, S. & Jung, C. (1974). *The Freud/Jung letters: The Correspondence Between Sigmund Freud and C. G. Jung.* Princeton: Princeton University Press.

Frith, C. & Johnstone, E. C. (2003). *Schizophrenia: A Very Short Introduction.* Oxford: Oxford University Press.

Frosh, S. (1991). *Identity Crisis: Modernity, Psychoanalysis and the Self.* London: Macmillan.

Fusar-Poli, P. & Politi, P. (2008). Paul Eugen Bleuler and the birth of schizophrenia (1908). *American Journal of Psychiatry,* **165**: 1407.

Gabel, J. (1976). *False Consciousness: An Essay on Reification*. New York: Harper and Row.

Gauntlett, D. (2002). *Media, Gender and Identity: An Introduction*. London and New York: Routledge.

Gawith, L. & Abrams, P. (2006). Long journey to recovery for Kiwi consumers: Recent developments in mental health policy and practice in New Zealand. *Australian Psychologist*, **41**: 140–8.

Geanellos, R. (2005). Adversity as opportunity: Living with schizophrenia and developing a resilient self. *International Journal of Mental Health Nursing*, **14**: 7–15.

Geddes, J., Freemantle, N., Harrison, P., & Bebbington, P. (2000). Atypical antipsychotics in the treatment of schizophrenia: Systematic overview and meta-regression analysis. *British Medical Journal*, **321**: 1371–6.

Geekie, J. & Read, J. (2009). *Making Sense of Madness: Contesting the Meaning of Schizophrenia*. London and New York: Routledge.

Georgaca, E. (2001). 'Poor girl': A case of active psychosis. *European Journal of Psychotherapy, Counselling and Health*, **4**: 175–88.

Gergen, K. J. (1991). *The saturated self: Dilemmas of identity in contemporary life*. New York: Basic Books.

Gilman, S. L. (1988). Constructing schizophrenia as a category of mental illness. *Disease and Representation: Images of Illness from Madness to Aids*. Ithaca: Cornell University Press.

Gilman, S. L. (1996). Judge dread (Daniel Paul Schreber's 'century'). *Artforum International*, **35**: 15–7.

Glass, J. M. (1987). Schizophrenia and rationality: On the function of the unconscious fantasy. In: Levin, D. M. (ed.) *Pathologies of the Modern Self: Postmodern Studies of Narcissism, Schizophrenia and Depression*. New York and London: New York University Press.

Glass, J. M. (1993). Postmodernism and the multiplicity of self. *Shattered Selves: Multiple Personality in a Postmodern World*. Ithaca and London: Cornell University Press.

Goffman, E. (1973). *Asylums: Essays on the Social Situation of Mental Patients and Other Inmates*. London: Penguin.

Goh, R. B. H. (2008). Myths of reversal: Backwards narratives, normative schizophrenia and the culture of causal agnosticism. *Social Semiotics*, **18**: 61–77.

Goldberg, A. (1999). *Sex, Religion, and the Making of Modern Madness: The Eberbach Asylum and German Society, 1815–1849*. New York: Oxford University Press.

Goldstein, J. M. & Lewine, R. R. J. (2000). Overview of sex differences in schizophrenia: Where have we been and where do we go from here? In: Castle, D. J., McGrath, J. & Kulkarni, J. (eds.) *Women and Schizophrenia*. Cambridge: Cambridge University Press.

Gordon, C. (1992). *Histoire de la Folie*: An unknown book by Michel Foucault. In: Still, A. & Velody, I. (eds.) *Rewriting the History of Madness: Studies in Foucault's Histoire de la Folie*. London and New York: Routledge.

Gordon, C. (2007a). Extreme prejudice: Notes on Andrew Scull's TLS review of Foucault's *History of Madness*. *Foucault Blog* [Online]. Available from: http://foucaultblog.wordpress.com/2007/05/20/extreme-prejudice/ [Accessed 17 December 2009].

Gordon, C. (2007b). *History of Madness* (review). *Notre Dame Philosophical Reviews* [Online]. Available: http://ndpr.nd.edu/review.cfm?id=8904 [Accessed 17 December 2009].

Gottesman, I. (1991). *Schizophrenia Genesis: The Origins of Madness*. New York: W. H. Freeman.

Gottschalk, S. (2000). Escape from insanity: 'Mental disorder' in the postmodern moment. In: Fee, D. (ed.) *Pathology and the Postmodern: Mental Illness as Discourse and Experience*. London: Sage.

Goulimari, P. (2004). 'Myriad little connections': Minoritarian movements in the postmodernism debate. *Postmodern Culture,* 14.

Green, M. F. (2003). *Schizophrenia Revealed: From Neurons to Social Interactions*. New York and London: Norton.

Greenberg, J. (1964). *I Never Promised You a Rose Garden, a Novel by Hannah Green*. New York: Holt, Rinehart and Winston.

Greene, T. (2007). The Kraepelinian dichotomy: The twin pillars crumbling? *History of Psychiatry,* **18**: 361–79.

Grigg, R. (1999). From the mechanism of psychosis to the universal condition of the symptom: On foreclosure. In: Nobus, D. (ed.) *Key Concepts of Lacanian Psychoanalysis*. New York: Other Press.

Grinker, R. R. (2010). In retrospect: The five lives of the psychiatry manual. *Nature,* **468**: 168–70.

Grossberg, L. (1988). Putting the pop back into postmodernism. In: Ross, A. (ed.) *Universal Abandon? The Politics of Postmodernism*. Minneapolis: University of Minnesota Press.

Guattari, F. (1996a). The divided Laing. In: Genosko, G. (ed.) *The Guattari Reader*. Oxford: Blackwell.

Guattari, F. (1996b). Franco Basaglia: Guerrilla psychiatrist. In: Genosko, G. (ed.) *The Guattari Reader*. Oxford: Blackwell.

Guattari, F. (1996c). *The Guattari Reader*. London: Blackwell.

Guattari, F. (1996d). Mary Barnes's 'trip'. In: Genosko, G. (ed.) *The Guattari Reader*. Oxford: Blackwell.

Guattari, F. (2006). *The Anti-Oedipus Papers*. New York: Semiotext(e).

Guattari, F. & Munster, A. (1977). Psycho-analysis and schizo-analysis: An interview with Félix Guattari. *Semiotext(e),* II: 77–85.

Hacking, I. (1999). *The Social Construction of What?* Cambridge, MA: Harvard University Press.

Haghgooie, S., Lithgow, B. J., Gurvich, C., & Kulkarni, J. (2009). Quantitative detection and assessment of schizophrenia using electrovestibulography. *4th International IEEE/ EMBS Conference on Neural Engineering, 2009*: 486–9.

Haghighat, R. (2008). Schizophrenia as social discourse: How do people use their diagnosis for social action? *European Psychiatry,* **23**: 549–60.

Haghighat, R. & Littlewood, R. (1995). What should we call patients with schizophrenia? A sociolinguistic analysis. *Psychiatric Bulletin,* **19**: 407–10.

Hammersley, P. & McLaughlin, T. (2010). *Introducing the Campaign for Abolition of the Schizophrenia Label* [Online]. Asylum. Available: http://www.asylumonline.net/ [Accessed 17 November 2010].

Haraway, D. (1985). A manifesto for cyborgs: Science, technology and socialist feminism in the 1980s. *Socialist Review,* **80**: 65–107.

Hardt, M. & Weeks, K. (eds.) (2000). *The Jameson Reader*. Oxford: Blackwell.

Hare, E. (1983). Was insanity on the increase? [The fifty-sixth Maudsley lecture, delivered before the Royal College of Psychiatrists, 19 November 1982]. *British Journal of Psychiatry*, **142**: 439–55.

Hare, E. (1988). Schizophrenia as a recent disease. *British Journal of Psychiatry*, **153**: 521–31.

Harland, R., Antonova, E., Owen, G. S., Broome, M. R., Landau, S., Deeley, Q., & Murray, R. (2009). A study of psychiatrists' concepts of mental illness. *Psychological Medicine*, **39**: 967–76.

Harvey, D. (1990). *The Condition of Postmodernity: An Enquiry into the Origins of Cultural Change*. Oxford: Blackwell.

Hayne, Y. & Yonge, O. (1997). The lifeworld of the chronic mentally ill: Analysis of 40 written personal accounts. *Archives of Psychiatric Nursing*, **11**: 314–24.

Healy, D. (2002). *The Creation of Psychopharmacology*. Cambridge, MA: Harvard University Press.

Heckers, S. (2008). Making progress in schizophrenia research. *Schizophrenia Bulletin*, **34**: 591–4.

Heinze, R. (2008). Violations of mimetic epistemology in first-person narrative fiction. *Narrative*, **16**: 279–99.

Helyer, R. (2009). *Glamorama*, cinematic narrative and contemporary fiction. In: Carroll, R. (ed.) *Adaptation in Contemporary Culture: Textual Infidelities*. London: Continuum.

Hill, P. (1997). *Lacan for Beginners*. New York: Writers and Readers Publishing.

Hinshelwood, R. D. (2004). *Suffering Psychosis: Psychoanalytic Essays on Psychosis*. Hovel and New York: Brunner-Routledge.

Hirsch, S. R. & Weinberger, D. R. (eds.) (2003). *Schizophrenia*. Malden, MA: Blackwell.

Hoenig, J. (1995). Schizophrenia—clinical section. In: Berrios, G. E. & Porter, R. (eds.) *A History of Clinical Psychiatry: The Origin and History of Psychiatric Disorders*. London: Athlone.

Hoff, P. (1995). Kraepelin: Clinical section, part I. In: Berrios, G. E. & Porter, R. (eds.) *A History of Clinical Psychiatry: The Origin and History of Psychiatric Disorders*. London: Athlone.

Holland, E. W. (1985–1986). The Anti-Oedipus: Postmodernism in theory; or, the post-Lacanian historical contextualization of psychoanalysis. *Boundary 2*, **14**: 291–307.

Holland, E. W. (1988). Schizoanalysis: The postmodern contextualization of psychoanalysis. In: Nelson, C. & Grossberg, L. (eds.) *Marxism and the Interpretation of Culture*. Chicago: University of Illinois Press.

Holland, E. W. (1998). From schizophrenia to social control. In: Kaufman, E. & Heller, K. J. (eds.) *Deleuze and Guattari: New Mapping in Politics, Philosophy and Culture*. Minneapolis: University of Minnesota Press.

Holland, E. W. (1999). *Deleuze and Guattari's Anti-Oedipus: Introduction to Schizoanalysis*. London and New York: Routledge.

Hooke, A. E. (2009). A moral logic to the archives of pain: Rethinking Foucault's work on madness. *Political Theory*, **37**: 432–41.

Hornstein, G. A. (2000). *To Redeem One Person is to Redeem the World: The Life of Frieda Fromm-Reichmann*. New York: The Free Press.

Hornstein, G. A. (2009). *Agnes's Jacket: A Psychologist's Search for the Meaning of Madness.* New York: Rodale.

Houen, A. (2004). Novel spaces and taking place(s) in the wake of September 11. *Studies in the Novel,* **26:** 419–38.

Houston, R. A. (2000). *Madness and Society in Eighteenth-Century Scotland.* Oxford: Clarendon Press.

Howes, O. D. & Kapur, S. (2009). The dopamine hypothesis of schizophrenia: Version III—the final common pathway. *Schizophrenia Bulletin,* **35:** 549–62.

Huffman, R. *This Is Baader-Meinhof* [Online]. Available: http://www.baader-meinhof.com [Accessed 26 October 2004].

Hutcheon, L. (1988). *A Poetics of Postmodernism.* London: Routledge.

Hutcheon, L. (1989). *The Politics of Postmodernism.* London and New York: Routledge.

Insel, T. R. (2010). Rethinking schizophrenia. *Nature,* **468:** 187–93.

Jaaro-Peled, H., Ayhan, Y., Pletnikov, M. V., & Sawa, A. (2010). Review of pathological hallmarks of schizophrenia: Comparison of genetic models with patients and nongenetic models. *Schizophrenia Bulletin,* **36:** 301–13.

Jameson, F. (1983). Postmodernism and consumer society. In: Foster, H. (ed.) *The Anti-Aesthetic: Essays on Postmodern Culture.* Port Townsend: Bay Press.

Jameson, F. (1984a). Periodizing the 60s. In: Sayres, S., Stephanson, A., Aronowitz, S., & Jameson, F. (eds.) *The 60s Without Apology.* Minneapolis: University of Minnesota Press.

Jameson, F. (1984b). Postmodernism, or the cultural logic of late capitalism. *New Left Review,* **146:** 53–92.

Jameson, F. (1988). Pleasure: A political issue (1983). *The Ideologies of Theory, Essays 1971–1986, Volume 2: The Syntax of History.* London: Routledge.

Jameson, F. (1991). *Postmodernism, or the Cultural Logic of Late Capitalism.* London: Verso.

Jameson, F. (2002). *A Singular Modernity: Essay on the Ontology of the Present.* London: Verso.

Jaspers, K. (1972). *General Psychopathology.* Manchester: Manchester University Press.

Jenkins, J. H. (2004). Schizophrenia as a paradigm case for understanding fundamental human processes. In: Jenkins, J. H. & Barrett, R. J. (eds.) *Schizophrenia, Culture, and Subjectivity: The Edge of Experience.* Cambridge: Cambridge University Press.

Jenkins, J. H. & Barrett, R. J. (2004a). Introduction. In: Jenkins, J. H. & Barrett, R. J. (eds.) *Schizophrenia, Culture, and Subjectivity: The Edge of Experience.* Cambridge: Cambridge University Press.

Jenkins, J. H. & Barrett, R. J. (eds.) (2004b). *Schizophrenia, Culture, and Subjectivity: The Edge of Experience.* Cambridge: Cambridge University Press.

Jervis, J. (1998). Sacred, secular, sublime: Modernity performs the death of God. *Exploring the Modern: Patterns of Western Civilization and Culture.* Oxford: Blackwell.

Johnstone, E. C., Humphreys, M. S., Lang, F. H., & Lawrie, S. M. (1999). *Schizophrenia: Concepts and Clinical Management.* Cambridge: Cambridge University Press.

Johnston, J. (1990). Ideology, representation, schizophrenia: Toward a theory of the postmodern subject. In: Shapiro, G. (ed.) *After the Future: Postmodern Times and Places.* Albany: State University of New York Press.

Johnstone, L. (2000). *Users and Abusers of Psychiatry: A Critical Look at Psychiatric Practice.* London: Routledge.

Jones, E. (1948). *Collected Papers on Psychoanalysis.* London: Bailliere, Tindall and Cox.

Judd, L. L. (1994). Introduction. In: Andreasen, N. C. (ed.) *Schizophrenia: From Mind to Molecule.* Washington: American Psychiatric Press.

Jung, C. (1944). *The Psychology of Dementia Praecox.* New York: Nervous and Mental Disease Monographs.

Kant, I. (1969). *The Critique of Judgement.* Oxford: Clarendon.

Katan, M. (1949). Schreber's delusion of the end of the world. *The Psychoanalytic Quarterly,* **18:** 60–6.

Katan, M. (1950a). Schreber's hallucinations about the little men. *International Journal of Psycho-Analysis,* **31:** 32–5.

Katan, M. (1950b). Structural aspects of a case of schizophrenia. *The Psychoanalytic Study of the Child,* **5:** 175–211.

Katan, M. (1952a). Further remarks about Schreber's hallucinations. *International Journal of Psycho-Analysis,* **33:** 429–32.

Katan, M. (1952b). Schreber's prepsychotic phase. *International Journal of Psycho-Analysis,* **33:** 429–32.

Kellendonk, C., Simpson, E. H., Polan, H. J., Malleret, G., Vronskaya, S., Winiger, V., Moore, H., & Kandel, E. R. (2006). Transient and selective overexpression of dopamine D2 receptors in the striatum causes persistent abnormalities in prefrontal cortex functioning. *Neuron,* **49:** 603–15.

Kellner, D. (1989). Introduction: Jameson, Marxism, and postmodernism. In: Kellner, D. (ed.) *Postmodernism/Jameson/Critique.* Washington: Maisonneuve Press.

Kendler, K. S. (2005). 'A gene for ...': The nature of gene action in psychiatric disorders. *American Journal of Psychiatry,* **162:** 1243–52.

Kerr, J. (1993). *A Most Dangerous Method: The Story of Jung, Freud, and Sabina Spielrein.* New York: Alfred A Knopf.

Kinney, D. K., Teixeira, P., Hsu, D., Napoleon, S. C., Crowley, D. J., Miller, A., Hyman, W., & Huang, E. (2009). Relation of schizophrenia prevalence to latitude, climate, fish consumption, infant mortality, and skin color: A role for prenatal vitamin D deficiency and infections? *Schizophrenia Bulletin,* **35:** 582–95.

Kirby, K. M. (1996). Re: Mapping subjectivity: Cartographic vision and the limits of politics. In: Duncan, N. (ed.) *Bodyspace: Destabilizing Geographies of Gender and Sexuality.* London and New York: Routledge.

Kirk, S. A. & Kutchins, H. (1992). *The Selling of DSM: The Rhetoric of Science in Psychiatry.* New York: Aldine de Gruyter.

Kittler, F. (1990). *Discourse Networks. 1800/1900.* Stanford: Stanford University Press.

Kleiman, R. (2003). Insane logic (lecture). Melbourne: The Freudian School of Melbourne.

Kleinman, A. (2004). Preface. In: Jenkins, J. H. & Barrett, R. J. (eds.) *Schizophrenia, Culture, and Subjectivity: The Edge of Experience.* Cambridge: Cambridge University Press.

Klein, M. (1952). Notes on some schizoid mechanisms. In: Riviere, J. (ed.) *Developments in Psycho-Analysis.* London: The Hogarth Press and the Institute of Psycho-Analysis.

Kotowicz, Z. (1997). *R. D. Laing and the Paths of Anti-Psychiatry*. London and New York: Routledge.

Kovel, J. (1987). Schizophrenic being and technocratic society. In: Levin, D. M. (ed.) *Pathologies of the Modern Self: Postmodern Studies of Narcissism, Schizophrenia and Depression*. New York and London: New York University Press.

Kraepelin, E. (1981). *Clinical Psychiatry*. New York, Scholars' Facsimiles & Reprints.

Kraepelin, E. (2000). Comparative psychiatry (1904). In: Littlewood, R. & Dein, S. (eds.) *Cultural Psychiatry and Medical Anthropology*. London: The Athlone Press.

Kraepelin, E. (2010). About the surveillance ward at the Heidelberg clinic for lunatics (1895). In: Eghigian, G. (ed.) *From Madness to Mental Heatlh: Psychiatric Disorder and Its Treatment in Western Civilization*. New Brunswick, NJ and London: Rutgers University Press.

Kreyenbuhl, J., Buchanan, R. W., Dickerson, F. B., & Dixon, L. B. (2010). The schizophrenia patient outcomes research team (PORT): Updated treatment recommendations 2009. *Schizophrenia Bulletin*, **36:** 94–103.

Lacan, J. (1966). On a question preliminary to any possible treatment of psychosis. *Écrits: A Selection*. New York and London: Norton.

Lacan, J. (1993). *The Seminar of Jacques Lacan: Book III The Psychoses 1955–1956*. New York: W W Norton.

LaCapra, D. (1992). Foucault, history and madness. In: Still, A. & Velody, I. (eds.) *Rewriting the History of Madness: Studies in Foucault's histoire de la folie*. London and New York: Routledge.

Laing, A. C. (1994). *R. D. Laing: A Biography*. London: Peter Owen.

Laing, R. D. (1967). *The Politics of Experience*. New York: Ballantine Books.

Laing, R. D. (1985). *Wisdom, Madness and Folly: The Making of a Psychiatrist*. London: Macmillan.

Laing, R. D. (1990). *The Divided Self: An Existential Study in Sanity and Madness*. London: Penguin.

Laing, R. D. & Esterton, A. (1964). *Sanity, Madness and the Family: Volume I, Families of Schizophrenics*. London: Tavistock.

Lasch, C. (1978). *The Culture of Narcissism: American Life in an Age of Diminishing Expectations*. New York: W W Norton.

Laugharne, R. (April 2002). Psychiatry, postmodernism and postnormal science. *Journal of the Royal Society of Medicine*, **95:** 207–10.

Laugharne, R. (2004). Psychiatry in the future, the next 15 years: Postmodern challenges and opportunities for psychiatry. *Psychiatric Bulletin*, **28:** 317–8.

Lawrie, S. M., Hall, J., McIntosh, A. M., Owens, D. G. C., & Johnstone, E. C. (2010). The 'continuum of psychosis': Scientifically unproven and clinically impractical. *British Journal of Psychiatry*, **197:** 423–5.

Lee, M. J. (ed.) (2000). *The Consumer Society Reader*. Malden, MA: Blackwell.

Levin, D. M. (1987a). Clinical stories: A modern self in the fury of being. In: Levin, D. M. (ed.) *Pathologies of the Modern Self: Postmodern Studies of Narcissism, Schizophrenia and Depression*. New York and London: New York University Press.

Levin, D. M. (ed.) (1987b). *Pathologies of the Modern Self: Postmodern Studies of Narcissism, Schizophrenia and Depression*. New York and London: New York University Press.

Levin, T. Y., Frohne, U., & Weibel, P. (2002). Editorial. In: Levin, T. Y., Frohne, U., & Weibel, P. (eds.) *Ctrl [space]: Rhetorics of Surveillance from Bentham to Big Brother.* Cambridge, MA: The MIT Press.

Lewin, M. (2009). Schizophrenia 'epidemic' among African Caribbeans spurs prevention policy change. *The Guardian* [Online]. Available: http://www.guardian.co.uk/society/2009/dec/09/african-caribbean-schizophrenia-policy [Accessed 9 December 2009].

Lewis, B. (2000). Psychiatry and postmodern theory. *Journal of Medical Humanities,* 21: 71–84.

Lieberman, J. A., Stroup, T. S., McEvoy, J. P., Swartz, M. S., Rosenheck, R. A., Perkins, D. O., Keefe, R. S. E., Davis, S. M., Davis, C. E., Lebowitz, B. D., Severe, J. & Hsiao, J. K. (2005). Effectiveness of antipsychotic drugs in patients with chronic schizophrenia. *New England Journal of Medicine,* 353: 1209–23.

Lothane, Z. (1992). *In Defense of Schreber: Soul Murder and Psychiatry.* Hillsdale, NJ: The Analytic Press.

Lotringer, S. (1977). Libido unbound: The politics of 'schizophrenia'. *Semiotext(e),* II: 5–10.

Lotringer, S. & Cohen, S. (2001). Introduction: A few theses on French theory in America. In: Lotringer, S. & Cohen, S. (eds.) *French Theory in America.* London and New York: Routledge.

Lyon, D. (2003). Surveillance technology and surveillance society. In: Misa, T. J., Brey, P., & Feenberg, A. (eds.) *Modernity and Technology.* Cambridge, MA: The MIT Press.

Lyotard, J. -F. (1977). Energumen capitalism. *Semiotext(e),* II: 11–26.

Lysaker, P. H. & Lysaker, J. T. (2008). *Schizophrenia and the Fate of the Self.* Oxford: Oxford University Press.

Lysaker, P. H. & Lysaker, J. T. (2010). Schizophrenia and alterations in self-experience: A comparison of 6 perspectives. *Schizophrenia Bulletin,* 36: 331–40.

Macalpine, I. & Hunter, R. A. (1955a). Discussion. *Memoirs of My Nervous Illness.* London: W M Dawson & Sons.

Macalpine, I. & Hunter, R. A. (1955b). Introduction. *Memoirs of My Nervous Illness.* London: W M Dawson & Sons.

MacDonald, A. W. & Schulz, S. C. (2009). What we know: Findings that every theory of schizophrenia should explain. *Schizophrenia Bulletin,* 35: 493–508.

Mann, S. (1994). *Psycho-Analysis and Society: An Introduction.* Sydney: UNSW Press.

Mannoni, O. (1988). Writing and madness: *Schreber als schreiber.* In: Allison, D. B., de Oliveira, P., Roberts, M. S. & Weiss, A. S. (eds.) *Psychosis and Sexual Identity: Towards a Post-Analytic View of the Schreber Case.* Albany: State University of New York Press.

Marini, M. (1992). *Jacques Lacan: The French Context.* New Brunswick, NJ: Rutgers University Press.

Marshall, P. D. (1997). *Celebrity and Power: Fame in Contemporary Culture.* Minneapolis: University of Minnesota Press.

Massumi, B. (1992). *A User's Guide to Capitalism and Schizophrenia: Deviations from Deleuze and Guattari.* Cambridge, MA: MIT Press.

Mathiesen, T. (1997). The viewer society: Michel Foucault's 'panopticon' revisited. *Theoretical Criminology,* 1: 215–34.

McDonald, C., Schulze, K., Murray, R. M., & Wright, P. (eds.) (2004). *Schizophrenia: Challenging the Orthodox*. London and New York: Taylor and Francis.

McGlashan, T. H. (2009). Psychosis as a disorder of reduced cathectic capacity: Freud's analysis of the Schreber case revisited. *Schizophrenia Bulletin,* **35:** 476–81.

McGuffin, P. (2004). Foreword. In: McDonald, C., Schulze, K., Murray, R. M., & Wright, P. (eds.) *Schizophrenia: Challenging the Orthodox*. London: Taylor and Francis.

McInerney, J. (1998). *Model Behavior: A Novel and 7 stories*. New York: Alfred A Kopf.

McKenna, P. J. (1994). *Schizophrenia and Related Syndromes*. Oxford: Oxford University Press.

McLean, A. (1995). Empowerment and the psychiatric consumer/ex-patient movement in the United States: Contradictions, crisis and change. *Social Science and Medicine,* **40:** 1053–71.

McLean, A. H. (2000). From ex-patient alternatives to consumer options: Consequences of consumerism for psychiatric consumers and the ex-patient movement. *International Journal of Health Services,* **30:** 821–47.

McLean, R. (2003). *Recovered not Cured: A Journey through Schizophrenia*. Melbourne: Allen and Unwin.

McNally, K. (2007). Schizophrenia as split personality/Jekyll and Hyde: The origins of the informal usage in the English language. *Journal of the History of the Behavioral Sciences,* **43:** 69–79.

Mendelsohn, D. (1999). Lesser than zero [Online]. *The New York Times*. Available: http://www.nytimes.com/books/99/01/24/reviews/990124.24mendelt.html [Accessed 24 February 2003].

Mental Health Division (2009). New horizons: A shared vision for mental health. London: Department of Health, Her Majesty's Government.

Metzl, J. (2009). *The Protest Psychosis: How Schizophrenia Became a Black Disease*. Boston: Beacon Press.

Meyer-Lindenberg, A. (2010). From maps to mechanisms through neuroimaging of schizophrenia. *Nature,* **468:** 194–202.

Michaels, W. B. (2003). Empires of the senseless: (The response to) terror and (the end of) history. *Radical History Review,* **85:** 105–13.

Miller, R. & Mason, S. E. (2002). *Diagnosis: Schizophrenia: A Comprehensive Guide for Patients, Families and Helping Professionals*. New York: Columbia University Press.

Mitchell, A. & Michalczuk, R. (2010). Monetary incentives for schizophrenia. *Schizophrenia Bulletin,* **36:** 24–5.

Mitchell, N., Sadler, J., & Robertson, M. (2009). Thomas Szasz: Psychiatrists respond. *All In the Mind*. ABC Radio National.

Mitchell, N. & Szasz, T. (2009a). Thomas Szasz speaks (part 1 of 2). *All In the Mind*. ABC Radio National.

Mitchell, N. & Szasz, T. (2009b). Thomas Szasz speaks (part 2 of 2). *All In the Mind*. ABC Radio National.

Moncrieff, J. (2009). *The Myth of the Chemical Cure: A Critique of Psychiatric Drug Treatment*. London: Palgrave Macmillan.

Morgan, A. (2010). Schizophrenia, reification and deadened life. *History of the Human Sciences,* **23:** 176–93.

Morgan, C. & Hutchinson, G. (2009). The social determinants of psychosis in migrant and ethnic minority populations: A public health tragedy. *Psychological Medicine,* **40**(5): 705–9.

Morse, M. (1990). An ontology of everyday distraction: The freeway, the mall, and television. In: Mellencamp, P. (ed.) *Logics of Television: Essays in Cultural Criticism.* London: BFI Books.

Mueser, K. T. & Jeste, D. V. (eds.) (2008). *Clinical Handbook of Schizophrenia.* New York: The Guilford Press.

Mullan, B. (1999). *R. D. Laing: A Personal View.* London: Duckworth.

Nasrallah, H. (2003). A review of the effect of atypical antipsychotics on weight. *Psychoneuroendocrinology,* **28**: 83–96.

Nasrallah, H. (2008). Atypical antipsychotic-induced metabolic side effects: Insights from receptor-binding profiles. *Molecular Psychiatry,* **13**: 27–35.

Nelson, G., Ochocka, J., Janzen, R., & Trainor, J. (2006). A longitudinal study of mental health consumer/survivor initiatives: Part I—literature review and overview of the study. *Journal of Community Psychology,* **34**: 247–60.

Nelson, G., Ochocka, J., Janzen, R., Trainor, J., Goering, P., & Lomotey, J. (2007). A longitudinal study of mental health consumer/survivor initiatives: Part V—outcomes at 3-year follow-up. *Journal of Community Psychology,* **35**: 655–65.

Niederland, W. G. (1984). *The Schreber Case: Psychoanalytic Profile of a Paranoid Personality.* Hillsdale, NJ: The Analytic Press.

Nielsen, H. S. (2004). The impersonal voice in first-person narrative fiction. *Narrative,* **12**: 133–50.

Nielsen, H. S. (2006). Telling doubles and literal-minded reading in Bret Easton Ellis's *Glamorama.* In: Durand, A.-P. & Mandel, N. (eds.) *Novels of the Contemporary Extreme.* London: Continuum.

Noll, R. (2006). The blood of the insane. *History of Psychiatry,* **17**: 395–418.

Noll, R. (2007). Kraepelin's 'lost biological psychiatry'? Autointoxication, organotherapy and surgery for dementia praecox. *History of Psychiatry,* **18**: 301–20.

O'Brien, B. (1960). *Operators and Things: The Inner Life of a Schizophrenic.* London: Elek Books.

O'Hara, M. (2010). Fightback over claims on mental illness and its prevalence among black people. *The Guardian* [Online]. Available: http://www.guardian.co.uk/society/2010/feb/03/mental-illness-bme-campaign [Accessed 3 February 2010].

O'Neill, J. (1989). Religion and postmodernism: The Durkheimian bond in Bell and Jameson. In: Kellner, D. (ed.) *Postmodernism/Jameson/Critique.* Washington: Maisonneuve Press.

O'Tuathaigh, C. M. P., Kirby, B. P., Moran, P. M., & Waddington, J. L. (2010). Mutant mouse models: Genotype–phenotype relationships to negative symptoms in schizophrenia. *Schizophrenia Bulletin,* **36**(2): 271–88.

Page, A. (dir.) (1977). *I Never Promised You a Rose Garden.* USA.

Parnas, J. & Sass, L. A. (2001). Self, solipsism, and schizophrenic delusions. *Philosophy, Psychiatry, Psychology,* **8**: 101–20.

Patientenkollektiv(H), P. S. *SPK Homepage* [Online]. Available: http://www.spkpfh.de/ [Accessed 26 October 2006].

Patton, P. (2001). Notes for a glossary. In: Genosko, G. (ed.) *Deleuze and Guattari: Critical Assessments of Leading Philosophers*. London and New York: Routledge.

Paulson, R. (1985). Versions of a human sublime. *New Literary History,* XVI: 427–37.

Pease, D. E. (1984). Sublime politics. *Boundary 2,* XII.**3–XIII.4:** 259–79.

Peters, J. D. (2010). Broadcasting and schizophrenia. *Media, Culture & Society,* 32: 123–40.

Petersen, P. S. (2005). 9/11 and the 'problem of imagination': *Fight Club* and *Glamorama* as terrorist pretexts. *Orbis Litterarum,* 60: 133–44.

Plant, S. (2001). Nomads and revolutionaries. In: Genosko, G. (ed.) *Deleuze and Guattari: Critical Assessments of Leading Philosophers*. London and New York: Routledge.

Poland, J. (2007). How to move beyond the concept of schizophrenia. In: Chung, M. C., Fulford, K. W. M. B., & Graham, G. (eds.) *Reconceiving Schizophrenia*. Oxford: Oxford University Press.

Porter, R. (2002). *Madness: A Brief History*. Oxford, Oxford University Press.

Porter, R. & Micale, M. S. (1994). Introduction: Reflections on psychiatry and its histories. In: Micale, M. S. & Porter, R. (eds.) *Discovering the History of Psychiatry*. Oxford: Oxford University Press.

Postel, J. & Allen, D. F. (1994). History and anti-psychiatry in France. In: Micale, M. S. & Porter, R. (eds.) *Discovering the History of Psychiatry*. Oxford: Oxford University Press.

Punter, D. (2003). E-textuality: Authenticity after the postmodern. *Critical Quarterly,* **43:** 68–91.

Rajchman, J. (1977). Analysis in power. *Semiotext(e),* II: 45–58.

Ramon, S., Healy, B., & Renouf, N. (2007). Recovery from mental illness as an emergent concept and practice in Australia and the UK. *International Journal of Social Psychiatry,* **53:** 108–22.

Ratcliffe, M. (2008). *Feelings of Being: Phenomenology, Psychiatry and the Sense of Reality*. Oxford: Oxford University Press.

Ratcliffe, M. (2010). Binary oppositions in psychiatry: For or against? *Philosophy, Psychiatry, & Psychology,* 17: 233–39.

Read, R. (2003). On delusions of sense: A response to Coetzee and Sass. *Philosophy, Psychiatry, Psychology,* 10: 135–41.

Reaume, G. (2002). Lunatic to patient to person: Nomenclature in psychiatric history and the influence of patients' activism in North America. *International Journal of Law and Psychiatry,* 25: 405–26.

Renee. (1970). *Autobiography of a Schizophrenic Girl, with an Analytic Interpretation by Marguerite Sechehaye*. New York: Signet.

Richardson, O. (1999). Glamorama [Online]. *The Age*. Available: http://www.theage.com.au/books/archives/easton.html [Accessed 5 November 2001].

Richardson, W. J. (1988). Lacan and the problem of psychosis. In: Allison, D. B., de Oliveira, P., Roberts, M. S. & Weiss, A. S. (eds.) *Psychosis and Sexual Identity: Towards a Post-Analytic View of the Schreber Case*. Albany: State University of New York Press.

Robbins, B. D. (2000). Schreber's soul-voluptuousness: Mysticism, madness and the feminine in Schreber's memoirs. *Journal of Phenomenological Psychology,* 31: 117–54.

Roberts, M. S. (1996). Schreber as machine, technophobe, and virtualist. *TDR (Cambridge, MA),* **40:** 31–47.

Romme, M. & Morris, M. (2007). The harmful concept of schizophrenia. *Mental Health Nursing*, **27**: 8–12.

Ronell, A. (1989). *The Telephone Book: Technology, Schizophrenia, Electric Speech*. Lincoln: University of Nebraska Press.

Rose, J. (1988). 'The man who mistook his wife for a hat' or 'a wife is like an umbrella'—fantasies of the modern and postmodern. In: Ross, A. (ed.) *Universal Abandon: The Politics of Postmodernism*. Minneapolis: University of Minnesota Press.

Rose, N. (1996). *Inventing Our Selves: Psychology, Power and Personhood*. Cambridge: Cambridge University Press.

Rose, N. (2006). *The Politics of Life Itself: Biomedicine, Power, and Subjectivity in the Twenty-First Century*. Princeton: Princeton University Press.

Rosenhan, D. L. (1975). On being sane in insane places. In: Scheff, T. J. (ed.) *Labeling Madness*. New Jersey: Prentice-Hall.

Roudinesco, E. (1997). *Jacques Lacan*. New York: Columbia University Press.

Russell, D. (1995). *Women, Madness and Medicine*. Cambridge: Polity Press.

Saks, E. (2007). *The Center Cannot Hold: My Journey Through Madness*. London: Virago.

Samuels, A. (1997). Jung and the post-Jungians. In: Young-Eisendrath, P. & Dawson, T. (eds.) *The Cambridge Companion to Jung*. Cambridge: Cambridge University Press.

Santner, E. L. (1996). *My Own Private Germany: Daniel Paul Schreber's Secret History of Modernity*. Princeton: Princeton University Press.

Sartorius, N. (2010). Short-lived campaigns are not enough. *Nature*, **468**: 163–65.

Sass, L. A. (1987a). Introspection, schizophrenia and the fragmentation of the self. *Representations*, **19**: 1–34.

Sass, L. A. (1987b). Schreber's panopticism: Psychosis and the modern soul. *Social Research*, **54**: 101–47.

Sass, L. A. (1988). The land of unreality: On the phenomenology of the schizophrenic break. *New Ideas in Psychology*, **6**: 223–42.

Sass, L. A. (1992). *Madness and Modernism: Insanity in the Light of Modern Art, Literature and Thought*. Cambridge, MA: Harvard University Press.

Sass, L. A. (1994a). Civilized madness: Schizophrenia, self consciousness and the modern mind. *History of the Human Sciences*, **7**: 83–120.

Sass, L. A. (1994b). *The Paradoxes of Delusion: Wittgenstein, Schreber, and the Schizophrenic Mind*. Ithaca: Cornell University Press.

Sass, L. A. (1996). 'The catastrophes of heaven': Modernism, primitivism, and the madness of Antonin Artaud. *Modernism/Modernity*, **3**: 73–91.

Sass, L. A. (1997). The consciousness machine: Self and subjectivity in schizophrenia and modern culture. In: Neisser, U. & Jopling, D. A. (eds.) *The Conceptual Self in Context: Culture, Experience, Self-Understanding*. Cambridge: Cambridge University Press.

Sass, L. A. (1998). Interpreting schizophrenia: Construal or construction? A reply to Robert J. Barrett. *Culture, Medicine and Psychiatry*, **22**: 495–503.

Sass, L. A. (2000). Schizophrenia, self-experience, and the so-called 'negative symptoms': Reflections on hyperreflexivity. In: Zahavi, D. (ed.) *Exploring the Self: Philosophical and Psychopathological Perspectives on Self-Experience*. Amsterdam and Philadelphia: John Bejamins Publishing Company.

Sass, L. A. (2000–2001a). Romanticism, creativity, and the ambiguities of psychiatric diagnosis: Rejoinder to Kay Redfield Jamison. *Creativity Research Journal,* **13:** 77–85.

Sass, L. A. (2000–2001b). Schizophrenia, modernism, and the 'creative imagination': On creativity and psychopathology. *Creativity Research Journal,* **13:** 55–74.

Sass, L. A. (2001). Self and world in schizophrenia: Three classic approaches. *Philosophy, Psychiatry, Psychology,* **8:** 251–70.

Sass, L. A. (2003). 'Negative symptoms', schizophrenia, and the self. *International Journal of Psychology and Psychological Therapy,* **3:** 153–80.

Sass, L. A. (2004a). 'Negative symptoms', commonsense, and cultural disembedding in the modern age. In: Jenkins, J. H. & Barrett, R. J. (eds.) *Schizophrenia, Culture, and Subjectivity: The Edge of Experience.* Cambridge: Cambridge University Press.

Sass, L. A. (2004b). Some reflections on the (analytic) philosophical approach to delusion. *Philosophy, Psychiatry, Psychology,* **11:** 71–80.

Sass, L. A. (2007). 'Schizophrenic person' or 'person with schizophrenia'? An essay on illness and the self. *Theory and Psychology,* **17:** 395–420.

Sass, L. A. & Parnas, J. (2001). Phenomenology of self-disturbances in schizophrenia: Some research findings and directions. *Philosophy, Psychiatry, Psychology,* **8:** 347–56.

Sass, L. A. & Parnas, J. (2003). Schizophrenia, consciousness, and the self. *Schizophrenia Bulletin,* **29:** 427–44.

Schatzman, M. (1971). Paranoia or persecution: The case of Schreber. *Family Process,* **10:** 117–207.

Schatzman, M. (1973). *Soul Murder: Persecution in the Family.* London: Allen Lane.

Scheff, T. J. (1975a). On reason and sanity: Some political implications of psychiatric thought. In: Scheff, T. J. (ed.) *Labeling Madness.* New Jersey: Prentice-Hall.

Scheff, T. J. (1975b). Schizophrenia as ideology. In: Scheff, T. J. (ed.) *Labeling Madness.* New Jersey: Prentice-Hall.

Schiller, L. & Bennett, A. (1994). *The Quiet Room: A Journey out of the Torment of Madness.* New York: Warner.

Schreber, D. P. (1955). *Memoirs of My Nervous Illness.* London: W M Dawson & Sons.

Schwarz, H. & Balsamo, A. (Spring 1996). Under the sign of 'semiotext(e)': The story according to Sylvère Lotringer and Chris Kraus. *CRITIQUE: Studies in Contemporary Fiction,* **37:** 205–21.

Scull, A. (1984). Was insanity increasing? A response to Edward Hare. *British Journal of Psychiatry,* **144:** 432–6.

Scull, A. (2007). The fictions of Foucault's scholarship: The frail foundations of the Foucaldian monument. *Times Literary Supplement,* May 21.

Sedgwick, P. (1982). *Psycho Politics.* London: Pluto Press.

Serres, M. (1994). The geometry of the incommunicable madness. In: Davidson, A. I. (ed.) *Foucault and His Interlocutors.* Chicago and London: Chicago University Press.

Shaw, P. (2006). *The Sublime.* Abingdon: Routledge.

Shean, G. D. (2004). *What is Schizophrenia and How Can We Fix It?* Lantham, MD: University Press of America.

Shorter, E. (1997). *A History of Psychiatry: From the Era of the Asylum to the Age of Prozac.* New York: John Wiley & Sons.

Shorter, E. & Healy, D. (2007). *Shock Therapy: A History of Electroconvulsive Treatment in Mental Illness*. New Brunswick, NJ and London: Rutgers University Press.

Showalter, E. (1987). *The Female Malady: Women, Madness and English Culture 1830–1980*. London: Virago.

Sica, A. (1995). Gabel's 'micro/macro' bridge: The schizophrenic process writ large. *Sociological Theory,* **13:** 66–99.

Simmons, P., Hawley, C. J., Gale, T. M., & Sivakumaran, T. (2010). Service user, patient, client, user or survivor: Describing recipients of mental health services. *The Psychiatrist,* **34:** 31–5.

Smart, B. (1993). *Postmodernity*. London and New York: Routledge.

Smith, A. C. (1982). *Schizophrenia and Madness*. London: George Allen & Unwin.

Smith, D. (1999). *Zygmunt Bauman: Prophet of Postmodernity*. Cambridge: Polity Press.

Snyder, K., Gur, R. E., & Andrews, L. W. (2007). *Me, Myself, and Them: A Firsthand Account of One Young Person's Experience with Schizophrenia*. New York: Oxford University Press.

Sontag, S. (1991). *Illness as Metaphor and Aids and Its Metaphors*. London: Penguin.

Speed, E. (2006). Patients, consumers and survivors: A case study of mental health service user discourses. *Social Science and Medicine,* **62:** 28–38.

Speed, E. (2007). Discourses of consumption or consumed by discourse? A consideration of what 'consumer' means to the service user. *Journal of Mental Health,* **16:** 307–18.

Stanghellini, G. (2004). *Disembodied Spirits and Deanimated Bodies: The Psychopathology of Common Sense*. Oxford: Oxford University Press.

Steele, R. S. (1982). *Freud and Jung: Conflicts of Interpretation*. London: Routledge & Kegan Paul.

Stephan, K. E., Friston, K. J., & Frith, C. D. (2009). Dysconnection in schizophrenia: From abnormal synaptic plasticity to failures of self-monitoring. *Schizophrenia Bulletin,* **35:** 509–27.

Stephanson, A. (1988). Regarding postmodernism—a conversation with Fredric Jameson. In: Ross, A. (ed.) *Universal Abandon? The Politics of Postmodernism*. Minneapolis: University of Minnesota Press.

Stephenson, W. (2007). 'A terrorism of the rich': Symbolic violence in Bret Easton Ellis's *Glamorama* and J. G. Ballard's *Super-Cannes*. *Critique,* **48:** 278–93.

Stevens, A. (1994). *Jung*. Oxford: Oxford University Press.

Strous, R. D. (2010). Psychiatric genocide: Reflections and responsibilities. *Schizophrenia Bulletin,* **36:** 208–10.

Swingewood, A. (1977). Review of *False Consciousness*. *The American Journal of Sociology,* **83:** 222–4.

Szasz, T. (1972). *The Myth of Mental Illness: Foundations of a Theory of Personal Conduct*. St Albans: Paladin.

Szasz, T. (1976). *Schizophrenia: The Sacred Symbol of Psychiatry*. New York: Basic Books.

Szasz, T. (2001). *Pharmacracy: Medicine and Politics in America*. Westport, CT: Praeger.

Szasz, T. (2004). Reply to Kendell. In: Schaler, J. A. (ed.) *Szasz under Fire: The Psychiatric Abolitionist Faces His Critics*. Chicago: Open Court.

Szasz, T. (2010). Psychiatry, anti-psychiatry, critical psychiatry: What do these terms mean? *Philosophy, Psychiatry, & Psychology,* **17:** 229–32.

Tai, S. & Turkington, D. (2009). The evolution of cognitive behavior therapy for schizophrenia: Current practice and recent developments. *Schizophrenia Bulletin,* **35**: 865–73.

Tausk, V. (1950). On the origin of the 'influencing machine' in schizophrenia (1919). In: Fliess, R. (ed.) *The Psycho-Analytic Reader: An Anthology of Essential Papers with Critical Introductions.* London: The Hogarth Press and the Institute of Pyscho-Analysis.

Taylor, B. (1987). *Modernism, Post-Modernism, Realism: A Critical Perspective for Art.* Winchester: Winchester School of Art Press.

Theweleit, K. (1990). *Object-choice (All You Need is Love . . .): On Mating Strategies & A Fragment of a Freud Biography.* London: Verso.

Thornton, T. (2007). *Essential Philosophy of Psychiatry.* Oxford: Oxford University Press.

Thurschwell, P. (2000). *Sigmund Freud.* London and New York: Routledge.

Torrey, E. F. (1988). Stalking the schizovirus. *Schizophrenia Bulletin,* **14**: 223–9.

Torrey, E. F. & Miller, J. (2001). *The Invisible Plague: The Rise of Mental Illness from 1750 to the Present.* New Brunswick, NJ: Rutgers University Press.

Torrey, E. F. & Yolken, R. H. (1995). Could schizophrenia be a viral zoonosis transmitted from house cats? *Schizophrenia Research,* **21**: 167–71.

Torrey, E. F. & Yolken, R. H. (2007). Editors' introduction: Schizophrenia and toxoplasmosis. *Schizophrenia Bulletin,* **33**: 727–28.

Torrey, E. F. & Yolken, R. H. (2009). Psychiatric genocide: Nazi attempts to eradicate schizophrenia. *Schizophrenia Bulletin* **36**: 26–32.

Tsuang, M. T., Nossova, N., Yager, T., Tsuang, M.-M., Guo, S.-C., Shyu, K. G., Glatt, S. J., & Liew, C. C. (2005). Assessing the validity of blood-based gene expression profiles for the classification of schizophrenia and bipolar disorder: A preliminary report. *American Journal of Medical Genetics Part B: Neuropsychiatric Genetics,* **133**: 1–5.

Turner, T. (1995). Schizophrenia—social section. In: Berrios, G. E. & Porter, R. (eds.) *A History of Clinical Psychiatry: The Origin and History of Psychiatric Disorders.* London: Athlone.

Ussher, J. (1991). *Women's Madness: Misogyny or Mental Illness?* Amherst: University of Massachusetts Press.

van Os, J., Kenis, G., & Rutten, B. P. F. (2010). The environment and schizophrenia. *Nature,* **468**: 203–12.

Vatz, R. E. & Weinberg, L. S. (1994). The rhetorical paradigm in psychiatric history: Thomas Szasz and the myth of mental illness. In: Micale, M. S. & Porter, R. (eds.) *Discovering the History of Psychiatry.* Oxford: Oxford University Press.

Velligan, D. I. (2009). Cognitive behavior therapy for psychosis: Where have we been and where are we going? *Schizophrenia Bulletin,* **35**: 857–8.

Vine, S. (ed.) (2005). *Literature in Psychoanalysis: A Reader.* New York: Palgrave Macmillan.

Viskerr, R. (1995). *Michel Foucault: Genealogy as Critique.* London: Verso.

Watters, E. (2010). *Crazy Like Us: The Globalization of the American Psyche.* New York: Free Press.

Weber, G. (1955). Medical expert's report to the court. *Memoirs of My Nervous Illness.* London: W M Dawson & Sons.

Weibel, P. (2002). Pleasure and the panoptic principle. In: Levin, T. Y., Frohne, U., & Weibel, P. (eds.) *Ctrl [space]: Rhetorics of Surveillance from Bentham to Big Brother*. Cambridge, MA: The MIT Press.

Wernicke, C. (1900). *Grundriss der psychiatrie*. Leipzig: Verlag von Georg Thieme.

Westphal, M. (1993). *Suspicion and Faith: The Religious Uses of Modern Atheism*. Grand Rapids, MI: William B. Eerdmans Publishing Company.

Whitaker, R. (2002). *Mad in America: Bad Science, Bad Medicine, and the Enduring Mistreatment of the Mentally Ill*. Cambridge, MA: Perseus Publishing.

Williamson, P. (2007). The final common pathway of schizophrenia. *Schizophrenia Bulletin*, **33**: 953–4.

Willick, M. S. (2001). Psychoanalysis and schizophrenia: A cautionary tale. *Journal of the American Psychoanalytic Association*, **49**: 27–56.

Woods, A. (2002). Subjectivity 'in crisis': Masculinity and schizophrenia in David Fincher's *Fight Club*. *antiTHESIS*, **13**: 76–95.

Woods, A. (2007). Schizophrenia's multiple refusals. In: Hamilton, C., Kelly, M., Minor, E., & Noonan, W. (eds.) *The Politics and Aesthetics of Refusal*. Newcastle: Cambridge Scholars Publishing.

Woods, A. (in press). Mathematics <> masculinity <> madness. In: Araoz, G. (ed.) *Madness in Con-text: Historical, Poetic and Artistic Pesrpectives*. Oxford: Interdisciplinary Press.

Woods, S. W., Addington, J., Cadenhead, K. S., Cannon, T. D., Cornblatt, B. A., Heinssen, R., Perkins, D. O., Seidman, L. J., Tsuang, M. T., Walker, E. F., & McGlashan, T. H. (2009). Validity of the prodromal risk syndrome for first psychosis: Findings from the North American prodrome longitudinal study. *Schizophrenia Bulletin*, **35**: 894–908.

World Heath Organisation. (2007). *International Statistical Classification of Diseases and Related Health Problems, 10th Revision* [Online]. Available: http://www.who.int/classifications/icd/en/ [Accessed 13 January 2010].

Xia, J. & Grant, T. J. (2009). Dance therapy for people with schizophrenia. *Schizophrenia Bulletin*, **35**: 675–6.

Young, E. (1999). Life in the lottery of cool. *The Guardian*, 16 January.

Žižek, S. (1999). *The Ticklish Subject: The Absent Centre of Political Ontology*. London: Verso.

Žižek, S. (2002). Big Brother, or, the triumph of the gaze over the eye. In: Levin, T. Y., Frohne, U., & Weibel, P. (eds.) *Ctrl [space]: Rhetorics of Surveillance from Bentham to Big Brother*. Cambridge, MA: The MIT Press.

Author Index

Abbott, A. 58
Abi-Rached, J. 20
Abraham, K. 65, 66, 68–9, 71–2, 75, 80, 166
Abrams, P. 60
Acker, K. 9, 131
Aldhous, P. 34
Allen, D. F. 130
American Psychiatric Association 34, 54, 55, 64
Andreasen, N. 13
Andrejevic, M. 180
Angermeyera, M. C. 59
Annesley, J. 204
Appignanesi, L. 68
Artaud, A. 23, 149, 151, 172, 204
Ayers, S. 205, 207, 209

Bailey, J. 186
Baker, C. 9
Balsamo, A. 131
Barham, P. 43
Barrett, R. J. 5–6, 36, 40, 60, 84, 164, 168, 171, 172, 183, 223
Barthes, R. 212
Basaglia, F. 151
Bateson, G. 140
Baudrillard, J. 7, 8, 176, 183, 184, 185, 186, 187–9, 190, 191, 195, 198, 199, 202, 203, 210, 211, 214, 215
Bauman, Z. 163, 176–7, 178–9, 181, 185, 202, 206, 214
Bebbington, P. 61
Beckett, A. 204
Beckett, S. 151, 156, 204
Beer, G. 5
Bennett, A. 222
Bentall, R. P. 2, 14, 39, 47, 50, 58, 59
Bentham, J. 97, 178, 180
Berger, B. 175
Berger, P. 175
Berman, J. 166
Berrios, G. E. 20–1, 35–6
Bin, K. 162
Binswanger, L. 70
Blackshaw, T. 179
Blankenburg, W. 162
Bleakley, A. 31
Bleuler, E. 1, 6, 7, 16, 34, 46–50, 51–2, 53, 54, 55, 56, 57, 59, 65, 68, 69, 70, 80, 133, 151

Bligh, J. 31
Blount, J. 204
Blume, H. 207
Bogue, R. 149, 152
Bolton, D. 4, 131, 165
Boroughs, W. 131
Bortle, S. 136
Boyers, R. 131
Boyle, M. 38–9, 48, 50
Bracken, P. J. 17, 58, 60, 132, 223
Braidotti, R. 150
Braun, J. 174
Breathnach, C. S. 33
Breggin, P. R. 58
Broome, M. R. 164–5
Buchanan, I. 145, 160
Buchanan, R. W. 58
Burke, E. 26–7, 28, 29, 32, 44, 138
Burroughs, W. S. 9
Burston, D. 130, 136
Busfield, J. 126
Butler, J. 189

Canetti, E. 91, 92–4, 101, 154
Caouette, J. 222
Carmichael, S. 130, 144
Carpenter, W. T. 34
Castle, D. J. 14
Charon, R. 223
Cheetham, M. A. 8, 15, 28, 29, 45, 99
Chesler, P. 125
Chung, M. C. 14
Cohen, S. 131
Colebrook, C. 150
Conley, J. 206, 210
Cooper, D. 130, 131, 140, 151
Cooper, R. 55, 165
COPE Initiative 127
Craddock, N. 39
Craig, T. K. J. 61
Crapanzano, V. 84, 98, 101, 106
Cresswell, M. 132
Crichton, P. 47, 49
Crossley, M. 6, 24, 127
Crossley, N. 6, 24, 127, 143–4, 223
Crow, T. J. 39, 54, 59
Currie, M. 183, 186, 196, 197
Cuthbert, B. N. 39
Cutting, G. 23

Davidson, L. 61, 223
de Certeau, M. 82, 94, 204
de Chirico, G. 200
de Man, P. 173
Delay, J. 130
Deleuze, G. 7, 9, 91, 131, 144, 145–61, 162,
    166, 167, 176, 185, 187, 188–9, 190, 193,
    194, 196, 200, 204, 210
Derrida, J. 21, 22, 23, 24, 25, 29, 32,
    158–9, 173
Deveson, A. 222
Dixon, L. B. 58
Dobbs, D. 34
Donnelly, M. 131
Due, R. 160
Dupont, J. 158

Eagleton, T. 27, 28, 192
Editor, Nature 14
Ehrenberg, A. 9, 184–5
Elliott, A. 150, 160, 197, 198
Ellis, B. E. 8, 202, 204–19, 222
Engstrom, E. J. 35, 40
Esquirol, J. E. D. 37
Estroff, S. E. 6, 40, 223
Ettler, J. 206
Evans, D. 115, 121

Fabrega, H. 40, 184
Farmer, A. E. 52
Farrell, J. 83, 92
Fatemi, S. H. 60
Fearne, P. 223
Fee, D. 197
Felman, S. 23, 24, 25, 32, 203
Ferns, P. 6
Fine, R. 65, 76, 84
Fink, B. 110, 112, 119, 120–1
Finlay, M. 197
Flechsig, P. E. 34, 76, 78–9, 90, 91, 94, 98,
    102, 103, 113, 127–8, 213
Fliess, W. 68
Folsom, T. D. 60
Foster, H. 186
Foucault, M. 9, 16–25, 29, 30–1, 32, 33, 34,
    41, 97, 125, 129, 131, 136, 148, 158, 160,
    162, 167, 175, 177–8, 180, 213, 214
Fraguas, D. 33
Frances, A. 34
Frank, M. 150
Frankland, G. 204
Freud, S. 7, 34, 63, 64, 65, 66, 67, 68, 69–70,
    71, 72, 75, 76–84, 85–6, 87, 88, 89, 98, 99,
    100–1, 104, 105, 108–10, 111, 113, 114,
    116, 121, 133, 138, 145, 151, 153, 154,
    155, 156, 158, 165, 166, 191, 203, 220
Frith, C. 33
Fromm-Reichmann, F. 166–7

Frosh, S. 183, 186, 193–4, 197–8
Fusar-Poli, P. 46

Gabel, J. 149–50, 185
Gauntlett, D. 176
Gawith, L. 60
Geanellos, R. 223
Geddes, J. 58
Geekie, J. 223
Geertz, C. 184
Genosko, G. 151–2
Georgaca, E. 112–13
Gergen 197
Giddens, A. 175
Gilman, S. L. 36, 46, 57, 95, 213
Ginsberg, A. 130
Glass, J. M. 150, 174, 197
Goffman, E. 42, 125, 126, 129, 135–6,
    137, 140, 209
Goh, R. B. H. 196, 221
Goldberg, A. 41, 57
Goldstein, J. M. 53
Gordon, C. 16, 17, 23
Gottesman, I. 60
Gottschalk, S. 197
Goulimari, P. 200
Grant, T. J. 58
Green, M. F. 15, 62
Greenberg, J. 166, 222
Greene, T. 39
Grigg, R. 110–11, 120
Grinker, R. R. 15
Grossberg, L. 195
Guattari, F. 7, 91, 131, 144, 145–61, 162,
    166, 167, 185, 187, 188–9, 190, 193,
    194, 196, 200, 204, 210

Hacking, I. 165
Hagan, W. 97
Haghgooie, S. 14
Haghighat, R. 6
Hammersley, P. 2
Haraway, D. 176
Hardt, M. 186
Hare, E. 33
Harland, R. 59
Harvey, D. 176, 183, 186, 195–6, 197
Hauser, R. 35
Hayne, Y. 223
Healy, D. 35, 40, 46, 48, 54, 57, 58, 59, 61,
    128, 130
Heckers, S. 39, 40
Heinze, R. 205
Helyer, R. 218
Hill, P. 112
Hinshelwood, R. D. 65
Hirsch, S. R. 54
Hoenig, J. 51

Hoff, P. 37
Holland, E. W. 150–1
Hollos, I. 158
Hooke, A. E. 17
Hornstein, G. A. 61, 166
Houen, A. 208
Houston, R. A. 16
Howes, O. E. 59
Huffman, R. 131
Hunter, R. A. 76, 81, 85–6
Hutcheon, L. 184
Hutchinson, G. 14

Insel, T. R. 21, 39, 62
Israëls, H. 87

Jaaro-Peled, H. 14
Jackson, H. 53
Jameson, F. 3, 7–8, 176, 181, 183, 184, 185,
        186, 189–96, 198–200, 201–2, 203, 204,
        206, 209, 210, 211, 214
Jaspers, K. 7, 16, 43, 45, 48, 50–1, 52, 56,
        60, 68, 75–6, 82, 116, 137, 138, 139,
        162, 164, 170, 219, 220
Jenkins, J. H. 40, 60, 171, 223
Jervis, G. 131
Jervis, J. 41
Jeste, D. V. 54
Johnston, E. C. 7, 33, 38, 47–8, 52, 53, 60
Johnston, J. 183, 186, 196–7
Johnstone, L. 223
Jones, E. 65
Judd, L. L. 13
Jung, C. 48, 65, 66, 67, 68–71, 72–5, 76, 83,
        84, 110, 151, 166

Kahlbaum, K. L. 44
Kant, I. 15, 27–8, 29, 30, 31, 51, 84,
        99, 107, 138
Kapur, S. 59
Karl, F. 173
Katan, M. 85, 100
Kellendonk, C. 14
Kellner, D. 189
Kendler, K. S. 59
Kermode, F. 173
Kerr, J. 70, 71, 72
Kinney, D. K. 14
Kirby, K. M. 198
Kirk, S. A. 55
Kittler, F. 90
Kleiman, R. 112
Klein, M. 117–18, 119, 137, 151, 166, 171
Kleinman, A. 15
Kotowicz, Z. 129, 131, 137, 142
Kovel, J. 174
Kraepelin, E. 7, 16, 34–46, 47, 48, 49, 50,
        51, 53, 54, 56, 59, 60, 61, 62, 65, 66,

68, 69, 71, 80, 84, 102, 133, 151, 152–3,
        157, 164, 219
Kreyenbuhl, J. 58
Kristeva, J. 173
Kutchins, H. 55

Lacan, J. 3, 7, 63, 64, 67, 81, 108–20, 121,
        138, 151, 152, 153–4, 156, 158, 166,
        185, 189, 193, 194, 203
LaCapra, D. 24
Laing, A. C. 130
Laing, R. D. 6, 7, 9, 17, 18, 88–9, 125, 126,
        129, 136–42, 143, 149, 151, 159, 162,
        167, 170
Lasch, C. 190
Laugharne, R. 223
Lawrence, D. H. 151
Lawrie, S. M. 39
Lee, M. J. 180
Levin, D. M. 174, 197
Levin, T. Y. 179
Lewin, M. 14
Lewine, R. R. J. 53
Lewis, B. 223
Lieberman, J. A. 58
Littlewood, R. 6
Lothane, Z. 88–90, 91, 92, 93–4, 101,
        128, 129
Lotringer, S. 131, 150
Luque, R. 20
Lyon, D. 179–80
Lyotard, J.-F. 131, 148, 173
Lysaker, J. T. 40, 223
Lysaker, P. H. 40, 223

Macalpine, I. 76, 81, 85–6, 108
MacDonald, A. W. 54
Mandel, E. 190
Mann, S. 119
Mannoni, O. 103
Marcuse, H. 130
Marini, M. 108, 112, 114, 120, 121
Marshall, P. D. 206
Marx, K. 145
Mason, S. E. 59, 121
Massumi, B. 150
Mathiesen, T. 179
McDonald, C. 13
McGlashan, T. H. 99
McGuffin, P. 15, 61
McInerney, J. 206
McKenna, P. J. 35, 52
McLaughlin, T. 2
McLean, A. H. 6, 127
McLean, R. 222
McNally, K. 47
Meinhof, U. 131
Mendelsohn, D. 204

Mental Health Division 61
Metzl, J. 3, 14, 144, 172, 187
Meyer-Lindenberg, A. 2
Micale, M. S. 128, 129
Michaels, W. B. 211, 221
Michalczuk, R. 58
Miller, H. 151
Miller, J. 14, 33
Miller, R. 59, 121
Minkowski, E. 149, 150, 162, 185
Mitchell, A. 58
Mitchell, N. 132
Moncrieff, J. 58
Morel, B.-A. 35
Morgan, A. 185
Morgan, C. 14
Morris, M. 39
Morse, M. 202
Mueser, K. T. 54
Munch, E. 191
Munster, A. 158

Nasrallah, H. 58
Nelson, G. 127
Niederland, W. G. 86–8, 89, 99, 114, 154
Nielsen, H. S. 205, 218
Nietzsche, F. 23, 200
Nijkinsky, V. 151
Noll, R. 14, 36

O'Brien, B. 222
O'Hara, M. 14
O'Neill, J. 192
O'Tuathaigh, C. M. P. 14
Orrill, R. 131
Orwell, G. 180
Owen, M. J. 39

Page, A. 166
Parnas, J. 163, 169, 170
Patientenkollektiv 131
Patton, P. 150
Paulson, R. 29
Pease, D. E. 31
Perelman, B. 204
Peters, J. D. 97, 208–9, 220–1
Petersen, P. S. 205
Pinel, P. 20
Plant, S. 146
Poland, J. 59
Politi, P. 46
Porter, R. 44, 128, 129
Postel, J. 130
Punter, D. 205, 218

Rajchman, J. 150
Ramon, S. 61
Ratcliffe, M. 4

Read, J. 223
Read, R. 171
Renee 166, 171, 172, 185, 193, 199–201, 204, 222
Richardson, O. 204
Richardson, W. J. 111
Robbins, B. D. 91–2
Roberts, M. S. 97
Romme, M. 39
Ronell, A. 74, 198
Rose, J. 194
Rose, N. 20, 41, 184
Rosenhan, D. L. 134
Roudinesco, E. 114
Rümke, H. C. 51
Russell, D. 126

Saks, E. 223
Samuels, A. 72
Santner, E. L. 87, 89, 91, 94–6, 114, 178, 213, 215
Sarraute, N. 172
Sartorius, N. 59
Sass, L. A. 7, 8, 9, 33, 63, 65, 84–5, 91, 94, 96–8, 101, 150, 162–75, 176, 177–8, 180–1, 183, 184, 199, 200–1, 202, 204, 205, 213, 214, 215–16, 218, 221
Schatzman, M. 88, 89, 90, 91, 93–4, 121, 154, 170
Scheff, T. J. 126, 135–6, 137, 140
Schiller, L. 222
Schneider, K. 34, 52, 53
Schreber, D. G. M. 86–7, 88, 89, 91, 93, 94, 97, 98, 114, 121, 213
Schreber, D. P. 5, 7, 34, 64, 65, 66–7, 68, 73, 75, 76–108, 110, 113–15, 118, 120, 121, 127, 128, 147, 151, 153–7, 158, 166, 170, 172, 173, 178, 193, 212–15, 219, 222
Schulz, S. C. 54
Schwarz, H. 131
Scull, A. 17, 33
Sechehaye, M. 166
Sedgwick, P. 129, 130, 133–4, 135, 142
Serres, M. 22
Shaw, P. 25
Shean, G. D. 13
Shorter, E. 35, 37, 46, 57, 68, 128
Showalter, E. 173, 222
Sica, A. 150
Smart, B. 175
Smith, A. C. 52
Smith, D. 178, 179
Snyder, K. 222–3
Sontag, S. 4–5
Speed, E. 6
Spencer, H. 133
Stanghellini, G. 4
Steele, R. S. 66

Stephan, K. E. 60
Stephanson, A. 191
Stephenson, W. 214
Stevens, A. 73
Stiller, B. 207
Strous, R. D. 46
Sullivan, H. S. 65
Swingewood, A. 150
Szasz, T. 7, 57, 62, 88–9, 125, 126, 129,
    131, 132–6, 137, 142–3, 162, 171

Tai, S. 58
Tausk, V. 151, 166, 172
Taylor, B. 200
Tester, K. 176, 177, 179
Theweleit, K. 68
Thomas, P. 58, 60, 132
Thornton, K. 4
Thurschwell, P. 82
Torrey, E. F. 14, 33, 46, 93
Tsuang, M. T. 14
Turkington, D. 58
Turner, T. 61

Ussher, J. 126

Van Gogh, V. 191
van Os, J. 2, 14
Vatz, R. E. 133
Velligan, D. I. 58

Villagrán, J. M. 20
Viskerr, R. 19, 20

Warhol, A. 173, 191, 211
Watters, E. 15
Weber, G. 77, 78, 90, 91, 103, 127–8, 213
Weber, M. M. 40
Weeks, K. 186
Weibel, P. 180
Weinberg, L. S. 133
Weinberger, D. R. 54
Wernicke, C. 37, 44
Westphal, M. 92
Whitaker, R. 129
Williamson, P. 59
Willick, M. S. 65, 119
Wittgenstein, L. 96, 97
Woods, A. 173, 222
Woods, S. W. 34, 199
Woolf, V. 172
World Health Organisation 15, 55

Xia, J. 58

Yolken, R. H. 14, 46, 93
Yonge, O. 223
Young, E. 207

Žižek, S. 116, 180, 189, 211

Subject Index

1968 student protests, Paris 130

advocacy groups 128
aetiology of schizophrenia 14, 46
  antipsychiatry 129
  biological accounts 59, 129, 164
  Bleuler's writings 49
  brain disease 36, 37, 49, 54, 59–60
  defective filter theories 53–4
  dopamine hypothesis 58–9
  ego boundaries, loss of 55, 64
  Freud's writings 78
  heredity 36, 58, 59, 129, 164
  homosexuality 79, 80, 81, 85–6, 91, 92, 93,
    98, 100, 104, 108–9, 110, 113, 129, 153
  impaired reality testing 55, 64
  institutional neurosis theories 53
  Jung's writings 70, 71
  Kraepelin's writings 36, 37, 38, 49
  parenting 119
  paternal function, failure of the 120–1, 129
  psychic structure 93, 112–13, 116–17,
    119, 120, 121, 194
  recency hypothesis 33
  regressive hypothesis 64–5, 72, 117–18,
    165, 166, 167
  Sass's writings 170
  toxin theory 65, 70, 71, 72, 73
  trauma 155
  and treatments 58–9
  viral hypothesis 33, 129
alienation and schizophrenia 108, 140, 170
Anti-Oedipus: Capitalism and Schizophrenia
  (Deleuze and Guattari) 7, 145–7
  Baudrillard's writings 188–9
  capitalism 148–9
  critical responses 150–3
  Jameson's writings 189, 193, 194
  politics of the sublime 157–61
  postmodernism 183, 185, 186
  Sass's writings 169
  and Schreber's *Memoirs* 153–7
antipsychiatry 4, 125–31, 143–4, 220, 223
  Deleuze and Guattari's *Anti-Oedipus* 146,
    147, 159
  Foucault's *Madness and Civilization* 17, 97,
    131
  Guattari 151–2
  Laing 88–9, 136–43
  literary texts 203–4
  metatheory 162

  postmodernism 183
  Sass 163, 167, 168
  Schreber's *Memoirs* 88, 89, 94
  Szasz 88–9, 132–6, 142–3
apophany 201
asylums and psychiatric institutions
  antipsychiatry 127, 128, 135
  Foucault's writings 19, 30–1
  Goffman 135
  Kraepelin's *Clinical Psychiatry* 41, 42, 44
  records 33
  Schreber 76, 77, 89, 90, 127
  symptomatic behaviour produced by 42,
    53, 135
autistic disorder 56
autobiographical accounts of
  schizophrenia 222–3
  *see also Autobiography of a Schizophrenic
    Girl* (Renee); *Memoirs of My Nervous
    Illness* (Schreber)
Autobiography of a Schizophrenic Girl
  (Renee) 166, 172, 185
  Jameson's analysis 193, 199–200,
    201–2, 204
  Sass's analysis 200–1, 204
auto-eroticism 66
  Abraham's writings 72, 80
  Freud's writings 68, 81

Babette S. (Jung's patient) 73–4, 75,
  76, 82, 83
Beat fiction 156
biographical accounts of
  schizophrenia 222–3
biological psychiatry *see* psychiatry: biological
bizarre, schizophrenia as 52, 55, 56,
  117, 139, 164
breakthrough and liberation,
  schizophrenia as 141, 167
Burghölzli clinic 68, 70, 71, 72, 73

capitalism 176
  see also consumerism
  Ellis's *Glamorama* 206, 209, 211, 213, 214
  and schizophrenia 129, 144, 197
    Baudrillard 186, 195
    Currie 196
    Deleuze and Guattari 146, 147–9, 158,
      160, 167, 190
    Goh 196
    Jameson 186, 190–2, 194, 195, 202

catatonia *see* sub-types of schizophrenia:
  catatonia
celebrity
  Ellis's *Glamorama* 204, 210, 215
  and psychotic discourse, resemblance
    between 208–9
  synopticon 179, 214
chlorpromazine 57, 128, 130
cinematic representations of
  schizophrenia 203–4
civil liberties and psychiatry 134
class consciousness 199
clinical picture of schizophrenia 223
  Kraepelin 36, 37–8, 39, 48, 49
Clinical Psychiatry (Kraepelin) 7, 16, 34–46
  and Bleuler's *Dementia Praecox* 48, 49, 50
  influence of 54
  and Jaspers's *General Psychopathology* 50
clinical theory, defined 3–4
Clinique de la Borde 152
cognitive dysfunction 67
cognitive mapping 195, 214
communication technologies 176, 187,
  190, 205
  and schizophrenia 188, 220–1
  see also media
complexity of schizophrenia 1–2
comprehensible, schizophrenia as 165,
  170, 171
consumer/survivor/ex-patient 6
consumerism 178–80, 182, 196, 197, 214
  see also capitalism
  Ellis's *Glamorama* 206, 210–11
consumers 6, 178–80, 202
contested language/vocabulary of
  schizophrenia 2, 3, 6, 126–7
continuum with normal experience,
  schizophrenia as on a 20, 39, 65
  antipsychiatry 126, 137
  Freud's writings 81
  Klein's writings 118
crisis of signification,
  schizophrenia as 192, 193
cultural factors in schizophrenia 60, 175
cultural theory, defined 3–4

defective filter theories of schizophrenia 53–4
delusions *see* symptoms of schizophrenia:
  delusions/delusional schema
degeneration 35–6, 168
dementia 47
  Schreber's *Memoirs* 101, 104, 106
dementia praecox 65–6
  Abraham 65–6, 68–9, 71–2, 80
  Freud 68, 75, 76–84
  Jung 65, 66, 68–71, 72–5, 76
  Kraepelin's *Clinical Psychiatry* 34–46, 48
  language 6

mental deterioration 164
  renaming as schizophrenia 34, 46–7
Dementia Praecox or The Group of
  Schizophrenias (Bleuler) 7, 16, 46–50
  first appearance in print of 'schizophrenia'
    term 1, 46
  and Jaspers's *General Psychopathology* 50
depression 90, 185
  see also manic-depressive psychosis
desire and schizophrenia 146
deterritorializing process,
  schizophrenia as a 158
Diagnostic and Statistical Manual
  (American Psychiatric Association) 34,
  54–6, 62
  aetiology of schizophrenia 59
  and indeterminacy of schizophrenia 61
diagnostic criteria for schizophrenia 49,
  53, 55–6
  and indeterminacy of schizophrenia 61
Dialectics of Liberation
  Conference 130, 144
disordered speech *see* symptoms of
  schizophrenia: disordered speech
disorganized schizophrenia *see*
  sub-types of schizophrenia:
  disorganized
Divided Self, The (Laing) 7, 126, 136–9, 140,
  141, 143, 159
dopamine hypothesis of schizophrenia 58–9
dreams 70, 74

Ecstasy of Communication, The
  (Baudrillard) 8, 185, 186–9, 210
ego
  antipsychiatry 142
  Klein's writings 117–18
  Lacan's writings 110
  Laing 142
  libido theory 80
  Schreber's *Memoirs* 98, 104
  word-association test 70
ego boundaries, loss of 167
ego-psychology 64, 65
  Klein's writings 119
  Schreber's *Memoirs* 98
electro-convulsive treatment 57
emancipation, schizophrenia as 159
embodiment and schizophrenia 144,
  173, 198–9
enlightenment, schizophrenia as 159
epidemiology of schizophrenia 14–15, 53
exigent introspection 163, 169, 181

fantasy, feminine 79
fascism 92, 93, 95
  see also psychiatry: and the Nazi regime
feminist movement 125–6

foreclosure
  Ellis's *Glamorama* 214
  Lacan's writings 110–11, 112, 113, 114,
    117, 119, 120, 193
free association 70
frontal lobe lobotomy 57

gender and schizophrenia 14, 53
  Baudrillard's writings 187
  Lacan's writings 119–21
  Sass's writings 172, 173
  see also feminist movement
General Psychopathology (Jaspers) 7, 16,
  50–2, 138, 139
Glamorama (Ellis) 8, 202, 204–5, 220
  postmodernism 205–15, 222
  and the schizophrenic sublime 215–19
governess psychosis 57

hallucinations *see* symptoms of schizophrenia:
  hallucinations
hebephrenia *see* sub-types of schizophrenia:
  hebephrenia
hermeneutic approach to schizophrenia 36,
  64, 82, 84
homosexuality 57
  aetiology of schizophrenia 79, 80,
    81, 85–6, 91, 92, 93, 98, 100, 104,
    108–9, 110, 113, 129, 153
  Schreber's *Memoirs* 85, 91, 92, 93, 104
  Freud's writings 80, 81, 86
hyperreflexivity and schizophrenia 163,
  168–71, 173, 174, 175
hypochondria 76, 86, 100, 101
hysteria 48, 64, 65, 120
  Abraham's writings 71
  Baudrillard's writings 187
  and 'the feminine' 121
  Jung's writings 69–70
  as privileged psychic disorder of
    psychoanalysis 68

idleness 19, 41
insanity 15, 33, 54
  Esquirol's taxonomies of 37
  Foucault's *Madness and
    Civilization* 16–25, 32, 41
  Freud's career 66
  Kraepelin's career 44
  Laing's writings 139, 142
  laws, Germany 128
  Morel 35
  Sass's writings 173
  Schreber 90, 127
institutional neurosis theories of
  schizophrenia 53
insulin coma therapy 57
interdisciplinary inquiry, importance of 2

International Classification of Diseases
  (WHO) 55
interpretive problem or puzzle,
  schizophrenia as 118
ipseity disturbance,
  schizophrenia as 163, 169

Kraepelinian classification of the
  psychoses 35

label, schizophrenia as a 129, 135, 136, 140
labour
  and schizophrenia 19, 40–1, 42–3, 56
  work ethic 177, 178, 179
language, identity as a function of 192
language/vocabulary of schizophrenia,
  contested 3, 6, 126–7
latent schizophrenia 50, 55
liberation, schizophrenia as 141, 167
libido 69, 75, 79–80, 86, 94, 98, 104, 113
liquid modernity 163, 176–7, 18
  Ellis's *Glamorama* 206
  see also postmodernity
literary representations of
  schizophrenia 203–4
literature, relevance to studies of
  psychopathology 203–4
lobotomy 57
loss of subjective depth, schizophrenia as 184

madness
  antipsychiatry 125, 129
  Laing 136, 141, 142
  crisis of representation 32
  'Dionysian' model of 167, 172
  feminist movement 126
  Foucault's writings 17, 18, 21–5, 29,
    32–3, 34
  and gender 173
  Guattari's writings 151–2
  Lacan's writings 109
  language 6
  Sass's writings 96
Madness and Civilization (Foucault) 16–25,
  29, 33, 97, 158–9
  antipsychiatry 17, 97, 131
Madness and Modernism (Sass) 7, 162,
  163–75, 176, 180–1, 200–1, 202
  literary texts 204, 205
manic-depressive psychosis
  Bentall 39
  Diagnostic and Statistical Manual 56
  Heckers 40
  Kraepelin 36, 39, 40, 49
Marxism and post-Marxism 14,
  176, 149–50
masturbatory insanity/psychosis 36, 57
  Schreber's *Memoirs* 85, 100, 101

media
  antipsychiatry 128
  celebrity and psychotic discourse,
    resemblance between 208–9
  Ellis's *Glamorama* 205, 215
  postmodernity 176, 179, 180, 202
  synopticon 179, 180, 215
  see also communication technologies
medical gaze 30–1
mega-vitamins 57
melancholia 184–5
Memoirs of My Nervous Illness (Schreber) 5,
    7, 64, 66–7, 84–5, 204
  criticism of psychiatry 127
  Deleuze and Guattari's *Anti-Oedipus* 147,
    154–7
  and Ellis's *Glamorama* 205, 212–15, 219
  Freud's analysis 65, 66, 73, 75, 76–84, 121,
    138, 153
  Klein's analysis 118
  Lacan's analysis 108–9, 110, 113–15, 120,
    153–4, 193
  power and politics 91–100, 154
  psychoanalytic and (psycho)biographical
    analyses 85–91, 154
  sublime 100–8
mental health policy 60, 223
mental health service users 6
Mental Illness and Psychology
    (Foucault) 17–18, 21, 24
metatheoretical framework 8, 162
  autobiographical and biographical accounts
    of schizophrenia 223
  Deleuze and Guattari's *Anti-Oedipus* 147,
    155, 157–8
  Sass 163, 167, 168, 216
  see also sublime
modernism 176
  Jameson's writings 191, 192
  and schizophrenia 181
  see also *Madness and Modernism* (Sass)
modernity 220
  Deleuze and Guattari's *Anti-Oedipus* 156
  Foucault's *Madness and Civilization* 24
  panopticon 97, 177–8
  and postmodernity 176–7, 180
  Sass's writings 171, 175
  and schizophrenia 33, 174, 175, 181
    recency hypothesis 33
  Schreber's *Memoirs* 95–6, 213, 215
mood disorder 56
moral choice, schizophrenia as a 133
multiple personality disorder 57
mystery of schizophrenia 15

Name-of-the-Father
  Ellis's *Glamorama* 214
  Jameson's writings 194

Lacan's writings 67, 111, 112, 113–14, 117,
    119, 120, 153–4, 193
narcissism
  Ellis's *Glamorama* 212
  Freud's writings 80, 81
  Klein's writings 117
narratives 222–3
neologisms
  Jung's writings 73–4
  Lacan's writings 111
  Schreber's 83
neuroscience 59
neurosis 64, 65
  Abraham's writings 71
  and dementia praecox, comparison
    between 69, 76
  Freud's 'Psycho-Analytic Notes' 66, 80, 81
  Lacan's writings 109, 110, 111
New Horizons strategy 61
normal experience and schizophrenia *see*
    continuum with normal experience,
    schizophrenia as on a
nosology
  Diagnostic and Statistical Manual 34
  Foucault's *Madness and Civilization* 21
  Freud's writings 81, 85
  Kraepelin's *Clinical Psychiatry* 35, 37, 39
  Lacan's writings 109
  psychoanalysis and biological psychiatry,
    differences between 68

object-relations theory 64, 119
Oedipal complex
  Lacan's writings 111
  Schreber's *Memoirs* 85–6
  *see also Anti-Oedipus: Capitalism and
    Schizophrenia* (Deleuze and Guattari)
Other to psychiatry, schizophrenia as 41, 164
over-diagnosis of schizophrenia 134

panopticon 177–8, 214
  and consumer society 179
  Ellis's *Glamorama* 215
  and postmodernism 180, 202, 214
  and schizophrenia 97
  see also synopticon
'paranoid', figure of the 147, 148, 149, 152,
    157, 159
paranoid–schizoid position 117, 119, 137
paranoid schizophrenia *see* sub-types of
    schizophrenia: paranoia
paraphrenia 6, 63
  Freud's writings 81, 108, 109, 121
pervasive developmental disorder 56
phenomenology
  of health and illness 5
  of mental illness 18
  of the postmodern 222

of psychopathology 4
of schizophrenia 3, 9, 181
    Gabel's writings 185
    Jaspers' *General Psychopathology* 50–1,
        138
    Laing's *The Divided Self* 126, 137, 138
    Sass's writings 163, 165, 172, 181, 183,
        199, 201
politics
    of psychoanalysis 67–8
    of schizophrenia 66
        antipsychiatry 130, 141
        Deleuze and Guattari's *Anti-
            Oedipus* 157–61
        Schreber's *Memoirs* 92–3
Politics of Experience, The (Laing) 7, 136, 138,
    140–2, 159
popular imaginary of schizophrenia 27, 64
postmodernism 3, 163, 221
    Deleuze and Guattari's *Anti-Oedipus* 146,
        160–1
    Ellis's *Glamorama* 204–16, 218, 219, 222
    paradoxical 184
    Sass's writings 173–4
    and schizophrenia 3, 181, 183–6,
        195–202, 203
        Ellis's *Glamorama* 205, 208, 209, 210–11,
            212, 216, 219
        figure of 'the postmodern
            schizophrenic' 186–9
        Jameson's 'Cultural Logic of Late
            Capitalism' 189–95
        stimmung 200–1, 202
*Postmodernism, or the Cultural Logic of Late
    Capitalism* (Jameson) 3, 7–8, 185, 186,
    189–95, 196, 201–2
postmodernity 175–82
    and schizophrenia 180–1, 186, 221
        Sass's writings 173, 175, 181
    see also liquid modernity
postpsychiatry 60
praecox feeling 51, 52, 170
projection 79, 111–12
psyche
    Baudrillard's *Ecstasy of Communication* 188
    Jaspers's *General Psychopathology* 51
    origins of dementia praecox 72
psychiatry 34–46
    antipsychiatry *see* antipsychiatry
    asylums *see* asylums and psychiatric
        institutions
    authority of 15
    biological 46, 50, 68, 223
        critiques 127–8
        and phenomenology 165
        Schreber's *Memoirs* 89, 90, 93, 94, 102–3
    and civil liberties 132, 134
    clinical encounter 52

critiques of 4, 39, 127–9
    see also antipsychiatry
    Deleuze and Guattari's *Anti-Oedipus* 148,
        158
    and the disciplinary sublime 8, 16, 29, 63,
        67, 84, 137
    history of 46
    institutions *see* asylums and psychiatric
        institutions
    medical gaze 30–1
    and the Nazi regime 46, 62, 72
        Schreber's *Memoirs* 92, 93, 94, 95
    philosophy of 4–5, 9
    and psychology, distinction between 66
    Sass's writings 168
    schizophrenia as defining problem for 15
    schizophrenia as Other to 41, 164
    and scientificity 39, 40, 128
    transcultural 60, 121, 174
psychic deterritorialization,
    schizophrenia as 146
psychoanalysis 118
    antipsychiatry 128, 137, 138
    Deleuze and Guattari's *Anti-Oedipus* 146,
        147, 154–5, 158–9
    dementia praecox and neurosis, similarities
        between 68–9
    Foucault's *Mental Illness and Psychology* 18
    Freud's writings 67–8, 69, 77–84
    hysteria 68, 75
    Jaspers's writings 116
    Jung's writings 69, 70, 73, 75, 76
    Klein's writings 117–18
    Lacan's writings 108, 114–15, 116, 117
    Laing's writings 137, 138
    politics 67–8
    and psychiatry, distinction between 66
    Sass's writings 165–6, 168
    Schreber's *Memoirs* 77–93, 99, 154–5
    social significance in schizophrenia 122
    textual sublime 63–4
'Psycho-Analytic Notes on an
    Autobiographical Account of a Case of
    Paranoia' (Freud) 7, 66, 76–84, 85–6, 87,
    88, 89, 99
    Jung's influence 75
    Lacan on 108–9, 138
    rationality, Schreber's crisis of 100–1
psychological accounts of schizophrenia 18,
    47, 143, 144, 162, 224
    Bleuler 46, 47, 50
    Jaspers 51
    Jung 65, 68, 69, 70, 73, 75
    Kraepelin 35, 45, 49
    Sass 163, 164, 175, 202, 204
    Schreber 84, 92, 93, 97
Psychology of Dementia Praecox, The
    (Jung) 65, 69–71, 73–4, 76

psychopathology, relevance of literature to
	studies of 203–4
psychopharmacology 57–8, 59, 61, 220
	antipsychiatry 128, 130
Psychoses, The (Lacan) 7, 108–17, 118
	sublime 114, 116–17, 118–19
psychosexual development 64–5
'Psycho-Sexual Differences between
	Hysteria and Dementia Praecox'
	(Abraham) 65–6, 71–2
psychosexual origins of paranoia 68
psychosis 65
	Abraham's writings 71
	antipsychiatry 125, 126, 134, 135, 140, 141
	and celebrity 208–9, 212
	dementia praecox and neurosis, similarities
		between 69
	Diagnostic and Statistical Manual 54–5
	Ellis's *Glamorama* 209
	Freud's writings 66, 81–5, 109
	hermeneutics 36
	Jameson's writings 193, 194
	Jung's writings 71
	Klein's writings 118
	Lacan's writings 63, 108–21, 193, 194
	Laing's writings 126, 138, 140, 141
	language 6
	and 'the masculine' 121
	psychoanalytic theory of 81, 83–4
	Schreber's *Memoirs* 81–8, 90–1, 94–6, 101,
		107–8, 115, 120
	substance-induced 56
	Szasz's writings 134, 135
psychosis risk syndrome 34

race and schizophrenia 3, 14, 96, 144, 172,
	173, 199
rebellion, schizophrenia as 158
recency hypothesis of schizophrenia 33
recovery approach to schizophrenia 61
regressive hypothesis of
	schizophrenia 64–5, 72
	Klein 117–18
	Sass 165, 166, 167
relevance of literature to studies of
	psychopathology 203–4
religious interpretations of schizophrenia 92,
	93, 102, 103, 104–7
repression 79–80, 81, 149
residual schizophrenia 34, 55
revolutionary, schizophrenia as 144, 146–7,
	149, 159, 197
romanticizing of schizophrenia 15

schizo, in Deleuze and Guattari's *Anti-
	Oedipus* 145–9, 152, 155–7, 159–61,
	188, 210, 211
schizoaffective disorder 56

schizoanalysis 158
Schizo-Culture 131
Schizo-Culture convention 131
schizoid states 137
Schizophrenia: The Sacred Symbol of Psychiatry
	(Szasz) 7, 132–5
schizophrenia
	aetiology *see* aetiology of schizophrenia
	alienation and 108, 140, 170
	autobiographical account 222–3
	as bizarre 52, 55, 56, 117, 139, 164
	as breakthrough and liberation 141, 167
	capitalism and *see* capitalism: and
		schizophrenia
	clinical picture 36, 37–8, 39, 48, 49, 223
	communication technologies and 188,
		220–1
	as comprehensible 165, 170, 171
	contested language/vocabulary of 2, 3,
		6, 126–7
	as on a continuum with normal experience
		see continuum with normal experience
	as crisis of signification 192, 193
	desire and 146
	diagnostic criteria 49, 53, 55–6, 61
	embodiment and 144, 173, 198–9
	epidemiology 14–15, 53
	gender and *see* gender and schizophrenia
	hyperreflexivity and 163, 168–71,
		173, 174, 175
	as interpretive problem or puzzle 118
	as ipseity disturbance 163, 169
	as a label 129, 135, 136, 140
	labour and 19, 40–1, 42–3, 56
	literary and cinematic
		representations 203–4
	as loss of subjective depth 184
	modernism and 181
		see also Madness and Modernism (Sass)
	modernity and 33, 174, 175, 181
	as Other to psychiatry 41, 164
	panopticon and 97
	phenomenology *see* phenomenology: of
		schizophrenia
	politics of *see* politics: of schizophrenia
	popular imaginary 27, 64
	postmodernism and *see* postmodernism
		and schizophrenia
	postmodernity and 173, 175,
		180–1, 186, 221
	as psychic deterritorialization 146
	psychological accounts *see* psychological
		accounts of schizophrenia
	race and 3, 14, 96, 144, 172, 173, 199
	religious interpretations 92, 93,
		102, 103, 104–7
	as revolutionary 144, 146–7, 149,
		159, 197

as scientific delusion 38
as social crisis 130
solipsism and 97–8
as sublime experience 8, 126, 136,
    139–42, 143
sub-types see sub-types of schizophrenia
symptoms see symptoms of schizophrenia
temporality 196, 198
as theoretic topos 3
as ununderstandable 50, 51–2, 56,
    139, 164, 170
'schizophrenic', figure of the 144
    antipsychiatry 125, 127, 130, 131, 144
    Laing 138
    Szasz 133, 135
    Deleuze and Guattari's Anti-Oedipus 147,
        148, 149, 152, 156–7, 159–60, 161
    postmodernity 181, 183, 186–9,
        196–7, 199
schizophrenogenic 64
    antipsychiatry 130, 131, 140–1
    Klein 119
    Laing 140–1
    Schreber's Memoirs 88
scientific delusion, schizophrenia as 38
scientificity and psychiatry 39, 40, 128
self 40, 164
    modern 41, 43
        Deleuze and Guattari's Anti-Oedipus 161
        Schreber's Memoirs 91
    postmodern 181–2
Semiotext(e) 131, 150, 186
sexuality 199
    see also homosexuality
shamanism, Schreber's Memoirs 91–2
signification, schizophrenia as
    crisis of 192, 193
simple schizophrenia 50, 55
social crisis, schizophrenia as 130
solipsism and schizophrenia 97–8
somatic symptoms 63, 67, 86, 87, 96,
    97, 155, 164
Sonnenstein asylum 76, 90, 93, 105, 155
soul murder 78–9, 90, 94, 98, 127
speech, disordered see symptoms of
    schizophrenia: disordered speech
SPK (Socialist Patients' Collective) 131,
    151–2
stigma 1, 15, 20, 47
    antipsychiatry 127, 128
    psychosis risk syndrome 34
    public education campaigns 59
stimmung 200–1, 202, 203
    Ellis's Glamorama 209, 210, 212
subjective depth, schizophrenia
    as loss of 184
subjectivity see self
sublimation 66

sublime 15–16, 25–9, 61–2, 65, 224
    antipsychiatry 125, 126, 131, 136, 162
        Laing 136, 137–9, 141–2, 143, 159
        Szasz 134, 135, 143
    Bleuler's Dementia Praecox 50
    definition 8
    Deleuze and Guattari's Anti-Oedipus 147,
        159, 160, 161
    Diagnostic and Statistical Manual 56, 57
    disciplinary sublime 8, 16, 25–9, 63,
        64, 67, 84, 137
    Jaspers's General Psychopathology 51
    Kraepelin's Clinical Psychiatry 43–6
    Lacan's The Psychoses 114, 116–17,
        118–19, 189
    paradoxical sublime 8, 183–5, 186
        Baudrillard's writings 188, 189
        Jameson's writings 190, 194
        postmodernism 183–4, 188, 197, 200
        Ellis's Glamorama 205, 209, 215–19
        Sass's writings 163, 165, 168, 170–1, 183,
            201
    schizophrenia as an experience of 8, 126
        Laing 136, 139–42, 143
    schizophrenic sublime 8, 29–34, 221,
        222, 223
        Ellis's Glamorama 215–19
        postmodernism 194, 197, 201
        Schreber's Memoirs 84, 99–108, 118, 154
    technological 194–5
    textual sublime 8, 63–5, 67
        Laing 137
        Schreber's Memoirs 84
sublime experience, schizophrenia as 8, 126
    Laing 136, 139–42, 143
substance-induced psychosis 56
sub-types of schizophrenia
    catatonia 34, 36, 49, 55
        Deleuze and Guattari's Anti-Oedipus 152
        Freud 68
        Jung 74
        Laing 137
        Schreber's Memoirs 157
    disorganized 34, 55
        Deleuze and Guattari's Anti-Oedipus
    hebephrenia 34, 36, 49, 55
        Deleuze and Guattari's Anti-
            Oedipus 152–3
        Freud 68
        Jung 73, 74
        Kraepelin 152–3
        Laing 137
        Schreber's Memoirs 157
    latent 50, 55
    paranoia 34, 36, 49, 55
        Deleuze and Guattari's Anti-Oedipus 152
        Freud 68, 75, 79, 80–3, 87
        Jung 74

sub-types of schizophrenia (*cont.*)
Lacan 108, 109
Laing 137
Schreber's *Memoirs* 64, 68, 79–83, 87,
90–1, 92, 93, 107, 157
residual 34, 55
simple 50, 55
undifferentiated 34, 55, 152
suffering 1, 4, 6, 14, 24–5, 57, 134, 168
surveillance 179–80
symptoms of schizophrenia 14, 48, 52, 53, 84
antipsychiatry 125, 135
Babette S. 74, 75
Bleuler's *Dementia Praecox* 48–9, 50,
52, 53
cognitive dysfunction 67
delusions/delusional schema 29, 36, 55, 56,
66, 73, 165, 220
Babette S. 74, 75
Deleuze and Guattari's *Anti-Oedipus* 155,
200
Ellis's *Glamorama* 209, 212, 216, 219
Jameson 194
Lacan 111, 113, 116, 154
Laing 159
Sass 169, 173
Schreber 75, 77–80, 83, 85–8, 92–108,
113, 115, 121, 153, 154, 156, 157,
170, 173, 212, 213
disordered speech 22, 24, 55, 63, 73, 75, 76,
111, 115, 117, 137
first rank 52
fundamental/accessory 48, 52, 53
hallucinations 36, 48, 52, 55, 56, 66, 73, 81,
84, 166
Deleuze and Guattari's *Anti-Oedipus* 155
Ellis's *Glamorama* 216
Johnston 197, 202
Lacan 111, 116
Sass 169
Schreber 83, 155
Kraepelin's *Clinical Psychiatry* 41, 42
negative 48, 53, 163, 169

positive 53
primary/secondary 48, 52
Schreber 66, 75, 77–80, 83, 85–8, 92,
94–108, 113, 115, 121, 153–7, 170,
173, 212, 213
somatic 63, 67, 86, 87, 96, 97,
155, 164
and technologies 220
textual approach 9, 64, 76, 77, 81, 84–5,
114, 115, 138, 222–3
synopticon 179, 214–15
Tarnation 222
temporarily of schizophrenia 196, 198
textual approach to schizophrenia 9, 64, 76,
77, 81, 84–5, 114, 115, 138, 222–3
see also hermeneutic approach to
schizophrenia
theoretical topos, schizophrenia as 3
therapeutic treatment *see* treatments and
therapy for schizophrenia
time–space compression 195–6
Time to Change campaign 61
toxin theory of schizophrenia 65, 70,
71, 72, 73
transference 66
transvestite fantasies, Schreber's
Memoirs 90, 173
treatments and therapy for schizophrenia 38,
57–8, 129
see also psychopharmacology
trema 200–1
undifferentiated schizophrenia 34, 55, 152
ununderstandable, schizophrenia as 50, 51–2,
56, 139, 164, 170
violence 29
in Ellis's *Glamorama* 205, 211, 212, 214
viral hypothesis of schizophrenia 33, 129
vocabulary of schizophrenia, contested 2, 3,
6, 126–7
word-association test 70
word salad 74
work ethic 177, 178, 179
see also labour